Prognostic and Predictive Factors in Breast Cancer

Prognostic and Predictive Factors in Breast Cancer

Edited by

Rosemary A Walker MBChB MD FRCPath
Professor of Pathology
University of Leicester
Department of Cancer Studies and Molecular Medicine
RKCSB
Leicester Royal Infirmary
Leicester
United Kingdom

Alastair M Thompson MBChB MD FRCSEd (Gen)
Professor of Surgical Oncology
Department of Surgery and Molecular Oncology
Ninewells Hospital and Medical School
University of Dundee
Dundee
Scotland

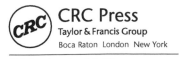
CRC Press
Taylor & Francis Group
Boca Raton London New York

CRC Press is an imprint of the
Taylor & Francis Group, an **informa** business

CRC Press
Taylor & Francis Group
6000 Broken Sound Parkway NW, Suite 300
Boca Raton, FL 33487-2742

First issued in paperback 2019

© 2008 by Taylor & Francis Group, LLC
CRC Press is an imprint of Taylor & Francis Group, an Informa business

No claim to original U.S. Government works

ISBN-13: 978-1-415-42225-3 (hbk)
ISBN-13: 978-0-367-38693-1 (pbk)

A CIP record for this book is available from the British Library.
Library of Congress Cataloging-in-Publication Data

**Visit the Taylor & Francis Web site at
http://www.taylorandfrancis.com**

**and the CRC Press Web site at
http://www.crcpress.com**

Contents

Contributors

Catherine Alix-Panabières
University Medical Center
Lapeyronie Hospital
Montpellier
France

Jan PA Baak
Department of Pathology
Stavanger University Hospital
Stavanger
Norway

JMS Bartlett
Edinburgh Cancer Research Centre
Western General Hospital
Edinburgh
Scotland

Pascale Cohen
ISPBL Faculty of Pharmacology
University of Lyon
Lyon
France

R Charles Coombes
Dept of Medical Oncology
Imperial College London
Hammersmith Hospital
London
United Kingdom

Gábor Cserni
Department of Pathology
Bacs-Kiskum County Teaching Hospital
Nyiriut
Kecskemet
Hungary

Johannes S de Jong
Department of Surgery
University Medical Center Groningen
Groningen
The Netherland

Paula HM Elkhuizen
Division of Radiation Oncology
Netherlands Cancer Institute
Amsterdam
The Netherlands

IO Ellis
Dept of Histopathology
Nottingham University Hospitals
Nottingham
United Kingdom

Chris W Elston
Former Consultant Histopathologist
City Hospital
Nottingham
and
Special Professor of Tumour Pathology
Nottingham University Medical School
Nottingham
United Kingdom

Julia MW Gee
Tenovus Centre for Cancer Research
Welsh School of Pharmacy
Cardiff University
Cardiff
United Kingdom

Sandra Ghayad
Faculty of Pharmacology
University of Lyon
Lyon
France

Gavin C Harris
Cantebury Health Laboratories
Christchurch Hospitals
Christchurch
New Zealand

Natasha Hava
Dept of Medical Oncology
Imperial College London
Hammersmith Hospital
London
United Kingdom

Deborah L Holliday
Postdoctoral Research Associate
Institute of Cancer
Barts, and
The London Queen Mary's School of Medicine
and Dentistry
Queen Mary
University of London
London
United Kingdom

Iain Hutcheson
Tenovus Centre for Cancer Research
Welsh School of Pharmacy
Cardiff University
Cardiff
United Kingdom

J Louise Jones
Tumour Biology Laboratory
CR-UK Clinical Cancer Centre
Queen Mary's School of Medicine & Dentistry
Barts and The London Hosptials
London
United Kingdom

Bas Kreike
Division of Radiation Oncology
Netherlands Cancer Institute
Amsterdam
The Netherlands

Sonia Lain
Department of Surgery and Molecular Oncology
University of Dundee
Dundee
United Kingdom

Rob JAM Michalides
Department of Cell Biology
Netherlands Cancer Institute
Amsterdam
The Netherlands

Volkmar Müller
Department of Gynecology
University Breast Center
University Medical Center Hamburg Eppendorf
Hamburg
Germany

Robert I Nicholson
Tenovus Centre for Cancer Research
Welsh School of Pharmacy
Cardiff University
Cardiff
United Kingdom

Karen Page
Department of Cancer Studies and Molecular
Medicine
Leicester Royal Infirmary
Leicester
United Kingdom

Klaus Pantel
Institute of Tumor Biology
Center of Experimental Medicine
University Medical Center Hamburg Eppendorf
Hamburg
Germany

Sarah E Pinder
Professor of Pathology
King's College London
Department of Academic Oncology
Guy's Hospital
London
United Kingdom

Lajos Pusztai
Department of Breast Medical Oncology
University of Texas MD Anderson Cancer Centre
Houston, TX
USA

Jacqueline A Shaw
Department of Cancer Studies and Molecular
Medicine
Leicester Royal Infirmary
Leicester
United Kingdom

Christos Sotiriou
Functional Genomics and Translational Research
Unit
Department of Medical Oncology
Jules Boldlt Institute
Brussells
Belgium

Oliver D Staples
Ninewells Hospital and Medical School
University of Dundee
Dundee
United Kingdom

Alastair M Thompson
Professor of Surgical Oncology
Department of Surgery and Molecular Oncology
Ninewells Hospital and Medical School
University of Dundee
Dundee
Scotland

Marc van de Vijver
Department of Pathology
Academic Medical Center
Amsterdam
The Netherlands

Elsken van der Wall
Department of Internal Medicine
University Medical Center Utrecht
Utrecht
The Netherlands

Paul J van Diest
Professor of Pathology
Head
Department of Pathology
UMC Utrecht
Utrecht
The Netherlands

Rosemary A Walker
Professor of Pathology
University of Leicester
Department of Cancer Studies and Molecular
Medicine
RKCSB
Leicester Royal Infirmary
Leicester
United Kingdom

Dorin Ziyaie
Ninewells Hospital and Medical School
University of Dundee
Dept of Surgery and Molecular Oncology
Dundee
United Kingdom

Prognostic and predictive factors in breast cancer: an overview

1

Rosemary A Walker and Alastair M Thompson

INTRODUCTION

It is well recognized that breast cancer is a heterogenous disease, with variation in clinical behavior, and that the biological nature of the disease and clinical outcome are closely interlinked. Management of the breast cancer patient is now a carefully planned exercise using a variety of factors which are associated with longer or shorter survival (prognostic factors), and/or can aid selection of relevant systemic therapy (predictive factors). The aim of this second edition of Prognostic and Predictive Factors in Breast Cancer is to provide up-to-date information and views on those factors used clinically and present data on approaches that are presently research but could be the tools for the future. The speed with which things progress is exemplified by microarrays; in the last edition (2003) these were discussed as newer approaches for the future, microarrays are now in clinical trials.

BACKGROUND

The baseline evidence for the variation in breast cancer behavior comes from studies from many years ago of women who had no treatment and of those that were before the advent of systemic (i.e. adjuvant) treatment following surgery. Bloom et al[1] reported on a series of 250 women seen at the Middlesex Hospital, London, UK between 1805 and 1933; 74% had advanced (stage IV) disease at the time of admission but 18% of these were still alive at 5 years without any treatment. The number of patients is small but this demonstrates the variation in the natural history of untreated breast cancer. The importance of having large series of patients to derive valid information was appreciated; it is from pre-adjuvant therapy studies that amassed information from one or more centers that data on the clinical importance of tumor size and node status comes.[2-7] A criticism of some of the studies, e.g. The National Cancer Institute Surveillance, Epidemiology and End Results (SEER) Program,[7] is that staging was based on a combination of clinical and pathological data, and that the reporting pathologists data was used with no review by one or a small number of individuals.

To gain important clinically relevant information about outcome it is necessary for studies to have sufficient numbers of pathologically staged patients who are categorized by age, surgical and adjuvant treatment, and whose cancers are assessed clinically and pathologically using standardized, clearly defined criteria. The derivation of the Nottingham Prognostic Index is an excellent example of this.[8] It was established by the long-term follow-up in a dedicated breast unit of patients who did not receive adjuvant therapy, had a standard management, and whose cancers were assessed using defined criteria[9,10] by a small number of pathologists.

The drive to find newer/different markers of breast cancer behavior has resulted in innumerable studies, many of limited value. Evaluation guidelines for breast cancer prognostic factors were proposed in 1991[11] and still apply today: the factor should possess clear biological significance; the study should be defined as a pilot, definitive or confirmatory; there should be an adequate sample size for meaningful calculations; the patient population must be defined and not biased, for example, in relation to size, node status or age; there must be methodological validation; clinical cut-off values must be defined; assays must be reproducible. Problems with tumor-marker prognostic studies (generally, not just breast) have been recognized in reporting recommendations (REMARK),[12] that were published simultaneously in US and European journals in 2005. These also emphasize the need for information about study design, preplanned hypotheses, patient and specimen characteristics, assay methods, and statistical analysis methods.

The American Society of Clinical Oncology first published evidence-based clinical practice guidelines for the use of tumor markers in breast cancer in 1996. In the 2007 update,[13] 13 categories of markers were considered, but not all had enough evidence to support routine use in clinical practice. Those that did included estrogen receptor (ER) and progesterone receptor (PR) (see Chapter 9) human epidermal growth factor receptor 2 (HER2) (see Chapter 13), and also certain gene expression assays (see Chapter 11).

USE OF PROGNOSTIC AND PREDICTIVE FACTORS IN CLINICAL PRACTICE

The standard prognostic factors such as tumor size and node status provide important information about likely patient outcome, but within the good prognosis groups such as axillary node-negative cases there can be differences in behavior. There is increasing emphasis on separating defined prognostic groups into low and high risk,[14] and using this, along with predictive markers, for the selection of adjuvant systemic therapy. Expert consensus meetings such as those held at St Gallen consider the primary therapy of early breast cancer and make recommendations which are published every 2 years or so.[15–17] The Early Breast Cancer Trialists' Collaborative Group undertake quinquennial overviews of the

randomized trials in breast cancer, with the last overview being published in 2005,[18] and these provide data on recurrence and mortality rates in relation to therapy. Using this, and in conjunction with the Nottingham Prognostic Index (NPI),[8] a prognostic table has been devised[19,20] and updated[21] to provide information about the benefit or not of polychemotherapy and endocrine therapy to individual patients. A National Health Service (NHS) R&D Health Technology Assessment[22] considered the NPI to be a useful clinical tool, and that additional factors may enhance its use.

Web-based tools are being used more extensively – www.adjuvantonline.com is one used by many clinicians for estimating the benefit of adjuvant therapy for women with stage I and II breast cancers. A population-based validation of the model (ADJUVANT!) showed it to perform reliably, although for women younger than 35 years of age, or with known adverse prognostic factors such as lymphovascular invasion, adjustments of risks were required.[23]

For these tools to be effective there is a need for the factors that form them to be derived accurately. Determination of tumor size, type, grade, node status, presence or not of lymphovascular invasion is the remit of the pathologists who are part of the breast multidisciplinary team, and this is discussed in Chapter 2. In order to ensure reproducibility, guidelines have been produced,[24] and quality assurance of the different parameters is undertaken in the UK. Pathologists are very much involved with the analysis of estrogen and progesterone receptors (Chapter 9) and HER2 (Chapter 13), which are the determinants for the selection of endocrine therapy and trastuzumab, respectively, now both used as adjuvant therapies as well as for metastatic disease. There are many factors which can affect performance of assays, and interpretation,[25,26] and whilst there are quality assurance schemes for the tests, quality assurance for interpretation has yet to be introduced.

Much of the above has related to the use of systemic therapy. However, local recurrence following conservative surgery for breast cancer is also important and the various therapeutic factors are discussed in Chapter 4, along with the surgical and pathological determinants of local recurrence.

MICROMETASTATIC AND METASTATIC DISEASE

The main reason for using adjuvant therapy after surgery is to treat micrometastatic disease, and so prevent metastases occurring at a later date. Our ability to monitor patients for micrometastases and understand their significance is still more restricted to research than open clinical application.

The introduction of sentinel node procedures has increased awareness of minimal spread (isolated tumor cells and micrometastases) to axillary lymph nodes, but its significance is still unresolved and this is discussed in Chapter 6.

The methods available for detection of disseminated and circulating tumor cells, and their clinical significance, are the focus of Chapter 7. Chapter 8 reviews progress in the investigation of the clinical utility of plasma DNA and RNA analysis for determining breast cancer behavior. It also describes how data from studies of tumor-specific alterations in circulating cell-free DNA indicate that analysis of nucleic acids in blood could become a diagnostic test.

BREAST CANCER BIOLOGY AND BEHAVIOR

Malignant cells are characterized by altered growth control (both proliferation and apoptosis), and the ability to invade and metastasize. Research into the many components of these processes could identify novel prognostic and predictive markers.

The prognostic value of proliferation, apoptosis, cell cycle and apoptotic proteins is discussed in Chapter 3, with the conclusion that although there are many ways to assess proliferation, mitosis counting in histological preparations is the most reproducible, with independent prognostic value. Methodological

fine-tuning and larger prospective trials are needed to establish the clinical value of other markers.

There is growing understanding of the importance of the interactions between cells, and between cells and the surrounding stromal environment. Breast cancers frequently exhibit altered cell adhesion molecule expression, have altered matrix protein expression, changes in the cellular components of the tumor microenvironment, and extensive remodeling of the stroma. Chapter 5 focuses on key changes in cell adhesion molecules and stromal components, which have been shown to modulate breast cancer cell function, the potential for such features to act as prognostic and predictive factors for behavior, and the opportunity to use such alterations as therapeutic targets.

p53 is well recognized as 'guardian of the genome', and alterations to the gene are common in cancers, including breast cancer. The precise clinical importance of p53 in breast cancer as a prognostic factor or predictor of disease response remains controversial and is discussed in Chapter 12, which concludes that substantial progress has been made in the understanding of p53 and therapeutic benefits are awaited.

ENDOCRINE RESPONSE AND RESISTANCE

As already indicated, determination of ER is critical for the selection of those patients who could benefit from endocrine treatment (Chapter 9). However, not all patients who have ER-positive cancers will obtain a response and a major clinical problem is the development of acquired resistance. Increased understanding of ER structure and function, knowledge of the two forms of ER (α and β) and their variant forms, and of the interactions between ER and growth factor receptors, and their signaling pathways (Chapters 9 and 10) is resulting in an important body of data which could result in the identification of clinically relevant predictors of endocrine response and resistance.

GENE EXPRESSION PROFILING

In the first edition, gene expression profiling was referred to in the Introduction, but now merits a chapter. The initial publications were concerned with subcategorization of breast cancers,[27-29] but soon the emphasis was on identifying expression profiles relating to prognosis and the prediction of response to endocrine therapy and chemotherapy, and these are discussed in Chapter 11. Genomic prognostic tests are now available. As the authors of Chapter 11 point out, no prospective randomized studies have been completed to demonstrate improved patient outcome by the use of these new tests and the two studies currently underway will not report for several years. They do point out that some forms of clinical benefit from novel tests may be more subtle than improvements to survival.

Gene expression profiling has also been used to examine tumors from patients who have developed local recurrence and those who have not (Chapter 4), and a gene set identified which may predict local recurrence, although studies of larger series are required.

For gene expression profiling to be widely applicable the arrays have to be able to use RNA isolated from fixed, embedded tissue, since this is what happens to most cancers.

CONCLUSIONS

The application of prognostic and predictive factors in the clinical setting has increased, and will continue to do so with advances in markers and therapies. The well-tested factors such as those forming the NPI and ER are still clearly important, and illustrate that all markers are only of value if determined reproducibly and accurately. There is great potential in many of the topics presented in this book, and the progression from research to the clinic should come, as shown by what has happened with gene expression profiling.

REFERENCES

1. Bloom H, Richardson W, Harries E. Natural history of untreated breast cancer (1805–1933). Br Med J 1962; 2: 213–21.

2. Fisher B, Slack NH, Bross IDJ et al. Cancer of the breast: size of neoplasm and prognosis. Cancer 1969; 24: 1071–80.

3. Adair F, Berg J, Joubert L, Robbins GF. Long-term follow-up of breast cancer patients: the 30-year report. Cancer 1974; 33: 1145–50.

4. Nemoto T, Vana J, Bedwani RN et al. Management and survival of female breast cancer: results of a national survey by the American College of Surgeons. Cancer 1980; 45: 2917–24.

5. Koscielny S, Tubiani M, Lê MG et al. Breast cancer: relationship between the size of the primary tumours and the probability of metastatic dissemination. Br J Cancer 1984; 49: 709–15.

6. Rosen PP, Groshen S, Saigo PE et al. A long term follow-up study of survival in stage I (T1N0M0) and stage II (T1N1M0) breast carcinoma. J Clin Oncol 1989; 7: 355–66.

7. Carter CL, Allen C, Henson DE. Relation of tumour size, lymph node status and survival in 24,740 breast cancer cases. Cancer 1989; 63: 181–7.

8. Galea MH, Blamey RW, Elston CW et al. The Nottingham Prognostic Index in primary breast cancer. Breast Cancer Res Treat 1992; 22: 207–19.

9. Elston CW, Ellis IO. Pathological prognostic factors in breast cancer. I. The value of histologcal grade in breast cancer: experience from a large study with long-term follow-up. Histopathology 1991; 19: 403–10.

10. Ellis IO, Galea M, Broughton N et al. Pathological prognostic factors in breast cancer. II. Histological type: relationship with survival in a large study with long-term follow-up. Histopathology 1993; 20: 479–89.

11. McGuire WL. Breast cancer prognostic factors: evaluation guidelines. J Natl Cancer Inst 1991; 83: 154–5.

12. McShane LM, Altman DG, Sauerbrei W et al. Reporting recommendations for tumor marker prognostic studies (REMARK). J Natl Cancer Inst 2005; 97: 1180–4.

13. Harris L, Fritsche H, Mennel R et al. American Society of Clinical Oncology 2007 update of recommendations for the use of tumor markers in breast cancer. J Clin Oncol 2007; 25: 5287–312.

14. McGuire WL, Clark GM. Prognostic factors and treatment decisions in axillary-node-negative breast cancer. New Engl J Med 1992; 326: 1756–61.

15. Goldhirsh A, Wood WC, Gelber RD et al. Meeting highlights: updated international expert consensus on the primary therapy of early breast cancer. J Clin Oncol 2003; 21: 3357–65.

16. Goldhirsh A, Glick JH, Gelber RD et al. Meeting highlights: international expert consensus on the primary therapy of early breast cancer 2005. Ann Oncol 2005; 16: 1569–83.

17. Goldhirsh A, Wood WC, Gelber RD et al. Progress and promise: highlights of the international expert consensus on the primary therapy of early breast cancer 2007. Ann Oncol 2007; 18: 1133–44.

18. Early Breast Cancer Trialists' Collaborative Group. Effects of chemotherapy and hormonal therapy for early breast cancer on recurrence and 15-year

survival: an overview of the randomized trials. Lancet 2005; 365: 1687–717.

19. Stotter A. A prognostic table to guide practitioners advising patients on adjuvant systemic therapy in early breast cancer. Eur J Surg Oncol 1999; 25: 341–3.

20. Feldman M, Stanford R, Catcheside A et al. The use of a prognostic table to aid decision making on adjuvant therapy for women with early breast cancer. Eur J Surg Oncol 2002; 28: 615–19.

21. Stotter A. Revised prognostic table to guide practitioners advising patients on adjuvant systemic therapy in early breast cancer. Eur J Surg Oncol 2007; 33: 1211–12.

22. Williams C, Brunskill S, Altman D et al. Cost-effectiveness of using prognostic information to select women with breast cancer for adjuvant systemic therapy. Health Technol Assess 2006; 10: 1–204.

23. Olivotto IA, Bajdik CD, Ravdin PM et al. Population-based validation of the prognostic model ADJUVANT!

24. for early breast cancer. J Clin Oncol 2005; 23: 2716–25.

24. Pathology reporting of breast disease. NHSBSP Publication No. 58, Sheffield: NHSBSP 2005.

25. Walker RA. Immunohistochemical markers as predictive tools for breast cancer. J Clin Pathol 2008 (in press).

26. Walker RA, Bartlett JMS, Dowsett M et al. HER2 Testing in the UK – further update to recommendations. J Clin Pathol 2008; in press.

27. Perou CM, Sorlie T, Eisen MB et al. Molecular portraits of human breast tumours. Nature 2000; 406: 747–52.

28. Hedenfalk I, Duggan D, Chen Y et al. Gene expression profiles in hereditary breast cancer. New Engl J Med 2001; 344: 539–48.

29. Sorlie T, Perou CM, Tibshirani R et al. Gene expression patterns of breast carcinomas distinguish tumour subclasses with clinical implications. Proc Natl Acad Sci USA 2001; 98: 10,869–74.

The role of the pathologist in assessing prognostic factors for breast cancer

2

Sarah E Pinder, Gavin C Harris and Christopher W Elston

INTRODUCTION

The assessment of prognostic factors, in order to provide a prediction of outcome, has become an essential part of the histopathologist's role in the handling and histological reporting of invasive breast carcinomas.[1] Only with this information available can the clinical team select the most appropriate treatment for the management of patients; those with an excellent prognosis can avoid unnecessary adjuvant treatment,[2] and women with a very poor prognosis can receive more aggressive therapies. In addition, factors which assist in the identification of patients who may respond or be resistant to specific therapies, i.e. predictive factors, can be identified. Such evaluation of predictive factors is an increasing part of the histopathologist's function and practice. Markers may be examined with techniques such as immunohistochemistry and fluorescence in situ hybridization, and include estrogen receptor (ER), progesterone receptor (PR) and human epidermal growth factor receptor 2 (HER2) for prediction of response to hormone agents and trastuzumab, respectively (see Chapters 9 and 13). Nevertheless, a large variety of robust and important prognostic features can be assessed using traditional hematoxylin and eosin (H&E) light microscopy. In this chapter, factors are described which have prognostic implications for breast cancer patients and an indication of their relative importance is also described. Table 2.1 indicates some of the range of assessable prognostic factors.

Table 2.1 Prognostic factors in breast cancer

Traditional morphological factors:

- tumor size
- lymph node stage
- tumor grade
- tumor type
- lymphovascular invasion

Miscellaneous factors
Hormone receptors
Molecular markers

MORPHOLOGICAL FACTORS

Tumor size

The prognostic importance of tumor size is well recognized; patients with larger invasive breast carcinomas have a poorer outcome than those with smaller lesions.[3–6] Many years ago, Rosen and Groshen[4] predicted 20-year relapse-free survival rates for women with tumors <10 mm, 11–13 mm, 14–16 mm and 17–22 mm in diameter of 88%, 73%, 65% and 59%, respectively. However, the clinical evaluation of tumor size is inaccurate, clinical–pathological agreement is seen in only 54% of cases.[7] Radiological assessment, particularly magnetic resonance imaging (MRI) and ultrasonography, which are both more accurate than mammographic estimate of tumor size,[8] is more precise than the clinical determination, but breast carcinomas should always be measured histopathologically. A macroscopic measurement can be performed for large lesions in three planes in the fresh state and then confirmed after fixation but, for small and in situ lesions in particular, the maximum size should be determined microscopically, e.g. using the Vernier scale on the microscope stage.

Smaller tumors are less frequently node-positive than larger lesions, but there is a risk of metastatic lymph node disease even for lesions <10 mm in size; Carter et al[9] reported nodal metastases in approximately 20% of patients with breast cancers <10 mm. Some have reported that 12% of breast carcinomas ≤5 mm in diameter are associated with lymph node metastases,[10] whilst others have suggested that nodal metastases are unlikely in tumors of this size range.[11] Because of the clear prognostic significance of breast cancer size, it is one of the lynchpins of data collection for radiology quality assurance (QA) in mammographic breast screening programs. Specifically, it is recommended that half of the invasive carcinomas detected by mammographic screening in the UK National Health Service Breast Screening Programme should be ≤15 mm in size. It is, therefore, essential for QA of breast screening programs that pathologists measure tumors as accurately as possible to the nearest millimeter, and do not "round up" or "round down" the size of tumors.

Lymph node stage

The presence or absence of locoregional lymph node metastases is one of the most important features in the prediction of disease-free and overall survival in breast cancer patients. Whilst lymph node metastasis is, at least in part, a time-dependent factor, i.e. a carcinoma is more likely to have lymph node metastases the longer it has been present, it is also a marker of a more intrinsically aggressive phenotype.[12,13] The average 10-year survival is 75% for node-negative patients compared to 25–30% for those with nodal disease.[14] Five-year survival rates for patients with node-negative disease have been documented to range from 98% (<0.5 cm) to 82% (>5.0 cm).[9] Prognosis also worsens with increasing numbers

of involved lymph nodes bearing metastatic deposits;[14] patients with four or more positive lymph nodes (lymph node stage 3 disease) have a poorer 5-year survival than those with three or fewer lymph nodes containing metastatic carcinoma (lymph node stage 2).[9,12]

The prognostic significance of extranodal extension of metastatic deposits is somewhat controversial, but there is reported to be an increased rate of recurrence when this feature is seen.[15] Some research has shown a worse overall survival, disease-specific survival and disease-free survival rates in those patients with extranodal spread; in particular, multivariate analysis of disease-specific survival in patients with 1–3 involved lymph nodes has shown independent prognostic significance.[16] Other reports have also shown an association with overall survival but, interestingly, no relation to local recurrence in the axilla.[17]

The TNM (tumor size, lymph node stage, presence of distant metastasis) staging system was initially proposed in 1954, and has been modified several times.[18] As noted above, the clinical assessment of tumor size is not accurate. Similarly, the clinical determination of lymph node size does not necessarily reflect the underlying pathology: nodes reactive to, for example, previous breast biopsy, may be enlarged without evidence of metastatic disease, whilst nodes containing metastatic carcinoma may be impalpable. Thus, the clinical TNM system is unreliable. The pathological TNM (pTNM) staging system incorporates the histological details of size and nodal disease, whilst metastasis is not, in general, assessed histologically and this component corresponds to the clinical "M" category.

Some breast units have historically undertaken routine lymph node clearance,[19] whilst others, especially in the UK, have performed four-lymph-node sampling. The latter groups have argued that node sampling provides sufficient and equivalent prognostic data, with less morbidity in the form of lymphoedema and reduced shoulder mobility.[20,21] There is evidence that a similar proportion of patients will be found to have metastatic disease with either surgical procedure.[20] However, this argument has, to a large extent, been superseded by the widespread acceptance and routine application of the theory and practice of the sentinel lymph node (SLN) biopsy procedure. This targeted procedure is based on the principle that injection of blue dye and/or radioisotope into the breast tissue can be used to identify the first lymph node draining to the axilla, and, therefore, that if disease has spread that this is the node that will bear metastatic tumor. There is a small false-negative rate,[22] and any potential long-term effect on survival is not established. However, as with four-node sampling, there is significantly less axillary morbidity with SLN biopsy than axillary dissection/clearance, and the value in patient management is now established as a standard of care.

Present UK histopathological practice regarding examination of lymph nodes is based on the premise that one should maximize the chance of identifying metastatic disease with simple, cost-effective techniques.[23] Whilst a very large number of pathology protocols for examination of SLNs are in use,[24] many require significant laboratory resources. At present, the UK guidelines recommend thin slicing of the node, embedding each lymph node separately, and histological examination of one level of the multiple slices of each lymph node with hematoxylin and eosin (H&E) stains. Examination of additional levels, immunohistochemistry and reverse transcriptave-polymerase chain reaction (RT-PCR) are not regarded as routine, nor is intraoperative assessment (e.g. by touch imprint cytology or frozen section),[23] although some groups in the UK and elsewhere undertake some, or all, of these additional procedures. As discussed in Chapter 6, the prognostic significance of micrometastases and isolated tumor cells remains uncertain, but it is recommended that these deposits should be reported as per UICC/TNM and AJCC Guidelines,[18,23,25] and categorized as isolated tumor cells, micrometastases or macrometastatic tumor. However, it should also be noted that there is some variation in application of these terms, particularly regarding the classification of very small deposits in the parenchyma, and further clarification of guidelines is awaited.

Three broad groups can be described according to the number of nodes with established metastatic deposits in the axilla. Thus, patients with no metastatic disease are classified as lymph node stage 1, those with 3 or fewer nodes containing metastatic carcinoma as nodal stage 2, and those with 4 or more nodes involved as lymph node stage 3; this should not be confused with the TNM staging system.[18] In some units, patients with primary invasive cancer within the inner half of the breast historically had internal mammary node sampling. If this is performed, and if this lymph node contains metastatic tumor without axillary deposits, the stage of disease is classified as nodal stage 2, but if any axillary node *and* the internal mammary node contain metastatic cancer the disease is categorized as stage 3. In addition, it is well recognized that the level within the axilla of the involved nodes is of prognostic value; those women with metastatic disease at the apex have a significantly poorer outcome[26] and are classified as having stage 3 disease, even if this is apparently the only axillary lymph node which is identified as bearing metastasis.

Histological grade

In many series, lymph node stage is the most important factor in predicting survival of patients with breast cancer but, in some centers, multivariate analyses have shown that histological grade is of similar weight. Indeed, histological grading has been repeatedly shown to predict for overall survival and disease-free survival (Figure 2.1).[27–29]

Grading must be performed with precision and care on tumor samples that are well fixed. All should ideally be received fresh in the laboratory and incised to obtain optimum fixation. A significant decrease in mitotic count, and hence mitotic score, is noted after a delay in fixation of only 1 hour.[30,31] It is vital to note that formalin penetrates fatty tissue slowly, and it seems likely that tumors which have not been incised (and are thus surrounded by several centimeters of tissue) may suffer a similar fate. Thus, histological grade, which incorporates an assessment of mitotic count, may be

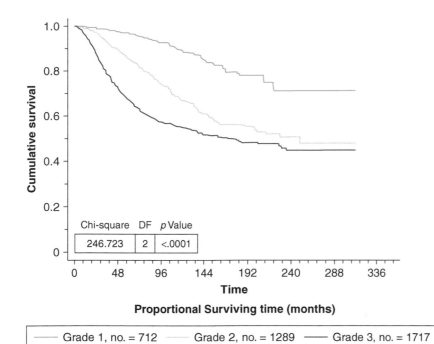

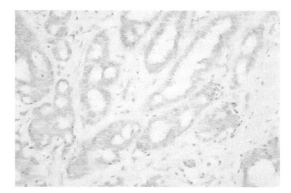

Figure 2.1 Overall survival for patients with primary operable breast carcinoma in the Nottingham Tenovus Primary Breast Carcinomas Series by histological grade.

Figure 2.2 Hematoxylin and eosin section showing tubule formation.

artificially low (e.g. grade 3 lesions may incorrectly be categorized as histological grade 2) if the lesion is poorly fixed; this may have significant treatment implications.

Histological grading of breast carcinomas is performed by a combined evaluation of three factors: gland/tubule formation; atypia/pleomorphism/nuclear size; and mitotic count. Although still described by some as the Bloom and Richardson grade[32] of an invasive breast cancer, the system was amended significantly by the Nottingham Group,[27] and it is this modified system which is recommended by the UK[23] and the European Breast Screening Pathology Groups, the US Directors of Anatomic and Surgical Pathology,[33] as well as the UICC[18] and WHO.

The assessment of glandular differentiation requires evaluation of the proportion of the whole of the tumor which is forming acini with a definite lumen; those carcinomas which show <10% tubule formation score 3, those between 10 and 75% score 2, and tumors forming tubules in >75% score 1 (Figure 2.2). Glandular spaces within more solid islands of invasive carcinoma, such as may be encountered within some "no special type" (NST) or mucinous tumors, should be included in this assessment. Nuclear size/pleomorphism/atypia is scored from 1 to 3

corresponding to mild, moderate and marked pleomorphism/nuclear size. The assessment of pleomorphism should be performed at a high magnification and involves a comparison with normal epithelial cells in the same sections. If there is significant variation in pleomorphism in different areas of a carcinoma, the highest pleomorphism score is recorded. The mitotic count of the tumor is also scored from 1 to 3; the precise number of mitoses per 10 high-power fields depends on the field area of the 40× lens, and varies significantly between microscopes;[23] thus, appropriate calibration of the microscope is essential. Breast carcinomas are notoriously heterogeneous, particularly with regard to mitotic figures, and the area of highest frequency of proliferation/mitoses is selected for assessment. This is often at the periphery of the tumor.[34,35] It must be noted that only unequivocal mitoses are included, and apoptotic and hyperchromatic nuclei should be ignored; only nuclei with definite features of metaphase, anaphase or telophase are counted.

The values of the three elements are then added, and the sum of the scores is used to classify the breast cancer as histological grade 1 (scores of 3, 4 and 5), grade 2 (scores of 6 or 7) or grade 3 (sum of scores of 8 or 9). With experience this procedure can be performed rapidly and is of significant importance for predicting patient survival; a patient with a grade 1 tumor will have an 85% chance of surviving 10 years, but patients with a grade 3 tumor have only a 45% 10-year survival rate (Figure 2.1).

In the past there has been considerable suspicion regarding the reproducibility of histological grading procedures. However, several studies have assessed the reproducibility of histological grading, with up to 80–87% agreement, due to the more objective criteria of the Nottingham modifications when compared to the original methodology.[36-38]

Previously, some pathologists have also questioned the application of histological grading to tumor types other than ductal/NST lesions. Although some tumor types are by definition of a specified grade (e.g. tubular carcinoma is of histological grade 1), others, such as lobular carcinoma, may vary. Whilst typically of histological grade 2 (scoring 3 for tubules, 2 for nuclear atypia and 1 for mitoses), occasionally these lesions may be of histological grade 1 (3, 1, 1) or grade 3 (3, 3, 2), and patients with these variants have outcomes as for the appropriate histological grade.

Histological type

In addition to histological grade, the "differentiation" of a tumor can be determined by an assessment of the histological type.[39]

Histological typing provides additional information to grade in predicting prognosis but in multivariate analysis the absolute effect of this is shown to be small.[40] However, histological typing does provide further biological information. Different tumor types may typically express particular markers; lobular carcinomas, for example, frequently show estrogen receptor (ER) expression and are cathepsin-D, E-cadherin and vimentin negative.[41,42] It is also well recognized that lobular carcinoma may show a different pattern of metastatic spread to other breast carcinomas,[43] although this is also true of histological grade.[44] Invasive micropapillary carcinomas have been shown to present with a high lymph node stage with increased frequency and often show definite vascular invasion.[13]

Many breast carcinoma types have been described, the most common being that of NST, which was previously known as ductal. However, over 18 different morphological types can be applied;[39] clearly, it is not appropriate to describe the diagnostic features of each here.

In order to improve reproducibility of typing, stricter criteria for classification have been described in the UK.[23] When no or <50% of the tumor shows special type characteristics the lesion is regarded as NST (ductal). When another morphological pattern is also present (between 50% and 90% of the tumor) the lesion is categorized as of mixed type. Thus, for example, a tumor may be classified as mixed NST and mucinous appearance. This is of importance as tumors of combined NST and "special type" have a better prognosis than NST alone, whilst other mixed types such as lobular with NST have a significantly poorer prognosis.[39] When a special type component constitutes ≥90% of the carcinoma, it is regarded as being of pure special type.

Some tumors of so-called special type are seen with increased frequency as a result of mammographic breast screening, for example, tubular, invasive cribriform and mucinous subtypes. These are usually of grade 1 morphology and have a good prognosis. However,

Table 2.2 Prognostic groups according to histological type (adapted from reference 40)

Excellent group: >80% 10-year survival
Tubular
Invasive cribriform
Mucinous
Tubulolobular

Good group: 60–80% 10-year survival
Tubular mixed
Alveolar lobular
Mixed ductal no special type (NST) and special type

Moderate group: 50–60% 10-year survival
Medullary
Atypical medullary
Invasive papillary
Classical lobular

Poor group: <50% 10-year survival
Mixed lobular
Solid lobular
Ductal NST
Mixed ductal NST/lobular

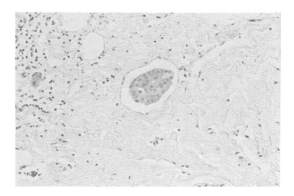

Figure 2.3 Hematoxylin and eosin section showing lymphovascular invasion.

some special type tumors, such as pure mucinous cancers, may, less commonly, be of histological grade 2 with a correspondingly poorer outcome. As noted above, lobular carcinoma may be formed from cells of large and pleomorphic appearance (pleomorphic lobular carcinoma variant). Table 2.2 summarizes prognostic data according to tumor type.

The histopathological features of tumors associated with mutations of the BRCA1 and BRCA2 genes have been described.[45,46] Carcinomas in patients with BRCA1 mutations are more likely to exhibit a pushing margin, high mitotic count and a lymphoid infiltrate on multivariate analysis, but not necessarily have a true medullary or atypical medullary morphology.[46] More recently, there has been considerable interest in the immunohistochemical profile of such subtypes; it has been shown that these carcinomas are one of the subgroup of 'basal-type' cancers and are frequently ER-negative, PR-negative, HER2-negative, p53-positive and have a high proliferation index.[47,48] BRCA2-associated breast carcinomas, conversely, whilst tending to be of higher grade than sporadic age-matched controls do not appear to have a specific immunoprofile,

although some reports suggest that these too have a low frequency of HER2 expression.[48]

Lymphovascular invasion

The presence of tumor emboli in vascular spaces is of prognostic significance in predicting survival of patients with breast carcinoma, which has been found by some groups to be independent of other variables.[49] It has been suggested that this feature is as strong a predictor of outcome as lymph node stage.[50] However, one of the main values of the assessment of this feature lies in predicting local recurrence in women who have had conservation surgery, and flap recurrence in those who have had mastectomy.[51] Thus, in some centers, the presence of vascular invasion is recognized as a risk factor for local recurrence of invasive carcinoma, and if present in addition to other features (such as young age and large tumor size) is regarded as a contraindication to breast-conserving surgery. More recently,[52] it has been shown in a large series of lymph node-negative patients that the assessment of lymphovascular invasion is of independent prognostic significance along with histological grade and tumor size, and it has been suggested that this feature should be considered in decisions about adjuvant treatment in this group of node-negative women. Finally, in rare cases where no lymph nodes have been excised and examined, the presence of vascular invasion can be used as a surrogate for lymph node stage.[14]

It had not previously been possible to distinguish accurately blood vessels from lymphatic spaces, and "lymphovascular invasion" is generally taken to mean tumor emboli within any endothelial-lined space at the periphery of the main mass of the tumor. In order for the diagnosis of lymphovascular invasion to be useful, strict criteria must be used so that artefactual shrinkage (e.g. around foci of ductal carcinoma in situ (DCIS)) is not misdiagnosed as tumor within a vascular space.[49] Immunohistochemical assessment may prove helpful in distinguishing those cases that show artefactual shrinkage from true vascular invasion by the positive immunoreactivity of the endothelial cell lining in the latter with, for example, CD31 antibody. More recently described lymphatic endothelial-specific antibodies have been applied to seek to distinguish blood vessels from lymphatic channels, and have proven to be of interest.[53] However, the prognostic value of such immunohistochemical assessment of lymphovascular invasion for patient survival is not yet clear.

MISCELLANEOUS AND MOLECULAR FACTORS

Extensive tumor necrosis appears to be associated with an aggressive clinical course.[54] However, where strict criteria have been applied, and multivariate analysis performed, an association with tumor size, histological grade and proliferation, as well as lymph node status, has been described, but there has been no independent prognostic value to this feature.[55] There is some evidence that the presence and relative size of fibrotic areas in breast carcinoma can be correlated with an early relapse.[56,57] However, whether these morphological features are robust enough to be included in a routine histopathology dataset remains controversial.

Many molecular markers have been assessed by groups and reported to be potential prognostic markers in invasive breast carcinoma. C-erbB-2/HER2-/neu is an oncogene and member of the epidermal growth factor receptor (EG-FR) family.[58] Amplification of the gene is one of the commonest genetic abnormalities occurring in breast carcinoma, although in a small proportion of cases (approximately 5%) overexpression appears to be the result of increased transcription.[58] In terms of prognostic significance, amplification of this gene appears to be associated with an aggressive phenotype, i.e. high histological grade, estrogen and progesterone negativity, and reduced overall and metastasis-free survival.[58,59] The significance of HER2 assessment, and the need for strict quality assurance methodology, now largely relates to the development of targeted monoclonal antibody therapies such as Herceptin (trastuzumab),[60] and this is discussed in Chapter 13.

Overexpression of EGFR correlates with estrogen receptor negativity and resistance to tamoxifen,[6] and clinical trials are underway to assess its therapeutic potential. Although there are some promising data from results of trials of the dual HER2 and EGFR tyrosine kinase inhibitor, lapatinib, in HER2-positive breast cancer, to date some other EGFR inhibitors have proven somewhat disappointing. In particular, there are difficulties with methodology for selection of those patients most likely to respond to these new drugs.[61]

Other molecular markers have been widely described. For some, changes are common in invasive breast cancer; p53 is mutated in nearly one-third of breast carcinomas and an association with an aggressive clinicopathological phenotype has long been recognized (see Chapter 12).[6] Evaluation of proliferation markers MIB1/Ki67 antigen,[62,63] proliferating cell nuclear antigen (PCNA) and S-phase fraction have shown a correlation with prognosis (see Chapter 3). Other molecular markers whose over- or underexpression have been reported as showing a correlation with prognosis include, not exclusively, transforming growth factor alpha, bcl-2, p16[INK4a], parathyroid hormone-related protein, metalloproteinases, integrins, E-cadherin, pS2 and cathepsin-D.[6,64–70] However, validation of their robustness as independent prognostic factors is disputed, and many have not withstood close scrutiny and repeat analysis.

But, most recently researchers have begun to examine invasive breast carcinomas with more advanced methodologies such as gene expression profiling and other "omics" techniques (see Chapter 11). There has been increasing recognition that breast carcinoma is not a single disease but a biological (as well as morphological) heterogeneous group of lesions, and using such approaches molecular methods of subclassification have been described. Gene expression profiling utilizing microarray analysis has identified breast cancer signatures which appear to be related to prognosis and potentially for treatment. Different molecular subtypes, designated luminal (either 2 or 3 groups), normal-like, HER2+/ER−, and basal-like have been proposed. Interestingly, such groupings have been confirmed with more commonly available immunohistochemical techniques, and confirmed to have prognostic value.[72] At present, there is increasing interest in the overlap between the "basal-type" of invasive breast carcinoma and the so-called "triple negative" (i.e. ER-negative, PR-negative and HER2-negative) breast cancers, partly because of the poor prognosis of these patients and partly because of the therapeutic conundrum they present clinically.

However, differences in design of study, patient groups included, array technology/ different platforms, and methods of analysis make correlation and interpolation of many of the omics study's results difficult.[74] Nevertheless, there are now a large number of studies which report, albeit differing, prognostic gene signatures. Indeed, clinical trials based on such signatures are planned and underway, although not without significant logistically and interpretive difficulties, as recognized by the trial group concerned.[74]

It is clear that breast cancer is a complex and heterogeneous disease, clinically and biologically. Although in the recent past a myriad of putative prognostic and predictive markers of breast cancer have been examined, very few have proven useful. Studies which have found a variable to be of independent importance have not generally been replicated by other groups. At present, the variables which have been shown repeatedly, and by different groups, to be of independent prognostic significance remain those routine histological factors which can be assessed using H&E stains. Such "routine" variables should not, however, be dismissed as "simple" biologically. Such histological features are a complex combination of time and tumor-dependent factors. For example, the presence of lymphovascular invasion or metastatic disease is likely to be a result of interaction of features involving cell–cell and cell–matrix adhesion, degradation/ infiltration, cell proliferation, tumor surface markers, and other specific genetic abnormalities.

PATIENT MANAGEMENT BASED ON PROGNOSTIC AND PREDICTIVE FACTORS

Although lymph node stage is a well-recognized predictor of outcome, it remains a relatively poor discriminator; neither a group of patients with close to 100% survival nor one with 100% mortality can be identified. Histological grade alone is similarly insufficiently robust. Maximal use of the known prognostic factors can be made when they are combined in a prognostic index identifying groups with a very good and a very poor outcome. With appropriate weighting from the beta values of multivariate analysis, the Nottingham Prognostic Index (NPI) has been formed, and confirmed[3] in studies from Nottingham and other groups,[75–78] as providing robust information for patients with operable primary breast carcinoma. In this index, the lymph node stage scored from 1 to 3, as described above, is added to histological grade (1, 2 or 3) and to 0.2× tumour size (in centimeters). Cut-off points of 2.4, 3.4, 4.4, 5.4 and 6.4 can be used to stratify the patients into groups (excellent, good, moderate I, moderate II, poor and very poor).[30] Based on the NPI score, decisions can be made regarding likelihood of survival and thus the appropriateness of adjuvant therapy. Those women with an extremely good predicted survival (e.g. those in the excellent prognostic group have a 96% 10-year survival) are unlikely to suffer further from their disease whilst in all probability gaining little from adjuvant systemic therapy. More recently, a method for predicting more precisely the likely outcome for an individualized NPI score for each patient has also been described.[80] Following such calculations of the patient's NPI score and selection of those patients who require adjuvant therapy, predictive markers can be applied in order to personalize treatment as much as possible.

Developments in the detection of predictive markers in tissue sections means that the histopathologist is now intimately involved in their assessment. ER acts as a predictive factor to determine the likelihood of response to hormone treatments such as tamoxifen or aromatase inhibitors (discussed in Chapter 9).[81,82] The nuclear immunoreactivity seen with ER antibodies can be assessed either in the form of an assessment of the percentage of immunostaining seen, or a combination of the intensity and percentage reactivity in a histochemical ("H") score,[83] or in a simplified method (the "Allred" score)[23,84] incorporating adding a score for the proportion of tumor cell nuclei staining: 0 = no nuclear staining; 1 = <1% nuclei staining; 2 = 1–10% nuclei staining; 3 = 10–33% nuclei staining; 4 = 33–66% nuclei staining; 5 = 66–100% nuclei staining to a score for staining intensity: 0 = no staining; 1 = weak staining; 2 = moderate staining; 3 = strong staining. Thus, summation gives a maximum value of 8.[84] A level of score predicts response to hormone therapy, and a score of 3 or more is regarded as ER-positive.

It is noteworthy that studies of interlaboratory immunohistochemistry for ER have shown a false-negative rate of between 30 and 60% for tumors expressing a low level of receptor.[85] In particular, it should be remembered that ER is a highly labile protein and rapid fixation, as well as adequate antigen retrieval, is vital for accurate assessment of ER status, as well as for determination of other histological prognostic factors.[23]

HER2 (see Chapter 13) is also most frequently assessed in the first instance immunohistochemically,[86] and this forms the basis for selection for treatment with the therapeutic monoclonal antibody trastuzumab (Herceptin), which is now routinely used in both metastatic and adjuvant setting for patients with tumors which are HER2-positive following clinical trials in the latter group of patients.[87] A scoring system is established for immunohistochemistry of 0, +1, +2, +3.[86] Cases scoring +3 have been shown to correlate with amplified HER2/neu.[88] Cases scoring +2 are subsequently assessed by fluorescent in situ hybridization to check whether there is genetic amplification. Tumors scoring +1 or 0 are considered negative.

The features that have been shown to predict for local recurrence include histological grade 3 tumors and young age, as well as the presence of definite lymphovascular invasion.[89] The presence of lymphovascular invasion is thus utilized clinically in some units, although not all. Patients who have features which are predictive of a high risk of local recurrence after breast conservation surgery may be advised to convert to mastectomy. If they have already have mastectomy they are advised to have radiotherapy to the skin flaps.

CONCLUSIONS

At present, the histological features of greatest weight in predicting the behavior of primary breast carcinomas are lymph node stage, histological grade and tumor size, and the presence of lymphovascular invasion. When combined, with each other and with clinical data, they can be used as a basis for selection of the most appropriate treatments, both surgical and systemic. Additional "predictive" markers provide invaluable information in the choice of the optimum treatment for patients with breast cancer who require adjuvant therapy. The assessment of ER status is essential in avoiding a time delay for patients who are unlikely to respond to hormone treatments, and patients with tumors that are HER2 negative will not benefit from trastuzumab. In summary, the histopathologist has a major role to play, not only in the diagnosis of breast cancer but in forming a part of the multidisciplinary management team, and providing vital prognostic and predictive data to enable the patient to receive the optimum treatment.

REFERENCES

1. Clark GM. Do we really need prognostic factors for breast cancer? Breast Cancer Res Treat 1994; 30: 117–26.
2. Page DL. Prognosis and breast cancer. Recognition of lethal and favourable prognostic types. Am J Surg Pathol 1991; 15: 334–49.
3. Galea MH, Blamey RW, Elston CE et al. The Nottingham Prognostic Index in primary breast cancer. Breast Cancer Res Treat 1992; 22: 207–19.
4. Rosen PP, Groshen S. Factors influencing survival and prognosis in early breast carcinoma (T1N0M0-T1N1M0). Assessment of 644 patients with median follow-up of 18 years. Surg Clin North Am 1990; 70: 937–62.
5. Rosen PP, Groshen S, Saigo PE et al. Pathological prognostic factors in stage I (T1N0M0) and stage II (T1N1M0) breast carcinoma: a study of 644 patients with median follow-up of 18 years. J Clin Oncol 1989; 7: 1239–51.
6. Fitzgibbons PL, Page DL, Weaver D. Prognostic factors in breast cancer – College of American Pathologists consensus statement 1999. Arch Pathol Lab Med 2000; 124: 966–78.
7. Yorkshire Breast Cancer Group. Critical assessment of the clinical TNM system in breast cancer. Br J Med 1980; 281: 134–6.
9. Carter CL, Allen C, Henson D. Relation of tumour size, lymph node status, and survival in 24,740 breast cancer cases. Cancer 1989; 63: 181–7.
10. Kollias J, Murphy CA, Elston CW et al. The prognosis of small primary breast cancers. Eur J Cancer 1999; 35: 908–12.
11. Siaz E, Toonkel R, Poppiti Jr RJ et al. Infiltrating breast carcinoma smaller than 0.5 centimeters – is lymph node dissection necessary? Cancer 1999; 85: 2206–11.
12. Jatoi I, Hilsenbeck SG, Clark GM et al. Significance of axillary lymph node metastasis in primary breast cancer. J Clin Oncol 1999; 17: 2334–40.
13. Nassar H, Wallis T, Andea A et al. Clinicopathologic analysis of invasive micropapillary differentiation in breast carcinoma. Mod Pathol 2001; 14: 836–41.
14. Rampaul RS, Pinder SE, Elston CW et al. Prognostic and predictive factors in primary breast cancer and their role in patient management; The Nottingham Breast Team. Eur J Surg Oncol 2001; 27: 229–38.
15. Ragaz J, Jackson SM. Significance of axillary lymph node extranodal soft tissue extension and indications for postmastectomy irradiation. Cancer 2000; 89: 223–4.
16. Bucci JA, Kennedy CW, Burn J et al. Implications of extranodal spread in node positive breast cancer: a review of survival and local recurrence. Breast 2001; 10: 213–19.
17. Donegan WL, Stine SB, Samter TG. Implications of extracapsular nodal metastases for treatment and prognosis of breast cancer. Cancer 1993; 72: 778–82.
18. UICC International Union Against Cancer. TNM Classification of Malignant Tumours, sixth edn. Eds Sobin LH, Wittekind Ch. New York: Wiley-Less, 2002: 131–41.
19. Cabanes PA, Salmon RJ, Vilcoq JR et al. Value of axillary dissection in addition to lumpectomy and radiotherapy in early breast cancer. The Breast Carcinoma Collaborative Group of the Institut Curie. Lancet 1992; 339: 1245–8.
20. Steele RJG, Forrest APM, Gibson T. The efficacy of lower axillary sampling in obtaining lymph node status in breast cancer: a controlled randomized trial. Br J Surg 1985; 72: 368–9.
21. Dixon JM, Dillon P, Anderson TJ et al. Axillary node sampling in breast cancer: an assessment of its efficacy. The Breast 1998; 7: 206–8.
22. Weaver DL. Sentinel lymph node biopsy in breast cancer: creating controversy and defining new standards. Adv Anat Path 2001; 8: 65–73.
23. National Coordinating Group for Breast Screening Pathology. Pathology Reporting of Breast Disease. NHSBSP Publication No 58. Sheffield: NHS Cancer Screening Programmes and The Royal College of Pathologists, 2005.
24. Cserni G, Amendoeira I, Apostolikas N et al. Discrepancies in current practice of pathological evaluation of sentinel lymph nodes in breast cancer. Results of a questionnaire based survey by the European Working Group for Breast Screening Pathology. J Clin Pathol 2004; 57: 695–701.
25. Singletary SE, Connolly JL. Breast cancer staging: working with the sixth edition of the AJCC Cancer Staging Manual. CA Cancer J Clin 2006; 56: 37–47.
26. Veronesi U, Galimberti V, Zurrida S et al. Prognostic significance of number and level of axillary node metastases in breast cancer. The Breast 1993; 3: 224–8.
27. Elston CW, Ellis IO. Pathological prognostic factors in breast cancer. I. The value of histological grade in breast cancer: experience from a large study with long-term follow-up. Histopathology 1991; 19: 403–10.
28. Simpson JF, Gray R, Dressler CD et al. Prognostic value of histologic grade and proliferative activity in axillary node-positive breast cancer: results from the Eastern Cooperative Oncology Group Companion Study EST 4189. J Clin Oncol 2000; 18: 2059–69.
29. Davis BW, Gelber RD, Goldhirsch A et al. Prognostic significance of tumour grade in clinical trials of adjuvant therapy for breast cancer with axillary lymph node metastasis. Cancer 1986; 58: 2662–70.
30. Brearley N, Kumah P, Bell JA et al. Delay to fixation of invasive breast carcinoma: effect on mitotic count,

MIB1, ER and p53 expression. Eur J Cancer 2001; 37 (Suppl): 2662–70 (abstract).

31. Cross SS, Start RD. Estimating mitotic activity in tumours. Histopathology 1996; 29: 485–8.

32. Bloom HJ, Richardson WW. Histological grading and prognosis in breast cancer. A study of 1409 cases of which 359 have been followed for 15 years. Br J Cancer 1957; 11: 359–77.

33. Connolly JL, Fechner RE, Kempson RL et al. Recommendations for the reporting of breast carcinoma. Hum Pathol 1996; 27: 220–4.

34. Thunnissen FBJM, Ambergen AW, Koss M et al. Mitotic counting in surgical pathology: sampling bias, heterogeneity and statistical uncertainty. Histopathology 2001; 39: 1–8.

35. Connor AJM, Pinder SE, Elston CW et al. Intra-tumoural heterogeneity of proliferation in invasive breast carcinoma evaluated with MIB1 antibody. The Breast 1997; 6; 171–6.

36. Robbins P, Pinder S, de Klerk N et al. Histological grading of breast carcinomas: a study of interobserver agreement. Hum Pathol 1995; 26: 873–9.

37. Frierson HF, Wolber RA, Berean KW et al. Interobserver reproducibility of the Nottingham modification of the Bloom and Richardson histologic grading system for infiltrating ductal carcinoma. Am J Clin Pathol 1995; 103: 195–8.

38. Dalton LW, Page DL, Dupont WD. Histologic grading of breast carcinoma. A reproducibility study. Cancer 1994; 73: 2765–70.

39. Ellis IO, Galea M, Broughton N et al. Pathological prognostic factors in breast cancer. II. Histological type. Relationship with survival in a large study with long-term follow-up. Histopathology 1992; 20: 479–89.

40. Pereira H, Pinder SE, Sibbering DM et al. Pathological prognostic factors in breast cancer IV. Should you be a typer or grader? A comparative study of two prognostic variables in operable breast cancer. Histopathology 1995; 27: 219–26.

41. Domagala W, Markiewski M, Kubiak R et al. Immunohistochemical profile of invasive lobular carcinoma of the breast: predominantly vimentin and p53 protein negative, cathepsin D and oestrogen receptor positive. Virchows Arch A Pathol Anat Histopathol 1993; 423: 497–502.

42. Domagala W, Wozniak L, Lasota J et al. Vimentin is preferentially expressed in high-grade ductal and medullary, but not in lobular breast carcinomas. Am J Pathol 1990; 137: 1059–64.

43. Lamovec J, Bracko M. Metastatic pattern of infiltrating lobular carcinoma of the breast: an autopsy study. J Surg Oncol 1991; 48: 28–33.

44. Porter GJR, Evans AJ, Pinder SE et al. Patterns of metastatic breast carcinoma: influence of tumour histological grade. Clin Radiol 2004; 59: 1094–8.

45. Lakhani SR, Easton DF, Stratton MR et al. Pathology of familial breast cancer: differences between breast cancers in carriers of BRCA1 or BRCA2 mutations and sporadic cases. The Lancet 1997; 349: 1505–10.

46. Lakhani SR, Jacquemier J, Sloane JP et al. Multifactorial analysis of differences between sporadic breast cancers involving BRCA1 and BRCA2 mutations. J Natl Cancer Inst 1998; 90: 1138–45.

47. Jacquemier J, Padovani L, Rabayrol L et al. European Working Group for Breast Screening Pathology; Breast Cancer Linkage Consortium. Typical medullary breast carcinomas have a basal/myoepithelial phenotype. J Pathol 2005; 207: 260–8.

48 Honrado E, Benítez J, Palacios J. Histopathology of BRCA1- and BRCA2-associated breast cancer. Crit Rev Oncol Hematol 2006; 59: 27–39.

49. Pinder SE, Ellis IO, Galea M et al. Pathological prognostic factors in breast cancer. III. Vascular invasion: relationship with recurrence and survival in a large study with long-term follow-up. Histopathology 1994; 24: 41–7.

50. Bettelheim R, Penman HG, Thornton-Jones H et al. Prognostic significance of peritumoral vascular invasion in breast cancer. Br J Cancer 1984; 50: 771–7.

51. O'Rourke S, Galea MH, Morgan D et al. Local recurrence after simple mastectomy. Br J Surg 1994; 81: 386–9.

52. Lee AHS, Pinder SE, Mitchell M et al. Prognostic value of lympho-vascular invasion in women with lymph node negative invasive carcinoma of the breast. Eur J Cancer 2006; 42: 357–62.

53. Van den Eynden GG, Van der Auwera I, Van Laere SJ et al. Distinguishing blood and lymph vessel invasion in breast cancer: a prospective immunohistochemical study. Br J Cancer 2006; 94: 1643–9.

54. Colpaert C, Vermeulen P, Jeuris W et al. Early distant relapse in 'node-negative' breast cancer patients is not predicted by occult axillary lymph node metastases, but by the features of the primary tumour. J Pathol 2001; 193: 442–9.

55. Ikpatt O, Ndoma-Egba R, Collan Y. Prognostic value of necrosis in Nigerian breast cancer. Adv Clin Path 2002; 6: 31–7.

56. Colpaert C, Vermeulen P, van Beest P et al. Intratumoral hypoxia resulting in the presence of a fibrotic focus is an independent predictor of early distant relapse in lymph node-negative breast cancer patients. Histopathology 2001; 39: 416–25.

57. Van den Eynden GG, Colpaert CG, Couvelard A et al. A fibrotic focus is a prognostic factor and a surrogate marker for hypoxia and (lymph)angiogenesis in breast cancer: review of the literature and proposal on the criteria of evaluation. Histopathology 2007; 51: 440–451.

58. Sahin AA. Biologic and clinical significance of Her-2/neu (cerbB-2) in breast cancer. Adv Anat Pathol 2000; 7: 158–66.

59. Ferrero-Pous M, Hacene K, Bouchet C et al. Relationship between c-erbB-2 and other tumour characteristics in breast cancer prognosis. Clin Cancer Res 2000; 6: 4745–54.

60. Dhesy-Thind B, Pritchard KI, Messersmith H et al. HER2/neu in systemic therapy for women with breast cancer: a systematic review. Breast Cancer Res Treat 2007 (in press; e-pub ahead of print).

61. O'Donovan N, Crown J. EGFR and HER-2 antago-nists in breast cancer. Anticancer Res 2007; 27: 1285–94.

62. Veronese SM, Gambacorta M, Gottardi O et al. Proliferation index as a prognostic marker in breast cancer. Cancer 1993; 71: 3926–31.

63. Pinder SE, Wencyk P, Sibbering DM et al. Assessment of the new proliferation marker MIB1 in breast carcinoma using image analysis: associations with other prognostic factors and survival. Br J Cancer 1995; 71: 146–9.

64. Gui GPH, Wells CA, Browne PD et al. Integrin expression in primary breast cancer and its relation to axillary nodal status. Surgery 1995; 117: 102–8.

65. Hui R, Macmillan D, Kenny F et al. INK4a gene expression and methylation in primary breast can-cer: overexpression of p16^{INK4a} messenger RNA is a marker of poor prognosis. Clin Cancer Res 2000; 6: 2777–87.

66. Henderson MA, Danks JA, Moseley JM et al. Parathyroid hormone-related protein production by breast cancers, improved survival and reduced bone metastases. J Nat Cancer Inst 2001; 93: 234–7.

67. Duffy MJ, Maguire TM, Hill A et al. Metallo-proteinases: role in breast carcinogenesis, invasion and metastasis. Breast Cancer Res 2000; 2: 252–7.

68. Jones JL, Royall JE, Walker RA. E-cadherin relates to EGFR expression and lymph node metastasis in pri-mary breast carcinoma. Br J Cancer 1996; 74: 1237–41.

69. Gillett CE, Miles DW, Ryder K et al. Retention of the expression of E-cadherin and catenins is associated with shorter survival in grade III ductal carcinoma of the breast. J Pathol 2001; 193: 433–41.

70. Gonzalez MA, Pinder SE, Wencyk PM et al. An immunohistochemical examination of the expression of E-cadherin, alpha- and beta/gamma-catenins, and alpha 2- and beta 1-integrins in invasive breast cancer. J Pathol 1999; 187: 523–9.

71. Sørlie T, Perou CM, Tibshirani R et al. Gene expres-sion patterns of breast carcinomas distinguish tumor subclasses with clinical implications. Proc Natl Acad Sci USA 2001; 98: 10,869–74.

72. Abd El-Rehim DM, Ball G, Pinder SE et al. High-throughput protein expression analysis using tissue microarray technology of a large well-characterised series identifies biologically distinct classes of breast cancer confirming recent cDNA expression analyses. Int J Cancer 2005; 116: 340–50.

73. Naderi A, Teschendorff AE, Barbosa-Morais NL et al. A gene-expression signature to predict survival in breast cancer across independent data sets. Oncogene 2007; 26: 1507–16.

74. Bogaerts J, Cardoso F, Buyse M et al. TRANSBIG con-sortium. Gene signature evaluation as a prognostic tool: challenges in the design of the MINDACT trial. Nat Clin Pract Oncol 2006; 3: 540–51.

75. Brown JM, Benson EA, Jones M. Confirmation of a long-term prognostic index in breast cancer. The Breast 1993; 2: 144–7.

76. Balslev I, Axelsson CK, Zedelev K et al. The Nottingham Prognostic Index applied to 9,149 patients from studies of the Danish Breast Cancer Cooperative Group (DBCG). Breast Cancer Res Treat 1994; 32: 281–90.

77. Sundquist M, Thorstenson S, Brudin L et al. Applying the Nottingham Prognostic Index to a Swedish breast cancer population. Br Cancer Res Treat 1999; 53: 1–8.

78. D'Eridita GD, Giardina C, Martellotta M et al. Prognostic factors in breast cancer: the predictive value of the Nottingham Prognostic Index in patients with long-term follow-up that were treated in a single institution. Eur J Cancer 2001; 37: 591–6.

79 Blamey RW, Ellis IO, Pinder SE et al. Survival of inva-sive breast cancer according to the Nottingham Prognostic Index in cases diagnosed in 1990–1999. Eur J Cancer 2007; 43: 1548–55.

80. Blamey RW, Pinder SE, Ball GR et al. Reading the prognosis of the individual with breast cancer. Eur J Cancer 2007; 43: 1545–7.

81. Robertson JFR, Ellis IO, Pearson D et al. Biological factors of prognostic significance in locally advanced breast cancer. Breast Cancer Res Treat 1994; 29: 259–64.

82. Goulding H, Pinder S, Cannon P et al. A new immunohistochemical antibody for the assessment of estrogen receptor status on routine formalin-fixed tissue samples. Hum Pathol 1995; 26: 291–4.

83. McCarty KSJ, Miller LS, Cox EB et al. Oestrogen receptor analyses: correlation of biochemical and immunohistochemical methods using monoclonal antibodies. Arch Pathol Lab Med 1985; 109: 16–721.

84. Harvey JM, Clark GM, Osborne CK et al. Estrogen receptor status by immunohistochemistry is superior to the ligand-binding assay for predicting response to adjuvant endocrine therapy in breast cancer. J Clin Oncol 1999; 17: 1474–81.

85. Rhodes A, Jasani B, Barnes DM et al. Reliability of immunohistochemical demonstration of oestrogen receptors in routine practice: interlaboratory vari-ance in the sensitivity of detection and evaluation of scoring systems. J Clin Pathol 2000; 53: 125–30.

86. Ellis IO, Bartlett J, Dowsett M et al. Best Practice No 176. Updated recommendations for HER2 testing in the UK. J Clin Pathol 2004; 57: 233–7.

87. Smith I, Procter M, Gelber RD et al. 2-year follow-up of Trastuzumab after adjuvant chemotherapy in HER2-positive breast cancer: a randomised con-trolled trial. Lancet 2007; 369: 29–36.

88. Dowsett M, Bartlett J, Ellis IO et al. Correlation between immunohistochemistry (HercepTest) and fluorescence in situ hybridization (FISH) for HER-2 in 426 breast carcinomas from 37 centres. J Pathol 2003; 199: 418–23.

89. Locker AP, Ellis IO, Morgan DA et al. Factors influ-encing local recurrence after excision and radio-therapy for primary breast cancer. Br J Surg 1989; 76: 890–4.

Prognostic value of proliferation and apoptosis in breast cancer

3

Paul J van Diest, Johannes S de Jong, Jan PA Baak,
Rob JAM Michalides and Elsken van der Wall

INTRODUCTION

Breast cancer is the leading cause of death among solid tumors in women, and the incidence is still increasing in the Western world, especially among younger women. In the Netherlands, there are close to 10,000 new cases every year in a population of 15 million people. At present, the disease will affect 12% of all women, and approximately 40% of patients will die from metastatic disease. Gain in survival can be expected from early detection and the use of adjuvant therapy. Mammographic screening strategies result in earlier diagnosis of breast cancer, and a 25–30% decrease in breast cancer mortality in woman over the age of 50 years.[1] However, mammographic screening is more likely to detect slower growing and better differentiated tumors (which inherently have a better prognosis) rather than rapidly growing aggressive tumors which often present as interval cancers.[2,3] Adjuvant chemo- and hormonal therapy have been shown to improve survival in breast cancer patients, but do have side-effects, and therefore selection of those patients who will gain the most benefit is critical. In addition to traditional prognostic factors (see Chapter 2) and predictive factors (such as steroid receptors (Chapter 9) and human epidermal growth factor receptor 2 (HER2)/neu (Chapter 13), other factors are required. There is a panoply of prognostic factors for breast cancer. Many of them are directly (e.g. cell cycle regulators[4]) or indirectly (e.g. through growth factors[5,6] or angiogenesis[7]) related to proliferation or apoptosis. This is no surprise, since growth of tumor cells is the net effect of an increase in cells due to proliferation and decrease in cell death due to apoptosis (and necrosis).

Although many studies evaluating the role of individual genes regulating these processes have greatly increased our knowledge of the complex processes of proliferation and apoptosis, the functional end-results of these – a cell dividing or going into apoptosis – have remained the most important prognostic factors.

The aim of this chapter is to review the prognostic value of proliferation and apoptosis for invasive breast cancer, primarily focusing on the clinical value of different methods to assess proliferation and cell death, and briefly evaluating the value of genes regulating proliferation and cell death.

PROLIFERATION

Assessment of proliferation

Different methods, based on the concept of the cell cycle, have become available for assessment of the rate of proliferation, and have been extensively reviewed.[8] Cellular proliferation takes place through a defined process in which several phases can be recognized. From the resting (G0) phase, they join the active cycling population after appropriate stimuli, and enter the first gap (G1) phase. Both phases have a highly variable duration.

In G1, the cell prepares for the synthesis (S) phase, in which DNA synthesis and doubling of the genome take place. The S phase is followed by a period of apparent inactivity known as the second gap (G2) phase, in which the cell prepares for further separation of chromatids during the mitotic (M) phase. After the M phase, each daughter cell may enter the G0 phase or move on to the G1 phase to repeat the cell cycle. The interphase, which comprises G1, S and G2 phases, forms the largest part of the cell cycle, but cells in these phases cannot be distinguished morphologically. Cells in the mitotic phase can, however, be easily identified because of the typical appearance of the chromosome sets during the different subphases of the M phase (Figure 3.1). This has been the basis for light microscopic counting of mitotic figures, the oldest form of assessing proliferation.

However, the duration of the mitotic phase can vary, especially in aneuploid tumors, so the number of mitoses is not linearly correlated to the rate of proliferation. Cell biologists, in particular, have therefore explored other methods. An optimal assessment of the proliferation rate of a tumor includes measurements of the growth fraction, as well as of the cell cycle time.[8] Cell cycle time is difficult to assess, but preliminary results have been described by assessment of argyrophylic nuclear organizer regions (AgNORs) in Ki67-positive cells, and these show promise.[9] Growth fraction can be more easily determined by immunohistochemical analysis of proliferation-associated antigens, such as Ki67, Ki-S1 topoisomerase IIα, proliferating cell nuclear antigen (PCNA), minichromosome maintenance protein 2 or phosphohistone H3, or DNA cytometric assessment of the percentage of S phase. Incorporation techniques (e.g. with bromodeoxyuridine (BrdU) and tritiated thymidine) theoretically provide the gold standard of cellular proliferation. All of these methods have their pros and cons from a cell biological or practical point of view.[8] The bottom line is that incorporation techniques are impractical, since fresh material is needed,

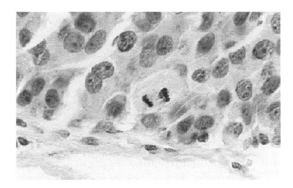

Figure 3.1 Mitotic figure as seen in hematoxylin and eosin (H&E)-stained section.

patients need to be injected intravenously and/or radioactivity is involved, and are therefore unattractive in daily practice. The percentage S phase is hampered by marked intratumor heterogeneity.[10] Minichromosome maintenance protein 2 and phosphohistone H3 are promising new proliferation markers. Mitosis counting and the Ki67 index therefore remain as practical and well-established methods. Mitosis counting has been well studied from a methodological point of view, and by large retrospective and prospective studies (see below).

Prognostic value of proliferation in breast cancer

The different methods for assessing proliferation have all been tested for their prognostic value in invasive breast cancer. Most studies have been performed on sporadic patients, and a few on BRCA1/2-related cases, which in general show higher proliferation compatible with their poorer prognosis.[11]

A high thymidine labeling index has been shown to be associated with poor prognosis in lymph node-positive and -negative breast cancer patients,[12–28] although not in all studies.[29] For BrdU, only a few clinical studies have been published. Thor et al[30] compared BrdU with the mitotic index and the Ki67 index, and found comparable prognostic values for all three techniques. Goodson et al[31] found BrdU to be slightly superior to Ki67. As stated above, these methods are, however, impractical for daily routine. For flow cytometry, most studies that used fresh/frozen material from a sufficient number of patients found a relationship between high percentage S phase and an unfavorable prognosis.[32–34] However, in view of the high intratumor heterogeneity of percentage S phase, it is difficult to use this as a marker for an individual patient.[32]

The monoclonal antibody Ki-S1 is believed to recognize a cell cycle-associated antigen, related to mitotic count,[35] but only a few clinical studies have been described, most revealing no prognostic value.[35–37]

Topoisomerase IIα is a recently established marker of proliferating cells. In one study, topoisomerase IIα and Ki67 scores closely paralleled each other,[38] indicating that the topoisomerase IIα labeling index also reflects the proliferative activity of tumor cells, and provided independent prognostic value in two studies.[38,39] Minichromosome maintenance protein 2 and phosphohistone H3 are promising markers, but as yet, only anecdotal data have been published.[40,41]

The Ki67 labeling index on frozen sections was prognostically relevant in several studies of invasive breast cancer.[42–44] The paraffin-reactive MIB1 antibody against Ki67 has confirmed the prognostic value of Ki67 on archival material,[27,28,38,39,42,45–60] including lymph node-negative patients,[61,62] with a good correlation between Ki67 and MIB1 staining.[44] In predominantly in situ cancers, even the Ki67 labeling index of the in situ parts seems to have prognostic value.[50] A marked decrease in the Ki67/MIB1 labeling index during or after treatment is associated with a good response to preoperative chemotherapy[63,64] and hormonal therapy.[65] However, not all studies on Ki67/MIB1 reached statistical significance.[34] It should be noted, though, that few studies have addressed methodological issues such as sampling strategies, intratumor heterogeneity, and reproducibility; most studies are retrospective, and thresholds vary.

Due to conflicting results, PCNA immunohistochemistry does not seem to provide a prognostically relevant assessment of proliferation in breast cancer.[66–71] Several studies have shown that mitotic count is the most important constituent of histological grade,[72,73] but there are well-known problems with reproducibility of grading due to lack of strict protocols.[74–80] In different studies from our group, we have shown that a highly protocol-driven way of assessing the mitotic activity index (MAI; counting at 400× magnification in an area of $1.6\,mm^2$ in the highest proliferative invasive area in the periphery of the tumor) results in it being a very strong prognostic factor, giving additional prognostic value to tumor size and lymph node status in several retrospective and prospective studies.[7,81–98] Several other groups from different countries have confirmed the prognostic value of mitosis counting in primary invasive breast cancer.[1,27,45,57,61,99–138] Elkhuizen et al[131] found that patients with a recurrence that had a high mitotic count following breast-conserving therapy after an interval >2 years had an equally poor prognosis to those patients with a local recurrence detected after a short interval. We have ourselves reported that mitosis counting in lymph node metastases offers some prognostic value.[88]

Table 3.1 provides an overview of the different studies on the MAI in breast cancer. The total number of patients investigated in these different studies is difficult to estimate, since not all of them used independent patient groups, but it is clear that the MAI has been studied in thousands of patients, and is usually of strong independent prognostic value. However, a few smaller studies have failed to reveal prognostic value.[108,114,133] In several studies, mitotic count has been shown to have specific additional prognostic value to tumor size and lymph node status – a combination denoted the morphometric prognostic index.[82,87,98,129,134]

For practical reasons, it would appear that the MAI by itself is preferable for clinical practice. The MAI has been proven to be reproducible in a multicenter study involving routine laboratories.[139] The prognostic value of the MAI holds for premenopausal lymph

Table 3.1 Overview of the different studies on the prognostic value of the mitoses counting in invasive breast cancer

Authors and ref*	n	Subgroup	Disease-free survival	Overall survival	Independent value?
			p value		
Aaltomaa et al[100]	293	LN–	0.005	–	yes
Aaltomaa et al[100]	224	LN+	0.004	–	yes
Aaltomaa et al[101]	106	all	<0.001	<0.001	yes
Aaltomaa et al[99]	281	LN–	0.0115	0.0007	yes
Aaltomaa et al[103]	688	all	<0.0001	<0.0001	yes
Aaltomaa et al[104]	611	all	<0.001	<0.001	yes
Baak et al[82]	271	ductal	–	<0.001	yes
Baak et al[83]	82	ductal	–	0.0254	yes
Baak et al[85]	576	LN–, <55 years	<0.0001	<0.0001	yes
Baak et al[138]	84	<1 cm	0.02	0.001	yes
	300	1–2 cm	<0.00001	<0.00001	yes
	124	2–3	0.0004	0.0008	yes
Barbareschi et al[106]	178	LN–	0.03	–	no
Biesterfeld et al[107]	104	all	–	<0.0001	yes
Biesterfeld and Reitmaier[45]	108	LN+	–	0.0093	yes
Bos et al[86]	153	all	0.046	0.017	yes
Chen et al[108]	255	LN–	n.s.	n.s.	no
Clahsen et al[61]	441	LN–	<0.01	–	–
Clayton[109]	378	LN–	–	<0.0001	yes
Clayton and Hopkins[110]	399	LN+	–	<0.0001	yes
Collan et al[87]	120	all	–	0.001	yes
Colpaert et al[111]	104	LN–	<0.0001	–	no
Eskelinen et al[112]	216	all	0.01	–	yes
Fiets et al[133]	164	LN	–		
Groenendijk et al[134]	387	all	<0.0001	–	–
Jannink et al[92]	186	all	–	<0.001	yes
Jannink et al[92]	189	all	–	<0.001	yes
Jalava et al[60]	265	all	–	0.0002	yes
Joensuu and Toikkanen[113]	311	all	–	<0.0001	–
De Jong et al[230]	112	all	–	0.0009	yes
Kato et al[114]	70	LN–	–	n.s.	no
Keshgegian and Cnaan[115]	126	all	0.0003	–	–
Kronqvist et al[116]	364	all	–	–	–
Kronqvist et al[117]	202	all	–	0.0001	yes
Ladekarl and Jensen[118]	71	ductal	–	0.1	yes
Ladekarl[119]	98	LN–	–	0.0005	yes
Laroye and Minkin[132]	76	all	–	n.s.	yes
Le Doussal et al[135]	1262	ductal	<0.0001	0.002	yes
Linden et al[94]	195	all	0.001	–	yes
Linden et al[95]	156	all	0.001	0.005	yes
Lipponen et al[120]	111	all	0.001	0.001	yes
Lipponen et al[136]	363	all	0.004	0.001	yes
Lipponen et al[121]	202	all	0.012	–	yes
Liu et al[122]	791	all	<0.0001	<0.0001	yes
Mandard et al[123]	281	LN–, premenopausal	<0.001	<0.001	yes

Table 3.1 (*Continued*)

Authors and ref*	n	Subgroup	p value Disease-free survival	Overall survival	Independent value?
Meyer et al[28]	631	LN–		0.0093	–
Offersen[137]	365	all		<0.0001	no[+]
Page et al[124]	311	LN–	n.s.	0.01	yes
Pietilainen et al[57]	191	all	–	0.0025	yes
Russo et al[68]	646	all	<0.0001	–	yes
Simpson et al[126]	560	LN+	0.004	–	yes
Theissig et al[127]	92	all	–	<0.0001	yes
Thor et al[30]	486	all	0.0001	0.007	yes
Toikkanen et al[128]	217	lobular	–	0.0001	yes
Tosi et al[129]	350	all	0.025	–	yes
Uyterlinde et al[96]	63	ductal	–	0.008	yes
Uyterlinde et al[97]	225	ductal	–	<0.0001	yes
Uyterlinde et al[98]	295	ductal	–	<0.0001	yes
Van Diest and Baak[88]	211	<55	–	<0.0001	yes
Van Diest et al[90]	20	LN+	–	0.004	–
Van Diest et al[91]	148	all	–	0.0001	yes
Younes et al[130]	300	ductal	–	0.0032	yes

* Note: Not all these studies use independent patient groups.
+ Multivariate analysis included, also grade at which it includes the mitotic activity index.
n.s., not significant.

node-negative patients,[89,92] which was confirmed in a nationwide prospective study in the Netherlands[85,140,141] (Figure 3.2).[85,139,140]

The College of American Pathologists Consensus Statement 1999 includes mitotic figure counting as a category I prognostic factor for breast cancer,[142] and mitotic count has also been recognized by the UICC as an 'essential prognostic factor'.[143] The MAI is not seriously affected by fixation delay, although poor fixation does lead to poorer morphology, which makes counting more difficult. It is therefore advisable to avoid delay in fixation whenever possible, and to keep fresh specimens in the refrigerator until fixation.[32] Mitosis should, in principle, be counted before chemotherapy, but even after chemotherapy, the mitotic index has prognostic value.[144,145] Counting should be done on excision specimens or mastectomies to avoid sampling error, but even counting of large core biopsies seem to be fairly representative.[146]

The advantage of a section-based morphological method to assess proliferation, such as mitosis counting, is that intratumor heterogeneity (e.g. central and peripheral tumor parts) is relatively easy to deal with.[147] The MAI has been criticized for not correcting for cellularity, but correction for volume percentage epithelium or cellularity does not lead to a relevant increase in prognostic value, although it does dramatically increase the time required for a proper assessment.[92]

Prediction of response to neoadjuvant therapy

High proliferation has also been associated with resistance to neoadjuvant therapy when measured by mitotic rate,[148,149] S-phase fraction[148] and the Ki67 index.[149,150] Cyclin A does not seem to correlate with neoadjuvant chemotherapy response.[151]

Summary

From the different methods available to assess proliferative activity in breast cancer, the MAI meets the criteria of well-established prospective prognostic value, stable thresholds, good reproducibility and practicality. It can therefore be used to stratify patients for adjuvant therapy. The Ki67 labeling index assessed with the MIB1 antibody is a good runner-up, and may become clinically applicable after further methodological

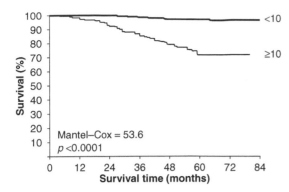

Figure 3.2 Survival of lymph node-negative breast cancer patients with low and high mitotic activity index (MAI) prospective results from the Dutch MMCP study.[85]

fine-tuning. The other methods are of biological rather than practical value.

Prognostic value of cell cycle-regulating genes

The prognostic value of expression patterns of cell cycle-regulating genes has been less well studied than, for example, MAI and MIB1. Some interesting data regarding cell cycle regulators have, however, been described which help us to understand changes in rate of proliferation in tumors, and some changes in expression seem to have some clinical value.

Cyclin A is expressed in the late phases of the cell cycle, and may thereby function as a marker of proliferating cells. The cyclin A labeling index (not influenced by amplification[152]) is indeed positively correlated with proliferation.[59] In a few breast cancer studies, a high cyclin A labeling index was associated with poor prognosis.[59,151,153]

Cyclin B is also expressed in the late phases of the cell cycle, and has been found to increase in frequency from normal breast tissue to atypical ductal hyperplasia (ADH), ductal carcinoma in situ (DCIS), and invasive carcinoma.[154] In one study, high cyclin B levels predicted poor prognosis.[155]

Cyclin D1, mainly expressed in the G1 phase, seems to play a role in breast carcinogenesis, since mRNA and protein overexpression is quite often found in ductal hyperplasia and in situ carcinoma,[156,157] especially in high-grade DCIS, which recur more frequently than low-grade ones.[158,159] Overexpression of cyclin D1 protein or mRNA occurs in the vast majority of invasive lobular carcinomas, but not in lobular carcinoma in situ.[160]

Overexpression of cyclin D1 in invasive breast cancers occurs in 40–50% of all cases,[91,161,162] about half of which is due to amplification of the cyclin D1 gene (CCND1) on chromosome 11q13. This amplification, and corresponding overexpression, is associated with a more aggressive tumor phenotype and/or worse prognosis.[152,163–164] In contrast, overexpression of the cyclin D1 protein was negatively correlated with proliferation, and by itself was not indicative of prognosis in large series of patients with stage I/II breast cancer,[91,162,167–169] whereas mRNA studies gave contradictory results.[170,171]

This apparent contradiction between the clinical impact of gene amplification and protein overexpression may be explained by the finding that approximately only half of the cases with overexpression of the cyclin D1 protein have amplification of the CCND1 gene. Since overexpression of the cyclin D1 protein is significantly linked with estrogen receptor (ER) positivity,[91,162,167,172] and since cyclin D1 is turned on by activated ER, the other half of the cases with overexpression of the cyclin D1 protein in breast cancer may be due to 'normal' stimulation by estradiol. The strong association between cyclin D1 and ER may explain why cyclin D1-positive patients respond better to adjuvant therapy.[173] The ability of cyclin D1 to upregulate p21[WAF1] may explain the negative correlation between cyclin D1 and proliferation.[174]

For cyclin E, also mainly expressed in the G1 phase, overexpression is correlated with a more aggressive phenotype, including high proliferation[175,176] and reduced survival.[177–182]

Overexpression of p21[WAF1] (also known as p21[CIF1]), a cyclin-dependent kinase (CDK) inhibitor, was correlated with reduced disease-free survival in several studies,[105,106,183–185] but not in all.[168] In the study of Domagala et al,[186] no direct association was found between p21[WAF1] expression and overall survival. However, a significantly poorer survival was noted for p21[WAF1]-negative/p53-positive patients treated with adjuvant chemotherapy. Similar results were obtained by Caffo et al[183] and Thor et al.[185] These data indicate that the p21[WAF1]/p53 phenotype may predict therapeutic response to chemo- and hormonal therapy. This may relate to underlying mutations in p53 resulting in failure to induce p21[WAF1] and apoptosis. Also, the subcellular localization of p21[WAF1] may be important. Although p21[WAF1] should have its major function in the nucleus, p21[WAF1] cytoplasmic staining is often found, and seems to be associated with high p53 levels and poor prognosis.[155] These results are rather confusing, since p21[WAF1] is basically a cell cycle inhibitor.

Lack or loss of p27[Kip1], another CDK inhibitor, is usually associated with higher proliferation, and indicates poor prognosis in breast cancer in most studies,[54,176,178–180,187] especially when p27[Kip1] is lost in combination with overexpression of cyclin E.[180] Not all studies have confirmed the adverse prognostic effect of loss of p27[Kip1],[54,168] and in one study[188] high p27[Kip1] expression interestingly was an indicator of poor prognosis in node-negative cases. Loss of p16[INK4A] (CDKN2A) seems to have no impact in breast cancer: varying frequencies of p16[INK4A] loss have been described,[189,190] without prognostic impact.[191] Retinoblastoma protein (pRb) expression does not seem to be of prognostic significance either.[191–193]

There have been very many studies of p53 in breast cancer, as described in Chapter 12. Although there are many conflicting results,[194,195] the majority of studies show that p53 accumulation,[185,196,197] or mutation,[164] is correlated with increased proliferation,[198] and is associated with poor prognosis[38,49] and poor clinical response to primary chemotherapy.[199] CDK4 protein overexpression, as well as CDK4 gene amplification, have also been found in invasive breast carcinomas, but do not correlate with prognosis.[169] Although the catalytic form of telomerase (hTERT) is not strictly a cell cycle-regulating protein, hTERT levels are correlated with proliferative activity of breast cancer.[200–203] However, evaluation of its prognostic significance has yielded conflicting results.[200–202,204,205]

Summary

Different cell cycle regulators are implicated in increased proliferation, but the impact of single regulators is difficult to appreciate, since they are parts of complex pathways where other regulators may take over their functions or modulate effects. The functional endpoint of these complex pathways (i.e. cell division or not) is therefore more straightforward to interpret, and more easily used in practice than changes in expression or function of individual regulators.

APOPTOSIS

Assessment of apoptosis

The duration of the process of apoptotic cell death is estimated to be 12–24 hours.[206] Visible changes in cell morphology, which allow morphological identification, are present in the late apoptotic phase and last for 30 minutes to several hours. This is much longer than the rapid completion of mitosis.[207] Light microscopy has proven to be a powerful way to identify apoptotic cells.[208] Several other techniques have been developed to assess the number of apoptotic cells, some identifying apoptosis in an earlier phase. The most widely used methods are agarose gel electrophoresis, in situ labeling techniques and flow cytometry.

Light microscopy

Identification of apoptotic cells by light microscopy has been used in various cancers.[209] The identification has been described as subjective but, after a short learning period, it can be done reproducibly when strict protocols are used.[208] The apoptotic cells can be recognized in standard hematoxylin and eosin (H&E)-stained slides based on the specific morphological features that take place in the degradation phase. The process usually involves single cells. The apoptotic cell shrinks and separates from its neighbors, and is surrounded by a halo-like clear space. Retracted, often pink to orange,

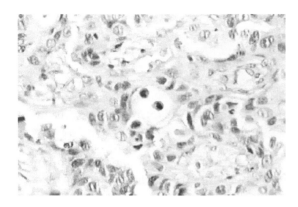

Figure 3.3 Apoptotic cells as they can be recognized in hematoxylin and eosin (H&E)-stained sections of a breast cancer.

cytoplasm is seen. The nuclear chromatin breaks up into irregular crescentic, beaded or nodular masses. Later in the process, small basophilic apoptotic bodies may be identified (Figure 3.3). Phagocytosis of apoptotic bodies occurs without release of proteolytic enzymes or generation of reactive oxygen metabolites, and therefore there is no acute inflammatory reaction.[208]

Counting apoptotic cells in H&E sections has the advantage that no additional staining or preparation is required, and the material is not lost after the measurement as with flow cytometry. Intratumor heterogeneity can be assessed. Large retrospective groups of patients can easily be evaluated, and other cell biological aspects of the tumor, such as proliferation (mitosis counting) and angiogenesis, can be determined in the same tumor section. Furthermore, automated assessments can be made using image analysis, providing a topographical relation between apoptosis, proliferation and angiogenesis.[210]

The number of apoptotic cells is usually expressed as the percentage of apoptotic tumor cells. Some authors, however, denote the number of apoptotic cells per 1000 tumor cells[211] or per defined area (e.g. 1.6 mm^2), as we do.[121,208] This saves tedious cell counts, and does not seem to make much difference. A magnification of 400× or 630× is appropriate.[208]

Immunohistochemistry of apoptosis-related proteins

M30 is a monoclonal antibody that recognizes a cytokeratin-18 cleavage product[212] which accumulates in apoptotic epithelial cells. M30 immunohistochemistry (or flow cytometry) is therefore useful to identify apoptotic cells in epithelial lesions. However, no clinical results have yet been described for breast cancer.

Different caspase enzymes are involved in the protein cleavage process during apoptosis. Caspase-3 activity is about the final step, and active caspase-3 is therefore the most useful immunohistochemical target to identify apoptotic cells. Few clinical studies have been described for breast cancer. The number of active caspase-3-positive cells correlates with morphological apoptosis counts and, not surprisingly, with high grade in one breast cancer study.[213]

Agarose gel electrophoresis

Apoptosis can be detected based on the principle that, owing to internucleosomal cleavage, chromosomal DNA is degraded into multimers of approximately 180–200 bp.[214] On an agarose gel, these fragments migrate electrophoretically at different speed according to their size, producing a characteristic ladder pattern. Larger 50–300 kbp fragments, which are the initial DNA fragments formed, require pulsed-field gel electrophoresis[215] or field-inversion gel electrophoresis[216] for their detection. Gel electrophoresis is widely used, but is not a morphological technique, which is a clear disadvantage. Further, it is difficult to use in a quantitative way.

In situ labeling techniques

In situ labeling techniques combine histochemical and immunohistochemical principles to label DNA strand breaks of apoptotic cells in situ, and are applicable to paraffin sections. In the terminal deoxyribonucleotidyl transferase (TdT)-mediated deoxyuridine triphosphate (dUTP)–biotin nick end-labeling

(TUNEL) method, TdT catalyses the addition of biotinylated dUTP to free 3′-OH ends of DNA fragments, with the synthesis of a polydeoxynucleotide polymer. The signal is amplified by avidin–biotin–peroxidase, and diaminobenzidine is used as chromogen.[217,218] The in situ end-labeling technique uses DNA polymerase for enzymatically mediated binding of biotinylated nucleotides to DNA breaks.[219] In situ labeling techniques identify apoptotic cells, including those with early nuclear chromatin margination. However, clearly recognizable apoptotic cells may remain unstained, whereas cells which lack the morphological features of apoptosis may be stained, including necrotic cells.[218,220] Also, the in situ labeling techniques depend greatly on tissue pretreatment, which usually includes acid (which may cause strand breaks itself), the concentration of the terminal transferase enzyme, and the type and concentration of the fixative. Comparisons with plain morphology by light microscopy do, however, show a good correlation with DNA end-labeling methods. Comparison of in situ nick translation and TUNEL shows that the latter is more sensitive.[218]

Altogether, in situ labeling techniques could be used to highlight apoptotic cells, but have the disadvantage of producing false-positive and -negative results when compared with light-microscopic assessment of the number of apoptotic cells. When apoptosis is a rare event, or when there are many apoptotic-like cells present (e.g. in the case of inflammation), labeling techniques may then, be useful.

Flow cytometry

In a flow cytometer, apoptotic cells can be identified by a decrease in forward light scatter, and subsequently in side scatter, because of cell shrinkage and subsequent decrease in light reflectiveness. When cells are incubated with a DNA-binding fluorochrome, apoptotic cells show reduced fluorescence. Flow cytometry can also be combined with in situ labeling techniques, as reviewed by Darzynkiewicz et al.[221] Flow cytometry is of great value for measuring the rate of apoptosis in cell cultures. It can also be combined with other apoptosis- or proliferation-related variables in the same measurement.

The disadvantages of flow cytometry are the loss of tumor material after measurement, the lack of visual control during the measurement, and the fact that it is less useful for detecting rare events such as apoptosis in human tumors. Active caspase-3 and M30 antibodies can also be used to detect apoptotic cells by flow cytometry.

Summary

For clinical studies, light-microscopic counting of apoptotic cells seems to be the most practical method. Immunohistochemistry for active caspase-3 and M30 are emerging methods that show promise.

Prognostic value of apoptosis in breast cancer

Several studies have been published regarding the clinical value of light-microscopic apoptosis counting in invasive breast cancer. In the studies by Vakkala et al,[221] Lipponen et al[122] and Zhang et al,[223] a high number of apoptotic cells was associated with a poor prognosis. A high apoptotic index was also associated with poor differentiation.[122] The number of apoptotic cells ranged from 0 to 138/mm^2. However, Lipponen et al[121] used five consecutive fields, while Zhang et al[222] used five randomly selected fields. In another larger series of patients, apoptosis counts were also significant in univariate survival analysis, but did not provide independent prognostic value.[123]

Our own study of 172 stage I and II invasive breast cancers, applying counting of apoptosis in H&E-stained sections according to a methodologically sound protocol (see Table 3.2),[208] showed the number of apoptotic cells per mm^2 (assessed in 10 high-power fields = 1.59 mm^2) to be positively correlated with the MAI ($p = 0.0001$) and histological grade ($p < 0.0001$). Patients with a high apoptotic index showed shorter overall survival than

Table 3.2 Univariate survival analysis results from a study evaluating the prognostic value of apoptosis counting in breast cancer in comparison with other prognostic features

Variable	Grouping	n	Survival	p value	Log rank
Tumor size	<2.5 cm	80	85	<0.0001	22.3
	∃2.5 cm	92	48		
Histologic type	Ductal, medullary	132	66	n.s.	0.4
	Others	40	65		
Histologic grade	I	73	81	0.0002	16.6
	II	61	57		
	III	38	49		
Lymph node status	Negative	86	77	0.001	10.7
	Positive	86	55		
Mitotic activity	<10	91	81	<0.0001	18.7
index (MAI)	∃10	81	50		
Apoptotic index	<10	80	78	0.0007	11.6
	∃10	92	55		

Modified from De Jong et al.[230]
n.s., not significant.

patients with a low apoptotic index, both in the total patient group as well as in the lymph node-positive group (Figure 3.4). Tumor size, MAI, lymph node status and apoptotic index were independent prognostic indicators in multivariate analysis. The apoptotic index was shown to be of additional prognostic value to the MAI in the total patient group as well as in the lymph node-positive group (Figure 3.5).[212] The value of the apoptotic index was confirmed by others,[224,225] but not by all,[226] and in one study a high apoptotic index indicated a favorable prognosis.[227]

Three studies have evaluated the prognostic value of the TUNEL technique for detecting apoptotic cells. Berardo et al[228] found no correlation with disease-free or overall survival in a series of 979 lymph node-positive breast cancer patients when patients were divided according to low or high rate of apoptosis. Further subdivision into four separate groups, based on the percentage of apoptotic cells, showed a trend towards worse survival as levels of apoptosis increased. Gonzalez-Campora et al,[229] studying 65 patients, did find the number of apoptotic cells to provide independent prognostic information.

Prognostic value of apoptosis-regulating genes in breast cancer

The apoptosis-regulating genes bcl-2, bcl-x, bak and bax are expressed in a subset of breast carcinomas. bcl-2 has been related to low rates of apoptotic cells and a favorable prognosis in invasive breast cancer.[195,232–235] The pro-apoptotic Bax protein, however, does not seem to show a strong relation to the number of apoptotic cells in invasive breast cancer,[236] and results on prognostic value are conflicting.[232,236]

High cytoplasmic expression of the apoptosis inhibitor survivin was associated with bcl-2 expression and the apoptotic index, and seems to indicate poor prognosis in breast cancer.[237–242] p53 is also implicated in apoptosis; its value in breast cancer is discussed in Chapter 12. p53 mutations correlate with increased apoptotic activity.[198]

CONCLUSIONS

Proliferation and apoptosis both play important roles in the clinical behavior of invasive breast cancer. Proliferation has been most widely

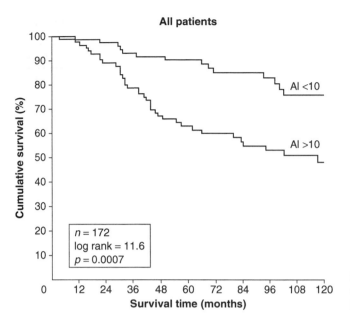

Figure 3.4   Survival curves for invasive breast cancer patients with low and high apoptotic indices (AI).[244]

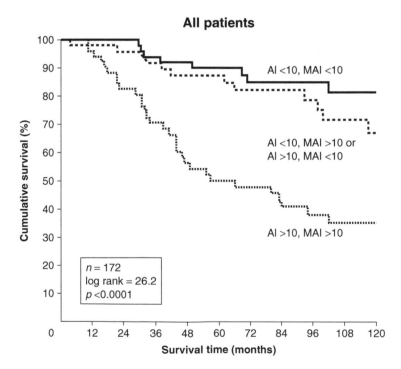

Figure 3.5   Survival curves for invasive breast cancer patients grouped according to the apoptotic index (AI) and the mitotic activity index (MAI).[244]

studied, and increased proliferation correlates strongly with poor prognosis, irrespective of the methodology used. However, from the different ways to assess proliferation, mitosis counting has most convincingly been proved to provide reproducible and independent prognostic value in invasive breast cancer. The MAI is therefore used in clinical practice in several European countries. The Ki67/MIB1 labeling index is a promising alternative, but needs further methodological fine-tuning. In general, it must be admitted that little attention has yet been paid to the value of these proliferation markers in predicting response to therapy. The apoptotic index is a new, promising prognostic factor. Further larger and prospective clinical studies are needed to establish its true clinical value.

Although much knowledge has been gained about genes implicated in the complex regulation processes of proliferation and apoptosis, analysis of individual genes is as yet clinically unsatisfactory, and analysis of the functional end-results of these complex processes – rate of proliferation and apoptosis – is far more important. This may, however, change when sophisticated statistical models become available to interpret complex microarray expression patterns.

REFERENCES

1. Kerlikowske K, Grady D, Rubin SM et al. Efficacy of screening mammography: a meta-analysis. JAMA 1995; 273: 149–54.
2. Groenendijk RP, Bult P, Tewarie L et al. Screen-detected breast cancers have a lower mitotic activity index. Br J Cancer 2000; 82: 381–4.
3. Cowan WK, Angus B, Gray JC, Lunt LG, al-Tamimi SR. A study of interval breast cancer within the NHS breast screening programme. J Clin Pathol 2000; 53: 140–6.
4. Van Diest PJ, Michalides RJ, Jannink I et al. Cyclin D1 expression in invasive breast cancer: correlations and prognostic value. Am J Path 1997; 150: 705–11.
5. Jong JS de, Van Diest PJ, Valk P van der, Baak JPA. Expression of growth factors, their receptors and growth inhibiting factors in invasive breast cancer I. An inventory in search of autocrine and paracrine loops. J Pathol 1998; 184: 44–52.
6. De Jong JS, Van Diest PJ, Valk P van der, Baak JPA. Expression of growth factors, their receptors and growth inhibiting factors in invasive breast cancer II. Correlations with proliferation and angiogenesis. J Pathol 1998; 184: 53–7.
7. De Jong JS, Van Diest PJ, Baak JPA. Hot spot microvessel density and the mitotic activity index are strong additional prognostic indicators in invasive breast cancer. Histopathology 2000; 36: 306–12.
8. Van Diest PJ, Brugal G, Baak JP. Proliferation markers in tumours: interpretation and clinical value. J Clin Pathol 1998; 51: 716–24.
9. Biesterfeld S, Farokhzad F, Kluppel D, Schneider S, Hufnagl P. Improvement of breast cancer prognostication using cell kinetic-based silver-stainable

10. Bergers E, Van Diest PJ, Baak JPA. Tumour heterogeneity of DNA cell cycle variables in breast cancer measured by flow cytometry. J Clin Path 1996; 49: 931–7.
11. Lakhani SR, Jacquemier J, Sloane JP et al. Multifactorial analysis of differences between sporadic breast cancers and cancers involving BRCA1 and BRCA2 mutations. J Natl Cancer Inst 1998; 90: 1138–45.
12. Cooke TG, Stanton PD, Winstanley J et al. Long-term prognostic significance of thymidine labelling index in primary breast cancer. Eur J Cancer 1992; 28: 424–6.
13. Courdi A, Hery M, Dahan E et al. Factors affecting relapse in node-negative breast cancer. A multivariate analysis including the labeling index. Eur J Cancer Clin Oncol 1989; 25: 351–6.
14. Daidone MG, Silvestrini R, Valentinis B et al. Proliferative activity of primary breast cancer and of synchronous lymph node metastases evaluated by [3H]-thymidine labelling index. Cell Tissue Kinet 1990; 23: 401–8.
15. Meyer JS, Friedman E, McCrate MM, Bauer WC. Prediction of early course of breast carcinoma by thymidine labeling. Cancer 1983; 51: 1879–86.
16. Meyer JS, McDivitt RW. Reliability and stability of the thymidine labeling index of breast carcinoma. Lab Invest 1986; 54: 160–4.
17. Meyer JS, Province M. Proliferative index of breast carcinoma by thymidine labeling: prognostic power independent of stage, estrogen and progesterone receptors. Breast Cancer Res Treat 1988; 12: 191–204.
18. Silvestrini R, Daidone MG, Di Fronzo G et al. Prognostic implication of labeling index versus estrogen receptors and tumor size in node-negative breast cancer. Breast Cancer Res Treat 1986; 7: 161–9.
19. Silvestrini R, Daidone MG, Valagussa P et al. 3H-thymidine-labeling index as a prognostic indicator in node-positive breast cancer. J Clin Oncol 1990; 8: 1321–6.
20. Silvestrini R, Daidone MG, Mastore M et al. Cell kinetics as a predictive factor in node-positive breast cancer treated with adjuvant hormone therapy. J Clin Oncol 1993; 11: 1150–5.
21. Silvestrini R, Daidone MG, Luisi A et al. Cell proliferation in 3,800 node-negative breast cancers: consistency over time of biological information provided by 3H-thymidine labeling index. Int J Cancer 1997; 74: 122–7.
22. Silvestrini R, Luisi A, Zambetti M et al. Cell proliferation and outcome following doxorubicin plus CMF regimens in node-positive breast cancer. Int J Cancer 2000; 87: 405–11.
23. Tubiana M, Pejovic MH, Chavaudra N, Contesso G, Malaise EP. The long-term prognostic significance of the thymidine labelling index in breast cancer. Int J Cancer 1984; 33: 441–5.

24. Tubiana M, Pejovic MH, Koscielny S et al. Growth rate, kinetics of tumor cell proliferation, and long-term outcome in human breast cancer. Int J Cancer 1989; 44: 17–22.

25. Volpi A, De Paola F, Nanni O et al. Prognostic significance of biologic markers in node-negative breast cancer patients: a prospective study. Breast Cancer Res Treat 2000; 63: 181–92.

26. Nio Y, Tamura K, Kan N et al. In vitro DNA synthesis in freshly separated human breast cancer cells assessed by tritiated thymidine incorporation assay: relationship to the long-term outcome of patients. Br J Surg 1999; 86: 1463–9.

27. Volpi A, Nanni O, De Paola F et al. HER-2 expression and cell proliferation: prognostic markers in patients with node-negative breast cancer. J Clin Oncol 2003; 21: 2708–12.

28. Meyer JS, Alvarez C, Milikowski C et al. Cooperative Breast Cancer Tissue Resource. Breast carcinoma malignancy grading by Bloom–Richardson system vs proliferation index: reproducibility of grade and advantages of proliferation index. Mod Pathol 2005; 18(8): 1067–78.

29. Bilir A, Ozmen V, Kecer M et al. Thymidine labeling index: prognostic role in breast cancer. Am J Clin Oncol 2004; 27: 400–6.

30. Thor AD, Liu S, Moore DH 2nd, Edgerton SM. Comparison of mitotic index, in vitro bromodeoxyuridine labeling, and MIB-1 assays to quantitate proliferation in breast cancer. J Clin Oncol 1999; 17: 470–7.

31. Goodson WH 3rd, Moore DH 2nd, Ljung BM et al. The prognostic value of proliferation indices: a study with in vivo bromodeoxyuridine and Ki-67. Breast Cancer Res Treat 2000; 59: 113–23.

32. Bergers E, Jannink I, Diest PJ van, Baak JPA. Influence of fixation delay on mitotic activity and flow cytometric %S-phase. Hum Pathol 1997; 28: 95–100.

33. Joensuu H, Toikkanen S, Klemi PJ. DNA index and S-phase fraction and their combination as prognostic factors in operable ductal breast carcinoma. Cancer 1990; 66: 331–40.

34. Pinto AE, Andre S, Pereira T, Nobrega S, Soares J. Prognostic comparative study of S-phase fraction and Ki-67 index in breast carcinoma. J Clin Pathol 2001; 54: 543–9.

35. Morris ES, Elston CW, Bell JA et al. An evaluation of the cell cycle-associated monoclonal antibody Ki-S1 as a prognostic factor in primary invasive adenocarcinoma of the breast. J Pathol 1995; 176: 55–62.

36. Bevilacqua P, Verderio P, Barbareschi M et al. Lack of prognostic significance of the monoclonal antibody Ki-S1, a novel marker of proliferative activity, in node-negative breast carcinoma. Breast Cancer Res Treat 1996; 37: 123–33.

37. Sampson SA, Kreipe H, Gillett CE et al. KiS1 – a novel monoclonal antibody which recognizes proliferating cells: evaluation of its relationship to prognosis in mammary carcinoma. J Pathol 1992; 168: 179–85.

38. Rudolph P, Olsson H, Bonatz G et al. Correlation between p53, c-erbB-2, and topoisomerase II alpha expression, DNA ploidy, hormonal receptor status and proliferation in 356 node-negative breast carcinomas: prognostic implications. J Pathol 1999; 187: 207–16.

39. Rudolph P, MacGrogan G, Bonichon F et al. Prognostic significance of Ki-67 and topoisomerase II alpha expression in infiltrating ductal carcinoma of the breast. A multivariate analysis of 863 cases. Breast Cancer Res Treat 1999; 55: 61–71.

40. Gonzalez MA, Pinder SE, Callagy G et al. Minichromosome maintenance protein 2 is a strong independent prognostic marker in breast cancer. J Clin Oncol 2003; 21: 4306–13.

41. Skaland I, Janssen EA, Gudlaugsson E et al. Phosphohistone H3 expression has much stronger prognostic value than classical prognosticators in invasive lymph node-negative breast cancer patients less than 55 years of age. Mod Pathol 2007; 20: 1307–15.

42. Sahin AA, Ro J, Ro JY et al. Ki-67 immunostaining in node-negative stage I/II breast carcinoma. Significant correlation with prognosis. Cancer 1991; 68: 549–57.

43. Veronese SM, Gambacorta M, Gottardi O et al. Proliferation index as a prognostic marker in breast cancer. Cancer 1993; 71: 3926–31.

44. Veronese SM, Maisano C, Scibilia J. Comparative prognostic value of Ki-67 and MIB-1 proliferation markers in breast cancer. Anticancer Res 1995; 15: 2717–22.

45. Biesterfeld S, Reitmaier M. Re-evaluation of prognostic mitotic figure counting in breast cancer: results of a prospective clinical follow-up study. Anticancer Res 2001; 21: 589–94.

46. Depowski PL, Brien TP, Sheehan CE et al. Prognostic significance of p34cdc2 cyclin-dependent kinase and MIB1 overexpression, and HER-2/neu gene amplification detected by fluorescence in situ hybridization in breast cancer. Am J Clin Pathol 1999; 112: 459–69.

47. Dettmar P, Harbeck N, Thomssen C et al. Prognostic impact of proliferation-associated factors MIB1 and S-phase in node-negative breast cancer. Br J Cancer 1997; 75: 1525–33.

48. Harbeck N, Dettmar P, Thomssen C et al. Prognostic impact of tumor biological factors on survival in node-negative breast cancer. Anticancer Res 1998; 18: 2187–97.

49. Beck T, Weller EE, Weikel W et al. Usefulness of immunohistochemical staining for p53 in the prognosis of breast carcinomas: correlations with established prognosis parameters and with the proliferation marker, MIB-1. Gynecol Oncol 1995; 57: 96–104.

50. Imamura H, Haga S, Shimizu T et al. Prognostic significance of MIB1-determined proliferative

activities in intraductal components and invasive foci associated with invasive ductal breast carcinoma. Br J Cancer 1999; 79: 172–8.

51. Jager JJ, Jansen RL, Arends JW et al. Anti-apoptotic phenotype is associated with decreased locoregional recurrence rate in breast cancer. Anticancer Res 2000; 20: 1269–75.

52. Jensen V, Ladekarl M, Holm-Nielsen P et al. The prognostic value of oncogenic antigen 519 (OA-519) expression and proliferative activity detected by antibody MIB-1 in node negative breast cancer. J Pathol 1995; 176: 343–52.

53. Kenny FS, Willsher PC, Gee JM et al. Change in expression of ER, bcl-2 and MIB1 on primary tamoxifen and relation to response in ER positive breast cancer. Breast Cancer Res Treat 2001; 65: 135–44.

54. Lau R, Grimson R, Sansome C, Tornos C, Moll UM. Low levels of cell cycle inhibitor p27^{kip1} combined with high levels of Ki-67 predict shortened disease-free survival in T1 and T2 invasive breast carcinomas. Int J Oncol 2001; 18: 17–23.

55. Locker AP, Birrell K, Bell JA et al. Ki67 immunoreactivity in breast carcinoma: relationships to prognostic variables and short term survival. Eur J Surg Oncol 1992; 18: 224–9.

56. Nakagomi H, Miyake T, Hada M et al. Prognostic and therapeutic implications of the MIB-1 labeling index in breast cancer. Breast Cancer 1998; 5: 255–9.

57. Pietilainen T, Lipponen P, Aaltomaa S et al. The important prognostic value of Ki-67 expression as determined by image analysis in breast cancer. J Cancer Res Clin Oncol 1996; 122: 687–92.

58. Pinder SE, Wencyk P, Sibbering DM et al. Assessment of the new proliferation marker MIB1 in breast carcinoma using image analysis: associations with other prognostic factors and survival. Br J Cancer 1995; 71: 146–9.

59. Michalides R, van Tinteren H, Balkenende A et al. Cyclin A is a prognostic indicator in early stage breast cancer with and without tamoxifen treatment. Br J Cancer 2002; 86: 402–8.

60. Jalava P, Kuopio T, Juntti-Patinen L et al. Ki67 immunohistochemistry: a valuable marker in prognostication but with a risk of misclassification: proliferation subgroups formed based on Ki67 immunoreactivity and standardized mitotic index. Histopathology 2006; 48: 674–82.

61. Clahsen PC, van de Velde CJ, Duval C et al. The utility of mitotic index, oestrogen receptor and Ki-67 measurements in the creation of novel prognostic indices for node-negative breast cancer. Eur J Surg Oncol 1999; 25: 356–63.

62. Lee AK, Loda M, Mackarem G et al. Lymph node negative invasive breast carcinoma 1 centimeter or less in size (T1a,bNOMO): clinicopathologic features and outcome. Cancer 1997; 79: 761–71.

63. Billgren AM, Rutqvist LE, Tani E et al. Proliferating fraction during neoadjuvant chemotherapy of primary breast cancer in relation to objective local response and relapse-free survival. Acta Oncol 1999; 38: 597–601.

64. Nole F, Minchella I, Colleoni M et al. Primary chemotherapy in operable breast cancer with favorable prognostic factors: a pilot study evaluating the efficacy of a regimen with a low subjective toxic burden containing vinorelbine, 5-fluorouracil and folinic acid (FLN). Ann Oncol 1999; 10: 993–6.

65. Chang J, Powles TJ, Allred DC et al. Prediction of clinical outcome from primary tamoxifen by expression of biologic markers in breast cancer patients. Clin Cancer Res 2000; 6: 616–21.

66. Aaltoma S, Lipponen P, Papinaho S, Syrjanen K. Proliferating-cell nuclear antigen (PC10) immunolabelling and other proliferation indices as prognostic factors in breast cancer. J Cancer Res Clin Oncol 1993; 119: 288–94.

67. Haerslev T, Jacobsen GK. Proliferating cell nuclear antigen in breast carcinomas. An immunohistochemical study with correlation to histopathological features and prognostic factors. Virchows Arch 1994; 424: 39–46.

68. Russo A, Bazan V, Morello V et al. Vimentin expression, proliferating cell nuclear antigen and flow cytometric factors. Prognostic role in breast cancer. Anal Quant Cytol Histol 1994; 16: 365–74.

69. Schoenborn I, Minguillon C, Moehner M et al. PCNA as a potential prognostic marker in breast cancer. The Breast 1994; 3: 97–102.

70. Tahan SR, Neuberg DS, Dieffenbach A et al. Prediction of early relapse and shortened survival in patients with breast cancer by proliferating cell nuclear antigen score. Cancer 1993; 71: 3552–9.

71. Thomas M, Noguchi M, Kitagawa H et al. Poor prognostic value of proliferating cell nuclear antigen labelling index in breast carcinoma. J Clin Path 1993; 46: 525–8.

72. Genestie C, Zafrani B, Asselain B et al. Comparison of the prognostic value of Scarff–Bloom–Richardson and Nottingham histological grades in a series of 825 cases of breast cancer: major importance of the mitotic count as a component of both grading systems. Anticancer Res 1998; 18: 571–6.

73. Le Doussal V, Tubiana-Hulin M, Friedman S et al. Prognostic value of histologic grade nuclear components of Scarff–Bloom–Richardson (SBR). An improved score modification based on a multivariate analysis of 1262 invasive ductal breast carcinomas. Cancer 1989; 64: 1914–21.

74. Boiesen P, Bendahl PO, Anagnostaki L et al. Histologic grading in breast cancer – reproducibility between seven pathologic departments. South Sweden Breast Cancer Group. Acta Oncol 2000; 39: 41–5.

75. Dalton LW, Page DL, Dupont WD. Histologic grading of breast carcinoma. A reproducibility study. Cancer 1994; 73: 2765–70.

76. Delides GS, Garas G, Georgouli G et al. Intralaboratory variations in the grading of breast carcinoma. Arch Pathol Lab Med 1982; 106: 126–8.

77. Frierson HF Jr, Wolber RA, Berean KW et al. Interobserver reproducibility of the Nottingham modification of the Bloom and Richardson histologic grading scheme for infiltrating ductal carcinoma. Am J Clin Pathol 1995; 103: 195–8.

78. Harvey JM, de Klerk NH, Sterrett GF. Histological grading in breast cancer: interobserver agreement, and relation to other prognostic factors including ploidy. Pathology 1992; 24: 63–8.

79. Tsuda H, Akiyama F, Kurosumi M, Sakamoto G, Watanabe T. Establishment of histological criteria for high-risk node-negative breast carcinoma for a multi-institutional randomized clinical trial of adjuvant therapy. Japan National Surgical Adjuvant Study of Breast Cancer (NSAS-BC) Pathology Section. Jpn J Clin Oncol 1998; 28: 486–91.

80. Theissig F, Kunze KD, Haroske G, Meyer W. Histological grading of breast cancer. Interobserver reproducibility and prognostic significance. Pathol Res Pract 1990; 186: 732–6.

81. Baak JPA, Kurver PHJ, Snoo-Nieuwlaat AJE et al. Prognostic indicators in breast cancer – morphometric methods. Histopathology 1982; 6: 327–39.

82. Baak JPA, Dop H van, Kurver PHJ et al. The value of morphometry to classic prognosticators in breast cancer. Cancer 1985; 56: 374–82.

83. Baak JPA, Chin D, Diest PJ van, Matze-Cok P, Bacus SS. Comparative long term prognostic value of quantitative Her2/Neu protein expression, DNA ploidy, morphometric and clinical features in paraffin-embedded invasive breast cancer. Lab Invest 1991; 64: 215–22.

84. Baak JPA, Wisse-Brekelmans ECM, Kurver PHJ et al. Regional differences in breast cancer survival are correlated with differences in differentiation and rate of proliferation. Hum Pathol 1992; 23: 989–92.

85. Baak JPA, van Diest PJ, Voorhorst FJ et al. Prospective multicentre evaluation of the independent prognostic value of mitotic activity index in lymph-node negative breast cancer patients aged less than 55. J Clin Oncol 2005; 23: 5993–6001.

86. Bos R, Groep P van der, Greijer AE et al. Levels of hypoxia-inducible factor-1a independently predict prognosis in lymph node-negative breast cancer patients. Cancer 2003; 97: 1573–81.

87. Collan Y, Kumpusalo L, Pesonen E et al. Prediction of survival in breast cancer: evaluation of different multivariate models. Anticancer Research 1998; 18: 647–50.

88. Van Diest PJ, Baak JPA. The morphometric Multivariate Prognostic Index (MPI) is the strongest prognosticator in premenopausal lymph node negative and lymph node positive breast cancer patients. Hum Pathol 1991; 22: 326–30.

89. Van Diest PJ, Matze-Cok E, Baak JP. Prognostic value of proliferative activity in lymph node metastases of patients with breast cancer. J Clin Pathol 1991; 44: 416–18.

90. Van Diest PJ, Baak JPA, Matze-Cok P, Bacus SS. Prediction of response to adjuvant chemotherapy in premenopausal lymph node positive breast cancer patients with morphometry, DNA flow cytometry and HER-2/neu oncoprotein expression: preliminary results. Path Res Pract 1992; 188: 344–9.

91. Van Diest PJ, Michalides RJ, Jannink I et al. Cyclin D1 expression in invasive breast cancer: correlations and prognostic value. Am J Path 1997; 150: 705–11.

92. Jannink I, Van Diest PJ, Baak JPA. Comparison of the prognostic value of Mitotic Activity Index (MAI), random MAI (rMAI), M/V-index, and random M/V-index (rM/V-index) in breast cancer patients. Hum Pathol 1995; 26: 1086–92.

93. Jannink I, Van Diest PJ, Baak JPA. Comparison of the prognostic value of mitotic frequency and mitotic activity index in breast cancer. The Breast 1996; 5: 31–6.

94. Linden JC van der, Baak JPA, Lindeman J et al. Prospective evaluation of the prognostic value of morphometry in primary breast cancer patients. J Clin Pathol 1987; 40: 302–6.

95. Linden JC van der, Lindeman J, Baak JPA et al. The multivariate prognostic index and nuclear DNA content are independent prognostic factors in primary breast cancer patients. Cytometry 1989; 10: 56–61.

96. Uyterlinde AM, Schipper NW, Baak JPA et al. Limited prognostic value of cellular DNA content to classical and morphometrical parameters in invasive ductal breast cancer. Am J Clin Pathol 1988; 89: 301–7.

97. Uyterlinde AM, Baak JPA, Schipper NW et al. Further evaluation of morphometric and flow cytometric features in breast cancer patients with long term follow-up. Int J Cancer 1990; 45: 1–7.

98. Uyterlinde AM, Baak JPA, Schipper NW et al. Prognostic value of morphometry and DNA flow cytometry features of invasive breast cancers detected by population screening: comparison with control group of hospital patients. Int J Cancer 1991; 48: 173–81.

99. Aaltomaa S, Lipponen P, Eskelinen M et al. Prognostic factors in axillary lymph node-negative (pN-) breast carcinomas. Eur J Cancer 1991; 27: 1555–9.

100. Aaltomaa S, Lipponen P, Eskelinen M et al. Prognostic scores combining clinical, histological and morphometric variables in assessment of the disease outcome in female breast cancer. Int J Cancer 1991; 49: 886–92.

101. Aaltomaa S, Lipponen P, Eskelinen M, Alhava E, Syrjanen K. Nuclear morphometry and mitotic indexes as prognostic factors in breast cancer. Eur J Surg 1991; 157: 319–24.

102. Aaltomaa S, Lipponen P, Eskelinen M et al. Prognostic factors after 5 years follow-up in female breast cancer. Oncology 1992; 49: 93–8.

103. Aaltomaa S, Lipponen P, Eskelinen M et al. Mitotic indexes as prognostic predictors in female breast cancer. J Cancer Res Clin Oncol 1992; 118: 75–81.

104. Aaltomaa S, Lipponen P, Eskelinen M et al. Predictive value of a morphometric prognostic index in female breast cancer. Oncology 1993; 50: 57–62.

105. Barbareschi M, Caffo O, Veronese S et al. Bcl-2 and p53 expression in node-negative breast carcinoma: a study with long-term follow-up. Hum Pathol 1996; 27: 1149–55.

106. Barbareschi M, Caffo O, Doglioni C et al. p21WAF1 immunohistochemical expression in breast carcinoma: correlations with clinicopathological data, oestrogen receptor status, MIB1 expression, p53 gene and protein alterations and relapse-free survival. Br J Cancer 1996; 74: 208–15.

107. Biesterfeld S, Noll I, Noll E, Wohltmann D, Bocking A. Mitotic frequency as a prognostic factor in breast cancer. Hum Pathol 1995; 26: 47–52.

108. Chen SC, Chao TC, Hwang TL et al. Prognostic factors in node-negative breast cancer patients: the experience in Taiwan. Changgeng Yi Xue Za Zhi 1998; 21: 363–70.

109. Clayton F. Pathologic correlates of survival in 378 lymph node-negative infiltrating ductal breast carcinomas. Mitotic count is the best single predictor. Cancer 1991; 68: 1309–17.

110. Clayton F, Hopkins CL. Pathologic correlates of prognosis in lymph node-positive breast carcinomas. Cancer 1993; 71: 1780–90.

111. Colpaert C, Vermeulen P, Jeuris W et al. Early distant relapse in 'node-negative' breast cancer patients is not predicted by occult axillary lymph node metastases, but by the features of the primary tumour. J Pathol 2001; 193: 442–9.

112. Eskelinen M, Lipponen P, Papinaho S et al. DNA flow cytometry, nuclear morphometry, mitotic indices and steroid receptors as independent prognostic factors in female breast cancer. Int J Cancer 1992; 51: 555–61.

113. Joensuu H, Toikkanen S. Identification of subgroups with favorable prognosis in breast cancer. Acta Oncol 1992; 31: 293–301.

114. Kato T, Kimura T, Miyakawa R et al. Clinicopathologic features associated with long-term survival in node-negative breast cancer patients. Surg Today 1996; 26: 105–14.

115. Keshgegian AA, Cnaan A. Proliferation markers in breast carcinoma. Mitotic figure count, S-phase fraction, proliferating cell nuclear antigen, Ki-67 and MIB-1. Am J Clin Pathol 1995; 104: 42–9.

116. Kronqvist P, Kuopio T, Collan Y. Morphometric grading in breast cancer: thresholds for mitotic counts. Hum Pathol 1998; 29: 1462–8.

117. Kronqvist P, Kuopio T, Collan Y. Quantitative thresholds for mitotic counts in histologic grading: confirmation in nonfrozen samples of invasive ductal breast cancer. Ann Diagn Pathol 2000; 4: 65–70.

118. Ladekarl M, Jensen V. Quantitative histopathology in lymph node-negative breast cancer. Prognostic significance of mitotic counts. Virchows Arch 1995; 427: 265–70.

119. Ladekarl M. Quantitative histopathology in ductal carcinoma of the breast. Prognostic value of mean nuclear size and mitotic counts. Cancer 1995; 75: 2114–22.

120. Lipponen P, Collan Y, Eskelinen MJ. Volume corrected mitotic index (M/V index), mitotic activity index (MAI), and histological grading in breast cancer. Int J Surg 1991; 76: 245–9.

121. Lipponen P, Aaltomaa S, Kosma VM et al. Apoptosis in breast cancer as related to histopathological characteristics and prognosis. Eur J Cancer 1994; 30A: 2068–73.

122. Liu S, Edgerton SM, Moore DH 2nd, Thor AD. Measures of cell turnover (proliferation and apoptosis) and their association with survival in breast cancer. Clin Cancer Res 2001; 7: 1716–23.

123. Mandard AM, Denoux Y, Herlin P et al. Prognostic value of DNA cytometry in 281 premenopausal patients with lymph node negative breast carcinoma randomized in a control trial: multivariate analysis with Ki-67 index, mitotic count, and microvessel density. Cancer 2000; 89: 1748–57.

124. Page DL, Gray R, Allred DC et al. Prediction of node-negative breast cancer outcome by histologic grading and S-phase analysis by flow cytometry: an Eastern Cooperative Oncology Group Study (2192). Am J Clin Oncol 2001; 24: 10–18.

125. Russo J, Frederick J, Ownby HE et al. Predictors of recurrence and survival of patients with breast cancer. Am J Clin Pathol 1987; 88: 123–31.

126. Simpson JF, Gray R, Dressler LG et al. Prognostic value of histologic grade and proliferative activity in axillary node-positive breast cancer: results from the Eastern Cooperative Oncology Group Companion Study, EST 4189. J Clin Oncol 2000; 18: 2059–69.

127. Theissig F, Baak JP, Schuurmans L et al. 'Blind' multicenter evaluation of the prognostic value of DNA image cytometric and morphometric features in invasive breast cancer. Anal Cell Pathol 1996; 10: 85–99.

128. Toikkanen S, Pylkkanen L, Joensuu H. Invasive lobular carcinoma of the breast has better short- and long-term survival than invasive ductal carcinoma. Br J Cancer 1997; 76: 1234–40.

129. Tosi P, Luzi P, Sforza V et al. Correlation between morphometrical parameters and disease free-survival in ductal breast cancer treated only by surgery. Appl Pathol 1986; 4: 33–42.

130. Younes M, Lane M, Miller CC, Laucirica R. Stratified multivariate analysis of prognostic markers in breast cancer: a preliminary report. Anticancer Res 1997; 17: 1383–90.

131. Elkhuizen PH, Hermans J, Leer JW, van de Vijver MJ. Isolated late local recurrences with high mitotic count and early local recurrences following breast-conserving therapy are associated with increased risk on distant metastasis. Int J Radiat Oncol Biol Phys 2001; 50: 387–96.

132. Laroye GJ, Minkin S. The impact of mitotic index on predicting outcome in breast carcinoma: a

comparison of different counting methods in patients with different lymph node status. Mod Pathol 1991; 4: 456–60.

133. Fiets WE, Bellot FE, Struikmans H et al. Prognostic value of mitotic counts of axillary node negative breast cancer patients with predominantly well-differentiated tumours. Eur Surg Oncol 2005; 31: 128–33.

134. Carbone A, Serra FG, Rinelli A et al. Morphometric prognostic index in breast cancer. Anal Quant Cytol Histol 1999; 21: 250–4.

135. Groenendijk RP, Bult P, Tewarie L et al. Screen-detected breast cancers have a lower mitotic activity index. Br J Cancer 2000; 82: 381–4.

136. Lipponen P, Papinaho S, Eskelinen M et al. DNA ploidy, S-phase fraction and mitotic indices as prognostic predictors of female breast cancer. Anticancer Res 1992; 12: 1533–8.

137. Offersen BV, Søresen FB, Knoop A et al. Danish Breast Cancer Cooperative Tumour Biology Committee. The prognostic relevance of estimates of proliferative activity in early breast cancer. Histopathology 2003; 43: 573–82.

138. Baak JP, van Diest PJ, Jaansen EA et al. Other collaborators of the Multicenter Morphometric Mammary Carcinoma Project (MMMCP) proliferation accurately identifies the high risk patients among small, low-grade, lymp node-negative invasive breast cancers. Ann Oncol 2007; Nov 27 (e-pub ahead of print).

139. Van Diest PJ, Baak JPA, Matze-Cok P et al. Reproducibility of mitosis counting in 2469 breast cancer specimens: results from the Multicenter Morphometric Mammary Carcinoma Project. Hum Pathol 1992; 23: 603–7.

140. Baak JPA, Kurver PHJ, Diest PJ van et al. Data processing and analysis in the Multicenter Morphometric Mammary Carcinoma Project (MMMCP). Path Res Pract 1989; 185: 657–63.

141. Baak JPA, Diest PJ van, Ariens ATh et al. The Multicenter Morphometric Mammary Carcinoma Project (MMMCP). A nationwide prospective study on reproducibility and prognostic power of routine quantitative assessments in the Netherlands. Path Res Pract 1989; 185: 664–70.

142. Fitzgibbons PL, Page DL, Weaver D et al. Prognostic factors in breast cancer. College of American Pathologists Consensus Statement 1999. Arch Pathol Lab Med 2000; 124: 966–78.

143. Gospodarowicz MK, Henson DE, Hutter RVP et al. UICC Prognostic Factors in Cancer, 2nd edn. New York: Wiley-Liss; 2001.

144. Akashi-Tanaka S, Tsuda H, Fukuda H, Watanabe T, Fukutomi T. Prognostic value of histopathological therapeutic effects and mitotic index in locally advanced breast cancers after neoadjuvant chemotherapy. Jpn J Clin Oncol 1996; 26: 201–6.

145. Honkoop AH, Pinedo HM, De Jong JS et al. Effects of chemotherapy on pathologic and biologic characteristics of locally advanced breast cancer. Am J Clin Pathol 1997; 107: 211–18.

146. Di Loreto C, Puglisi F, Rimondi G et al. Large core biopsy for diagnostic and prognostic evaluation of invasive breast carcinomas. Eur J Cancer 1996; 32A: 1693–700.

147. Jannink I, Risberg B, Diest PJ van, Baak JPA. Heterogeneity of mitoses counting in breast cancer. Histopathology 1996; 29: 421–8.

148. Aas T, Geisler S, Eide GE et al. Predictive value of tumour cell proliferation in locally advanced breast cancer treated with neoadjuvant chemotherapy. Eur J Cancer 2003; 39: 438–46.

149. Vincent-Salomon A, Rousseau A, Jouve M et al; Breast Cancer Study Group. Proliferation markers predictive of the pathological response and disease outcome of patients with breast carcinomas treated by anthracycline-based preoperative chemotherapy. Eur J Cancer 2004; 40: 1502–8.

150. Dowsett M, Smith IE, Ebbs SR et al; IMPACT Trialists Group. Prognostic value of Ki67 expression after short-term presurgical endocrine therapy for primary breast cancer. J Natl Cancer Inst 2007; 99: 167–70.

151. Poikonen P, Sjöström J, Amini RM et al. Cyclin A as a marker for prognosis and chemotherapy response in advanced breast cancer. Br J Cancer 2005; 93: 515–19.

152. Courjal F, Louason G, Speiser P et al. Cyclin gene amplification and over-expression in breast and ovarian cancers: evidence for the selection of cyclin D1 in breast and cyclin E in ovarian tumors. Int J Cancer 1996; 69: 247–53.

153. Bukholm IR, Bukholm G, Nesland JM. Over-expression of cyclin A is highly associated with early relapse and reduced survival in patients with primary breast carcinomas. Int J Cancer 2001; 93: 283–7.

154. Megha T, Lazzi S, Ferrari F et al. Expression of the G2-M checkpoint regulators cyclin B1 and P34^{CDC2} in breast cancer: a correlation with cellular kinetics. Anticancer Res 1999; 19: 163–9.

155. Winters ZE, Hunt NC, Bradburn MJ et al. Subcellular localisation of cyclin B, Cdc2 and p21(WAF1/CIP1) in breast cancer. Association with prognosis. Eur J Cancer 2001; 37: 2405–12.

156. Gillett CE, Lee AH, Millis RR, Barnes DM. Cyclin D1 and associated proteins in mammary ductal carcinoma in situ and atypical ductal hyperplasia. J Pathol 1998; 184: 396–400.

157. Mommers ECM, Van Diest PJ, Leonhart AM, Meijer CJLM, Baak JPA. Expression of proliferation and apoptosis related proteins in usual ductal hyperplasia of the breast. Hum Pathol 1998; 29: 1539–45.

158. Weinstat-Saslow D, Merino MJ, Manrow RE et al. Overexpression of cyclin D mRNA distinguishes invasive and in situ breast carcinomas from non-malignant lesions. Nat Med 1995; 1: 1257–60.

159. Simpson JF, Quan DE, O'Malley F, Odom-Maryon T, Clarke PE. Amplification of CCND1 and

expression of its protein product, cyclin D1, in ductal carcinoma in situ of the breast. Am J Pathol 1997; 151: 161–8.

160. Oyama T, Kashiwabara K, Yoshimoto K, Arnold A, Koerner FC. Frequent overexpression of the cyclin D1 oncogene in invasive lobular carcinoma of the breast. Cancer Res 1998; 58: 2876–80.

161. Hall M, Peters G. Genetic alterations of cyclins, cyclin-dependent kinases, and Cdk inhibitors in human cancer. Adv Cancer Res 1996; 68: 67–108.

162. Michalides R, Hageman Ph, van Tinteren H et al. A clinico-pathological study on overexpression of cyclin D1 and of p53 in a series of 248 patients with operable breast cancer. Br J Cancer 1996; 73: 728–34.

163. Seshadri R, Lee CS, Hui R et al. Cyclin D1 amplification is not associated with reduced overall survival in primary breast cancer but may predict early relapse in patients with features of good prognosis. Clin Canc Res 1996; 2: 1177–84.

164. Cuny M, Kramar A, Courjal F et al. Relating genotype and phenotype in breast cancer: an analysis of the prognostic significance of amplification at eight different genes or loci and of p53 mutations. Cancer Res 2000; 60: 1077–83.

165. Tsuda H, Hirohashi S, Shimosato Y et al. Correlation between long-term survival in breast cancer patients and amplification of two putative oncogene-coamplification units: hst-1/int-2 and cerbB-2/ear-1. Cancer Res 1989; 49: 3104–8.

166. Schuuring E, Verhoeven E, Tinteren H van et al. Amplification of genes within the chromosome 11q13 region is indicative of poor prognosis in patients with operable breast cancer. Cancer Res 1992; 52: 5229–34.

167. Nielsen NH, Emdin SO, Cajander J, Landberg G. Deregulation of cyclin E D1 in breast cancer is associated with inactivation of the retinoblastoma protein. Oncogene 1997; 14: 295–304.

168. Reed W, Fllrenes VA, Holm R, Hannisdal E, Nesland JM. Elevated levels of p27, p21 and cyclin D1 correlate with positive oestrogen and progesterone receptor status in node-negative breast carcinoma patients. Virchows Arch 1999; 435: 116–24.

169. Takano Y, Takenaka H, Kato Y et al. Cyclin D1 overexpression in invasive breast cancers: correlation with cyclin-dependent kinase 4 and oestrogen receptor overexpression, and lack of correlation with mitotic activity. J Cancer Res Clin Oncol 1999; 125: 505–12.

170. Kenny FS, Hui R, Musgrove EA et al. Overexpression of cyclin D1 messenger RNA predicts for poor prognosis in estrogen receptor-positive breast cancer. Clin Cancer Res 1999; 5: 2069–76.

171. Utsumi T, Yoshimura N, Maruta M et al. Correlation of cyclin D1 MRNA levels with clinico-pathological parameters and clinical outcome in human breast carcinomas. Int J Cancer 2000; 89: 39–43.

172. Hui R, Cornish AL, McClelland RA et al. Cyclin D1 and estrogen receptor messenger RNA levels are positively correlated in primary breast cancer. Clin Canc Res 1996; 2: 923–8.

173. Pelosio P, Barbareschi M, Bonoldi E et al. Clinical significance of cyclin D1 expression in patients with node-positive breast carcinoma treated with adjuvant therapy. Ann Oncol 1996; 7: 695–703.

174. De Jong JS, Van Diest PJ, Michalides RJAM, Baak JPA. Concerted overexpression of the genes encoding p21 and cyclin D1 is associated with growth inhibition and differentiation in various carcinomas. Mol Pathol 1999; 52: 78–83.

175. Scott KA, Walker RA. Lack of cyclin E immunoreactivity in non-malignant breast and association with proliferation in breast cancer. Br J Cancer 1997; 76: 1288–92.

176. Keyomarsi K, O'Leary N, Molnar G et al. Cyclin E, a potential prognostic marker for breast cancer. Cancer Res 1994; 54: 380–5.

177. Catzavelos C, Tsao MS, DeBoer G et al. Reduced expression of the cell cycle inhibitor p27[Kip1] in non-small cell lung carcinoma: a prognostic factor independent of Ras. Cancer Res 1999; 59: 684–8.

178. Tan P, Cady B, Wanner M et al. The cell cycle inhibitor p27 is an independent prognostic marker in small (T1a,b) invasive breast carcinomas. Cancer Res 1997; 57: 1259–63.

179. Fredersdorf S, Burns J, Milne AM et al. High level expression of p27(kip1) and cyclin D1 in some human breast cancer cells: inverse correlation between the expression of p27(kip1) and degree of malignancy in human breast and colorectal cancers. Proc Natl Acad Sci USA 1997; 94: 6380–5.

180. Porter PL, Malone KE, Heagerty PJ et al. Expression of cell-cycle regulators p27Kip1 and cyclin E, alone and in combination, correlate with survival in young breast cancer patients. Nat Med 1997; 3: 222–5.

181. Nielsen NH, Arnerlov C, Emdin SO, Landberg G. Cyclin E overexpression, a negative prognostic factor in breast cancer with strong correlation to oestrogen receptor status. Br J Cancer 1996; 74: 874–80.

182. Nielsen NH, Arnerlov C, Cajander S, Landberg G. Cyclin E expression and proliferation in breast cancer. Anal Cell Pathol 1998; 17: 177–88.

183. Caffo O, Doglioni C, Veronese S et al. Prognostic value of p21(WAF1) and p53 expression in breast carcinoma: an immunohistochemical study in 261 patients with long-term follow-up. Clin Cancer Res 1996; 2: 1591–9.

184. Mathoulin-Portier MP, Viens P, Cowen D et al. Prognostic value of simultaneous expression of p21 and mdm2 in breast carcinomas treated by adjuvant chemotherapy with antracyclin. Oncol Rep 2000; 7: 675–80.

185. Thor AD, Liu S, Moore DH 2nd, Shi Q, Edgerton SM. p21 (WAF1/CIP1) expression in breast cancers: associations with p53 and outcome. Breast Cancer Res Treat 2000; 61: 33–43.

186. Domagala W, Welcker M, Chosia M et al. p21/WAF1/ Cip1 expression in invasive ductal breast carcinoma: relationship to p53, proliferation rate, and survival at 5 years. Virchows Arch 2001; 439: 132–40.

187. Catzavelos C, Bhattacharya N, Ung YC et al. Decreased levels of the cell-cycle inhibitor p27[Kip1] protein: prognostic implications in primary breast cancer. Nature Med 1997; 3: 227–30.

188. Barbareschi M, van Tinteren H, Mauri FA et al. p27(kip1) expression in breast carcinomas: an immunohistochemical study on 512 patients with long-term follow-up. Int J Cancer 2000; 89: 236–41.

189. Xu L, Sgroi D, Sterner CJ et al. Mutational analysis of CDKN2 (MTS1/p16ink4) in human breast carcinomas. Cancer Res 1994; 54: 5262–4.

190. Dublin EA, Patel NK, Gillett CE et al. Retinoblastoma and p16 proteins in mammary carcinoma: their relationship to cyclin D1 and histopathological parameters. Int J Cancer 1998; 79: 71–5.

191. Pietilainen T, Lipponen P, Aaltomaa S et al. Expression of retinoblastoma gene protein (Rb) in breast cancer as related to established prognostic factors and survival. Eur J Cancer 1995; 31A: 329–33.

192. Berns EM, de Klein A, van Putten WL et al. Association between RB-1 gene alterations and factors of favourable prognosis in human breast cancer, without effect on survival. Int J Cancer 1995; 64: 140–5.

193. Sawan A, Randall B, Angus B et al. Retinoblastoma and p53 gene expression related to relapse and survival in human breast cancer: an immunohistochemical study. J Pathol 1992; 168: 23–8.

194. Bergh J. Clinical studies of p53 in treatment and benefit of breast cancer patients. Endocr Relat Cancer 1999; 6: 51–9.

195. Castiglione F, Sarotto I, Fontana V et al. Bcl2, p53 and clinical outcome in a series of 138 operable breast cancer patients. Anticancer Res 1999; 19: 4555–63.

196. Thor AD, Moore DH II, Edgerton SM et al. Accumulation of p53 tumor suppressor gene protein: an independent marker of prognosis in breast cancers. J Natl Cancer Inst 1992; 84: 845–55.

197. Andersen TI, Holm R, Nesland JM et al. Prognostic significance of TP53 alterations in breast carcinoma. Br J Cancer 1993; 68: 540–8.

198. Van Slooten HJ, van De Vijver MJ, Borresen AL et al. Mutations in exons 5–8 of the p53 gene, independent of their type and location, are associated with increased apoptosis and mitosis in invasive breast carcinoma. J Pathol 1999; 189: 504–13.

199. Bottini A, Berruti A, Bersiga A et al. p53 but not bcl-2 immunostaining is predictive of poor clinical complete response to primary chemotherapy in breast cancer patients. Clin Cancer Res 2000; 6: 2751–8.

200. Carey LA, Kim NW, Goodman S et al. Telomerase activity and prognosis in primary breast cancers. J Clin Oncol 1999; 17: 3075–81.

201. Clark GM, Osborne CK, Levitt D, Wu F, Kim NW. Telomerase activity and survival of patients with node-positive breast cancer. J Natl Cancer Inst 1997; 89: 1874–81.

202. Mokbel K, Parris CN, Ghilchik M, Williams G, Newbold RF. The association between telomerase, histopathological parameters, and KI-67 expression in breast cancer. Am J Surg 1999; 178: 69–72.

203. Poremba C, Bocker W, Willenbring H et al. Telomerase activity in human proliferative breast lesions. Int J Oncol 1998; 12: 641–8.

204. Hoos A, Hepp HH, Kaul S et al. Telomerase activity correlates with tumor aggressiveness and reflects therapy effect in breast cancer. Int J Cancer 1998; 79: 8–12.

205. Roos G, Nilsson P, Cajander S et al. Telomerase activity in relation to p53 status and clinico-pathological parameters in breast cancer. Int J Cancer 1998; 79: 343–8.

206. Leist M, Nicotera P. The shape of cell death (breakthroughs and views). Biochem Biophys Res Commun 1997; 236: 1–9.

207. Staunton MJ, Gaffney EF. Apoptosis: basic concepts and potential significance in human cancer. Arch Pathol Lab Med 1998; 122: 310–19.

208. Schepop HAM van de, Jong JS de, Van Diest PJ, Baak JPA. Apoptosis counting in breast cancer: a methodological study. Mol Pathol 1996; 49: 214–17.

209. Soini Y, Paakko P, Lehto VP. Histopathological evaluation of apoptosis in cancer. Am J Pathol 1998; 153: 1041–53.

210. Kong J, Ringer DP. Quantative in situ image analysis of apoptosis in well and poorly differentiated tumors from rat liver. Am J Pathol 1995; 147: 1626–32.

211. Shinohara T, Ohshima K, Murayama H. Apoptosis and proliferation in gastric carcinoma: the association with histological type. Histopathology 1996; 29: 123–9.

212. Leers MP, Kolgen W, Bjorklund V et al. Immunocytochemical detection and mapping of a cytokeratin 18 neo-epitope exposed during early apoptosis. J Pathol 1999; 187: 567–72.

213. Hadjiloucas I, Gilmore AP, Bundred NJ, Streuli CH. Assessment of apoptosis in human breast tissues using an antibody against the active form of caspase 3: relation to histopathological characteristics. Br J Cancer 2001; 85: 1522–6.

214. Wyllie AH. Glucocorticoid-induced thymocyte apoptosis is associated with endogenous endonuclease activation. Nature 1980; 284: 555–6.

215. Walker PR, Weaver VM, Lach B. Endonuclease activities associated with high molecular weight and internucleosomal DNA fragmentation in apoptosis. Exp Cell Res 1994; 213: 100–6.

216. Oberhammer FA, Hochegger K, Froschl G. Chromatin condensation during apoptosis is accompanied by degradation of lamin A+B without enhanced activation of cdc2 kinase. J Cell Biol 1994; 136: 827–37.

217. Gavrieli Y, Sherman Y, Ben-Sasson SA. Identification of programmed cell death in-situ via specific labeling of nuclear DNA fragmentation. J Cell Biol 1992; 119: 493–501.

218. Mundle SD, Gao XZ, Khan S. Two in situ labeling techniques reveal different patterns of DNA fragmentation during spontaneous apoptosis in vivo and induced apoptosis in vitro. Anticancer Res 1995; 15: 1895–904.

219. Wijsman JH, Jonker RR, Keijzer R. A new method to detect apoptosis in paraffin sections: in situ end-labeling of fragmented DNA. J Histochem Cytochem 1993; 41: 7–12.

220. Gaffney EF, O Neill AJ, Staunton MJ. In situ end-labeling, light microscopic assessment and ultrastructure of apoptosis in lung carcinoma. J Clin Pathol 1995; 48: 1017–21.

221. Darzynkiewicz Z, Juan G, Li X. Cytometry in cell necrobiology: analysis of apoptosis and accidental cell death (necrosis). Cytometry 1997; 27: 1–27.

222. Vakkala M, Lähteenmäki K, Raunio H, Pääkkö P, Soini Y. Apoptosis during breast carcinoma progression. Clin Cancer Res 1999; 5: 319–24.

223. Zhang GJ, Kimijima I, Abe R. Apoptotic index correlates to bcl-2 and p53 protein expression, histological grade and prognosis in invasive breast cancers. Anticancer Res 1998; 18: 1998–9.

224. Srinivas P, Abraham E, Ahamed I et al. Apoptotic index: use in predicting recurrence in breast cancer patients. J Exp Clin Cancer Res 2002; 21: 233–8.

225. González-Cámpora R, Galera Ruiz MR, Vázquez Ramírez F et al. Apoptosis in breast carcinoma. Pathol Res Pract 2000; 196: 167–74.

226. Sirvent JJ, Aguilar MC, Olona M et al. Prognostic value of apoptosis in breast cancer (pT1-pT2). A TUNEL, p53, bcl-2, bag-1 and Bax immunohistochemical study. Histol Histopathol 2004; 19: 759–70.

227. Schöndorf T, Göhring UJ, Becker M et al. High apoptotic index correlates to p21 and p27 expression indicating a favorable outcome of primary breast cancer patients, but lacking prognostic significance in multivariate analysis. Pathobiology 2004; 71: 217–22.

228. Berardo MD, Elledge RM, de Moor C et al. Bcl-2 and apoptosis in lymph node positive carcinoma. Cancer 1998; 82: 1296–302.

229. Gonzalez-Campora R, Galera Ruiz MR, Vazquez Ramirez F et al. Apoptosis in breast carcinoma. Pathol Res Pract 2000; 196: 167–74.

230. De Jong JS, Van Diest PJ, Baak JPA. Number of apoptotic cells as a prognostic marker in invasive breast cancer. Br J Cancer 2000; 82: 368–73.

231. Daidone MG, Veneroni S, Benini E et al. Biological markers as indicators of response to primary and adjuvant chemotherapy in breast cancer. Int J Cancer 1999; 84: 580–6.

232. Kymionis GD, Dimitrakakis CE, Konstadoulakis MM et al. Can expression of apoptosis genes, bcl-2 and bax, predict survival and responsiveness to chemotherapy in node-negative breast cancer patients? J Surg Res 2001; 99: 161–8.

233. Le MG, Mathieu MC, DoucRasy S et al. c-myc, p53 and bcl2, apoptosis-related genes in infiltrating breast carcinomas: evidence of a link between bcl-2 protein over-expression and a lower risk of metastasis and death in operable patients. Int J Cancer 1999; 84: 562–7.

234. Sierra A, Castellsagué X, Coll T et al. Expression of death-related genes and their relationship to loss of apoptosis in T1 ductal breast carcinomas. Int J Cancer 1998; 79: 103–10.

235. Slooten HJ van, Vijver MJ van de, Velde CJ van de et al. Loss of Bcl-2 in invasive breast cancer is associated with high rates of cell death, but also with increased proliferation activity. Br J Cancer 1998; 77: 789–96.

236. Veronese SM, Mauri FA, Caffo O et al. Bax immunohistochemical expression in breast carcinoma: a study with long-term follow-up. Int J Cancer 1998; 79: 13–18.

237. Tanaka K, Iwamoto S, Gon G et al. Expression of survivin and its relationship to loss of apoptosis in breast carcinomas. Clin Cancer Res 2000; 6: 127–34.

238. Yamashita S, Masuda Y, Kurizaki T et al. Survivin expression predicts early recurrence in early-stage breast cancer. Anticancer Res 2007; 27: 2803–8.

239. Al-Joudi FS, Iskandar ZA, Imran AK. Survivin expression correlates with unfavourable prognoses in invasive ductal carcinoma of the breast. Med J Malaysia 2007; 62: 6–8.

240. Hinnis AR, Luckett JC, Walker RA. Survivin is an independent predictor of short-term survival in poor prognostic breast cancer patients. Br J Cancer 2007; 96: 639–45.

241. Ryan BM, Konecny GE, Kahlert S et al. Survivin expression in breast cancer predicts clinical outcome and is associated with HER2, VEGF, urokinase plasminogen activator and PAI-1. Ann Oncol 2006; 17: 597–604.

242. Span PN, Sweep FC, Wiegerinck ET et al. Survivin is an independent prognostic marker for risk stratification of breast cancer patients. Clin Chem 2004; 50: 1986–93.

Risk factors for local recurrence following conservation therapy in breast cancer

4

Paula HM Elkhuizen, Bas Kreike and Marc J van de Vijver

INTRODUCTION

During recent decades, the surgical approach to treat breast cancer has changed. Throughout most of the 20th century the traditional surgical approach has been the radical or the modified radical mastectomy. The radical mastectomy was introduced by Halsted;[1] it included removal of the breast, including an ample amount of the overlying skin, the greater part of the underlying pectoral muscles, all axillary lymph nodes and, in later years, also the supraclavicular nodes in most cases. The Halsted mastectomy was readily accepted due to its good treatment results. In later years it was found that less mutilating surgery, with preservation of the pectoral major muscles or both pectoral muscles (the modified radical mastectomy) was equally effective with regard to locoregional control and survival. From the 1970s onwards, the modified radical mastectomy became the standard surgical treatment of early breast cancer.

Already early in the 20th century, attempts to treat breast cancer with local excision of the tumor were reported; after the 1970s, larger studies of breast-conserving treatment were started. With the presently used conservative treatment, the tumor is removed, ideally with a margin of 1–2 cm normal surrounding tissue. It was found that when a conservative surgical approach was used, radiation therapy is mandatory to achieve acceptable local control rates.[2–5] Six prospective randomized trials,[6–11] comparing mastectomy with conservative surgery and radiation for the treatment of stage I–II breast cancer, showed no significant difference in terms of locoregional control with limited follow-up, but publications of the same trials with longer follow-up data showed poorer local control after breast-conserving therapy (BCT) as compared to mastectomy.[12–15] However, these trials demonstrated no significant differences in distant metastasis or long-term survival between the treatment approaches. As a result of these large trials, the surgical approach has shifted from mastectomy to BCT. In June 1990 it was concluded at the Consensus Development Conference on the Treatment of Early Breast Cancer, convened by the National Cancer Institute in the USA, that BCT is an appropriate method of primary therapy for the majority of women with stage I and II breast cancer.[16]

PATIENT FOR BREAST-CONSERVING THERAPY AND FOR LOCAL RECURRENCE

In the initial years after the introduction of BCT, patients were selected mainly on the basis of small size of tumor and the absence of multifocal disease, as defined by mammography and physical examination. During the 1980s, a number of studies were performed to define subgroups of patient who were at high risk for local relapse (LR). It was found that risk factors for LR after BCT are different to risk factors for LR after mastectomy. For instance, tumor size and positive lymph nodes, well-known risk factors for LR after mastectomy, have not been identified as risk factors for LR after BCT. The difference in risk factors for LR after both modalities complicates the choice between mastectomy and BCT.

Renewed tumor growth in the treated breast is assumed to arise from microscopic tumor foci left behind after surgery. In studying mastectomy specimens from 282 patients with invasive primary breast cancers, Holland et al[17] found additional tumor foci of invasive and noninvasive carcinoma in the breast tissue around the reference mass in nearly two-thirds of the specimens. Of these tumor foci, 43% were located >2 cm from the reference mass. Also, there was no difference between primary tumors ≤2 cm and tumors >2 cm with respect to tumor foci in number or distance from primary tumors. In other words, regardless of primary tumor size, tumor cells are frequently left behind in the operated breast at a distance of >2 cm of the dominant tumor. Radiotherapy administered after local excision is aimed at eradicating these remaining tumor cells, and is of major importance.[2–5] However, in cases where the remnant tumor burden is too large for eradication by radiotherapy, or when the remaining tumor cells are radioresistant, patients will present with a LR. For instance, risk factors found for LR after BCT include positive tumor margins[18–27] and lymphangio-invasive growth;[18,21,28,29] both risk factors represent a higher risk for a significant tumor burden after conservative surgery.

Treatment-related factors which are associated with low risk of LR include the use of more extensive surgery. After quadrantectomy, a lower risk for LR is found compared to lumpectomy.[30] However, extended surgery reduces the LR rate, but at the cost of compromising the cosmetic result. Patients nowadays are considered candidates for BCT if an acceptable cosmetic result can be achieved and no significant risk for complications is present (i.e. a history of pre-existing collagen vascular disease, or previous radiation).

Margins

Margin status of the invasive tumor has been found in many studies to be of predictive value for LR after BCT, as summarized in Figure 4.1.[18–27] In practice, the most commonly used method to assess microscopic margins is inking of the breast specimen with subsequent sections taken perpendicular to the inked surface. The distance between the inked margin and cancer cells can then be assessed. Close margins have variably been defined as tumor within 1–2 mm of the margin. The definition of a negative margin has ranged from no cancer cells at the margin to a distance of >1–2 mm. Involvement of the margin may be focal (i.e. ≤3 low-power fields) or diffuse (>3 low-power fields).

Gage et al[22] showed no difference in the LR rate in patients with negative margins for those cases in which there are cancer cells within 1 mm of the inked margins compared to cases in which cancer cells are more distant from the resection margin. Patients with negative margins (>1 mm) had a 5-year risk of LR of 2%, and patients with close margins (negative ≤1 mm) had a similar risk for LR at 5 years of 3%. The authors showed that patients with only focally positive tumor margins had a considerable lower risk of LR than those with more than focally positive margins. The 5-year risk for LR for patients with focally positive tumor margins was 9%. Patients with tumor margins more than focally positive as assessed in 3 low-power fields, had a 28% risk for LR at 5 years. These data have been updated after prolonged follow-up showing similar results.[25]

As seen in Figure 4.1, most series demonstrate an increased incidence of LR in patients with positive resection margins, although the incidence of LR varies among the different studies. The variations in LR rates may be related to the extent of the surgical resection, the presence or absence of ductal carcinoma in situ, and the extent of the tumor-involved margin. In general, reexcision should be advised in cases of a tumor resection with margins that are more than focally positive.

Tumor features

Tumor size (T1 versus T2) and tumor location has not been found to be associated with a higher risk of local recurrence after BCT.

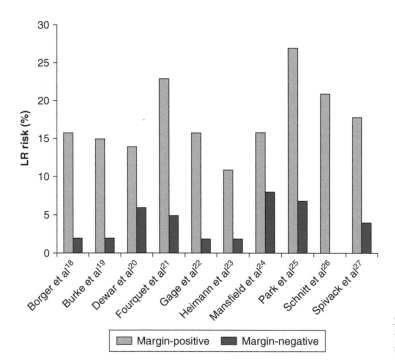

Figure 4.1 Microscopic margin status of invasive tumor and risk of local recurrence (LR).

There is no increased risk of breast recurrence in T2 tumors provided that an excision with tumor-negative margins has been performed.[31,32] Also, location of the tumor (outer quadrants, subareolar, or central tumors) does not predict a different risk for LR, as long as an excision with negative margins can be performed. Histologic type does not appear to be associated with risk of LR.[33] Invasive lobular carcinomas were found in two series[34,35] to be associated with increased risk for LR; however, additional series reported no increased risk.[29,31,33,36–40] Patients with lobular histology are now considered candidates for conservative surgery and radiation, provided that the tumor is not multifocal and that adequate excision can be performed with negative tumor margins. Data on tumors with medullary, colloid, or tubular histology are limited, but suggest that these patients do not have an increased risk for LR. Also, patients with positive axillary nodes do not have an increased risk for LR when treated with BCT,[29,31,32,41] in contrast to patients treated with mastectomy.[42,43]

In 15–30% of patients, the invasive breast carcinoma is accompanied by an extensive component of ductal carcinoma in situ (EDCIS). An important finding has been the identification of this EDCIS component as a risk factor for LR after BCT. In a study by Vicini et al,[44] and in a later update by Boyages et al,[45] it was found that patients with an EDCIS constituted 28% of the patients with infiltrating ductal carcinoma, and yet accounted for 60% of all local recurrences. Other studies have confirmed EDCIS as an important risk factor for LR after BCT.[19,21,26,29,40,46–48] In Figure 4.2, some of these data are summarized.[19,21,26,45–47] There have also been studies that did not find EDCIS as a risk factor for LR.[31,32,49,50] This may in part be the result of lack in reproducibility among pathologists in defining EDCIS. However, Vicini et al[44] did postulate that margin status may be of importance; and patients in the Boston series[44,45] underwent only a limited gross excision of the invasive tumor before radiotherapy, while no margin assessment for the EDCIS component was used to guide treatment.

The increased risk for LR for patients with EDCIS is a result of the growth pattern of DCIS. DCIS grows along the ducts in the

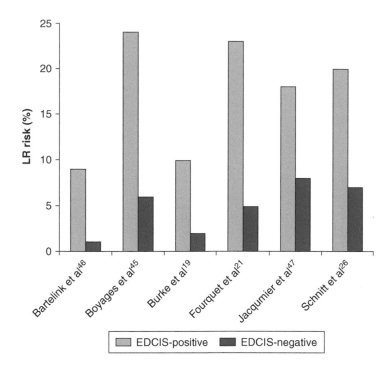

Figure 4.2 Presence of extensive component ductal carcinoma in situ (EDCIS) and risk of local recurrence (LR).

breast without invasion of the underlying tissue. This growth pattern results in a non-palpable lesion, which is difficult to remove with tumor-negative margins. When EDCIS is found in the pathologic specimen, it is possible that a significant tumor burden is still present in the breast. It has been found that when accurate margin assessment is done, and EDCIS is removed with negative margins, EDCIS loses its predictive value for a local recurrence.[19,22,26,46] For the EDCIS component, the same rules apply as for the invasive component: it should be attempted to achieve tumor-free margins; when the margins are more than focally positive for EDCIS, patients need to undergo re-excision to obtain free margins.[51–55]

Age and genetic factors

Of interest, a risk factor for LR after BCT found in several studies is young age.[18,21,29,32,40,41,56–67] In Figure 4.3, data on LR rates are presented for patients under and above 35 years of age at the time of BCT.[21,29,31,32,41,60–64,67] Young age is associated with the presence of other risk factors for LR,[68] but is in most studies also an independent

risk factor for LR. Apparently, an unknown biological factor is present in (relating to the tumors of) these young patients which results in a high risk for LR. It is estimated that 5–10% of women with breast cancer have hereditary breast cancer with an autosomal Mendelian pattern of inheritance. Twenty per cent of the patients have familial breast cancer, with one or more first- or second-degree relatives without an autosomal dominant pattern of inheritance. The identification of the BRCA1 and BRCA2 genes has directed increasing attention to the hereditary form of breast cancer and its treatment. Some physicians recommend mastectomy as the preferred surgical treatment for these women. There is no evidence that women with a positive family history of breast cancer have a higher risk of recurrence than those with a negative family history.[19,69–72] Most of the series have not distinguished between patients with hereditary and familial breast cancer. Pierce et al[73] studied the LR rate after BCT in women known to carry a germline BRCA1/2 mutation. In total, 71 patients with germline mutations were compared with sporadic controls. No difference in LR was found; at 5 years LR as a first event was found in 2% of the cohort with

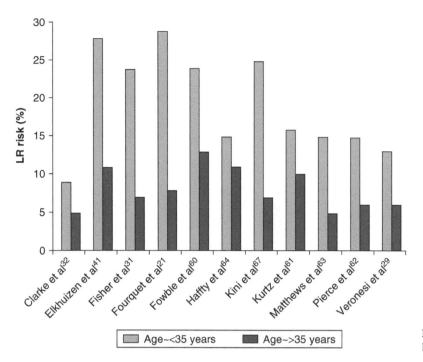

Figure 4.3 Age and risk of local recurrence (LR).

BRCA1/2 germline mutations versus 4% of the sporadic cohort.

Other factors

Tumor-related contraindications to conservative therapy include diffuse microcalcifications suspicious for malignancy seen on mammography or multiple gross lesions within the breast. Grossly positive or diffusely positive microscopic excision margins, which cannot be rendered negative by re-excision without producing excessive deformity, preclude conservative management. The above findings are highly predictive of a large residual tumor burden within the breast, which is difficult to control with irradiation and will result in an unacceptable high rate of LR.[74] It is still not possible to select *all* high-risk patients, despite the risk factors for LR after BCT that have been detected so far. To make a good selection for all patients when offering BCT, with acceptable LR risk, it is necessary to find additional risk factors for LR.

In recent decades, new molecular markers have been found to be of importance for prognosis in breast cancer patients. These markers, which are known to play a role in breast cancer growth, have not been extensively studied as risk factors for LR. For instance, it is known that overexpression of the human epidermal growth factor receptor 2 (HER2) gene (also known as c-erbB2/neu) is found in 50% of the cases of ductal carcinoma in situ of the breast, while overexpression in invasive tumors is only found in 20%.[75,76] Because of the association of EDCIS with LR risk after BCT, it can be hypothesized that patients with HER2 overexpression may be at risk for LR. Inactivation of the p53 tumor suppressor gene may also be associated with increased risk of LR. In experimental models, an intact p53 gene plays a role in the induction of apoptosis by radiation therapy.[77,78] Tumor cells with p53 mutations can therefore be hypothesized to be radioresistant, which in the case of BCT may result in higher LR rates.

More recently, microarray gene expression profiling techniques have been developed. These high-throughput techniques make it possible to study the association of the expression of thousands of genes with LR after BCT. Using this approach, Kreike et al[79] showed, in a study of 50 primary tumors, that there is not a large difference in the overall gene expression profile between tumors developing LR and those that do not. Nuyten et al[80] used a preselected set of genes that was constructed to predict metastasis-free survival in breast cancer patients. Using this gene set, they showed that it may possibly also predict LR based on the gene expression profile of the primary tumor.[80] Studies of large series of well-characterized breast carcinomas from patients undergoing BCT will be required to obtain reliable gene expression profiles associated with LR. Such predictive gene expression profiles are likely to help in understanding the mechanisms underlying LR after BCT; and to help in guiding optimal locoregional treatment in individual patients.

THE INFLUENCE OF RADIOTHERAPY ON LOCAL RECURRENCE

As outlined above, radiotherapy given after surgery is very important to eradicate microscopic tumor left in the breast after lumpectomy, and thus to achieve acceptable LR rates. Randomized trials[2–5,81,82] have demonstrated that adjuvant radiation therapy following conservative surgery reduces the risk of local recurrences remarkably compared to surgery alone.[2–5,81,82] In the nonirradiated lumpectomy cohort in the National Surgical Adjuvant Breast Program (NSABP)-B06 trial, a local recurrence rate of 39% was found, compared to 14% in the irradiated patients at 20 years of follow-up.[2] The local recurrence rates found in the other studies for the group of nonirradiated patients are similar to these results. A recent meta-analysis by the Early Breast Cancer Trialists' Collaborative Group, studied a group of 7300 patients that were treated with breast-conserving surgery in trials of radiotherapy. They showed a 5-year local recurrence risk of 7% versus 26% (absolute reduction 19%), and 15-year breast cancer mortality risks of 30.5% versus 35.9% (reduction 5.4%), all in favor of adjuvant radiotherapy following breast-conserving surgery.[81]

Studies have been performed in which radiotherapy was the only treatment for breast cancer. Pierquin et al[83] used combinations of external megavoltage irradiation with interstitial implants of radioactive sources to raise the combined dose in the primary tumor mass to 90–100 Gy. Doses of this magnitude provided control of all primary breast carcinomas <5 cm in diameter. In a retrospective analysis of 463 breast tumors with radiotherapy alone, Arriagada et al[84] demonstrated the independent influence of radiation dose for tumor control of primary breast cancer of various sizes. For tumors <4 cm a local control rate at 3 years of 25% was found when doses of 40–50 Gy were given. At 3 years, local control was obtained with 70–80 Gy in 81% of the cases, while doses >80 Gy resulted in local control for all breast carcinomas. For tumors of a larger size, the control rates were lower, but still a dose-effect on tumor control was seen. It should be noted, that high radiation doses on the breast will yield high risk for complications, especially severe fibrosis.[65,85]

Nowadays, following conservative surgery, radiation therapy is given to the whole breast to a total dose of 45–50 Gy in a period of 5 weeks. This is usually followed by a boost of 10–20 Gy to the original tumor bed. In this way, a moderate radiation dose is given, resulting in minimal adverse effects on the breast and surrounding tissues. Variations in the radiotherapy technique are found to have impact on the LR rate. Prolongations of the overall treatment time with <8 Gy/week was found to be associated with high LR rates.[86]

Also, during the interval of surgery and radiotherapy, repopulation of residual tumor cells may occur. A long delay between surgery and radiation therapy may therefore increase the rate of LR. Delay of radiation treatment is mostly studied in patients who received chemotherapy given during this interval. Few studies have been published about the effect of surgery–radiotherapy interval without chemotherapy given during this interval, and although higher LR rates are reported with increasing interval,[87,88] this has not been found in all studies.[32,89]

After radiation to the whole breast, usually a boost is given to the tumor bed. The treatment volume of the boost is determined by the diameter of the tumor with a safety margin of approximately 2–3 cm. Surgical clips placed in the tumor bed are very useful in accurately determining the boost localization. A radiation boost to the tumor bed can be given in different ways: by photons, electrons or iridium-192 implants. There is no correlation between the type of boost employed and the risk of LR.[90–93]

It has been demonstrated that for patients with unknown margins of tumor resection, the addition of a boost appears to decrease the risk of a breast recurrence.[94] For patients with negative margins, the value of an additional boost had been a subject of debate, which was ended with the results of the EORTC 22881 trial.[65] This prospective trial randomized patients with microscopically negative margins after tumor excision between a boost or no boost. In total, 5318 early stage breast cancer patients were randomized to an additional boost of 16 Gy or no boost following whole breast radiation of 50 Gy. At 10 years follow-up, the cumulative incidence of local recurrence was 10.2% versus 6.2% for the no boost and the boost group, respectively, resulting in a reduction of LR with a factor of 0.59. Also in this study, young age was the most important risk factor for LR. It was also shown that patients younger than 40 years of age show the largest absolute clinical benefit from the additional boost. The LR risk in this age group was reduced from 23.9% to 13.5% at 10 years. As a result, the number of salvage mastectomies has been reduced by 41%. The EORTC 22881 trial also randomized patients ($n=251$) with a microscopically incomplete excision between a boost dose of 10 Gy versus 26 Gy.[95] A higher boost dose of 26 Gy resulted in a nonsignificant trend towards a lower LR rate. At 10 years, the cumulative incidence of local recurrence was 17.5 % versus 10.8 %; however, at the cost of an increased risk of fibrosis.

LOCAL RECURRENCE AFTER BREAST-CONSERVING THERAPY IS ASSOCIATED WITH POOR PROGNOSIS

LR after mastectomy has been known to be associated with poor prognosis even in the absence of synchronous distant metastases.[96,97] It was considered in the initial period of BCT that prognosis after LR would be favorable because of the option of salvage mastectomy. In 1991, Fisher et al[98] first described LR as a predictor for distant metastasis; this was later confirmed in other studies.[29,99,100] It also appeared that after BCT a LR was found to be associated with poor prognosis. Whether LR is the cause of subsequent distant metastasis and poor prognosis or just an indicator of aggressive disease could not be resolved in these studies. Risk factors for distant metastasis after LR have only been studied in a few, very heterogeneous, studies.[21,99,101–108] A short interval between BCT and time of LR, mostly defined as <2–3 years, is found to be a prognosticator for poor survival after LR.[21,98–100,103–106] However, in most studies focusing on risk factors for survival after LR, patients are included who have distant metastasis diagnosed before or simultaneously with LR.

As already stated above, the results of the recently published Early Breast Cancer Trialists' Collaborative Group meta-analysis[81] postulate that adequate local treatment reducing local recurrence rates would, in the hypothetical absence of any other causes of death, avoid about one breast cancer death over the next 15 years for every four local recurrences avoided.

THE INFLUENCE OF ADJUVANT SYSTEMIC THERAPY ON LOCAL RELAPSE IN BREAST-CONSERVING THERAPY

Adjuvant chemotherapy has been shown to have impact on LR. Lumpectomy *without* radiation has been associated with a significant risk of breast cancer recurrence also if chemotherapy is given with 5-year LR rates of 30–40%.[7,82] However, when patients are treated with BCT including radiotherapy and adjuvant chemotherapy, a decreased incidence of LR is reported when compared to conservative surgery with radiation alone.[7,64,109–111] In the NSABP B-13 trial,[109] a total of 760 node-negative breast cancer patients with estrogen receptor-negative tumors were randomized between BCT followed by sequential methotrexate and fluorouracil or BCT alone. The risk for LR at 8 years among node-negative patients who had tumor-free margins after BCT was 2.6% for patients treated with adjuvant chemotherapy versus 13.4% for patients treated with BCT alone. Similar data were also found for adjuvant tamoxifen after BCT; in the NSABP-B-14 trial,[112] at 7 years the LR rate was 2.2% for node-negative patients who were randomized to receive tamoxifen versus 5.5% of the patients randomized to receive placebo. Postmenopausal node-negative patients treated in the Stockholm Adjuvant Tamoxifen Trial,[113] were randomized to receive either adjuvant tamoxifen or no further treatment. At 8 years follow-up, patients treated with BCT who received tamoxifen had an LR as first event of 3% versus 7% in patients who did not receive tamoxifen.

Thus, the use of adjuvant systemic therapy seems to potentiate the effects of breast irradiation after breast-conserving surgery for invasive breast cancer. It has also been shown that different chemotherapy regimes hold different effects on local control. In the NSABP B-19 protocol,[109] node-negative breast cancer patients treated with BCT were randomized between sequential methotrexate and fluorouracil versus CMF (cyclophosphamide, methotrexate, fluorouracil). At 8 years, LR were detected in 2.6% of the patients treated with the sequential regimen versus 0.6% of the patients treated with CMF.

With the increasing use of chemotherapy as adjuvant treatment, also for node-negative patients it is important to note that sequencing of chemotherapy and radiotherapy may impact on local control. Options for sequencing of radiotherapy and chemotherapy include: the delivery of all chemotherapy prior to radiotherapy or all radiotherapy prior to chemotherapy (sequential regimens); the simultaneous initiation of both modalities (concurrent regimens); or the initiation of radiotherapy in the midst of the chemotherapy program (sandwich regimens). Concurrent regimens have the theoretical advantage of initiating both modality treatments (for local and systemic therapy) without a delay in either modality, and is thereby likely not associated with increased risk for LR. However, concurrent regimens may be associated with increased risk of toxicity. Concurrent chemotherapy is not associated with an increased risk of symptomatic pneumonitis in patients treated with tangential fields only. However, in one study treatment to the breast and regional nodes with concurrent chemotherapy, an incidence of 9% of symptomatic pneumonitis was found compared to 1% in patients who were treated with a sequential regimen.[114] The concurrent use of chemotherapy has been associated with a less favorable cosmetic result in some series, but not in others.[85,115]

When using a sequential regimen there have been reports, mainly from nonrandomized studies, that delay of radiotherapy in favor of chemotherapy results in higher LR.[116–118] There has been one randomized trial,[119] unfortunately including only a relatively small number of patients, for which the initial analysis showed a 14% risk of local recurrence in the chemotherapy-first group versus 5% in the radiotherapy-first group at 5 years follow-up. However, systemic recurrence was more frequent when radiation therapy was given first. In subgroup analysis of this study, it was found that for patients with negative tumor margins no difference was found in local or distant recurrence rate whether they were treated with chemotherapy or radiotherapy first. Patients with close, positive or unknown tumor margins had higher incidence of LR in the chemotherapy-first regimen and the higher incidence of distant recurrences in the radiotherapy-first group persisted. An update of this study after a longer follow-up period failed to show any difference in disease outcome between the chemotherapy-first group and the radiotherapy-first group.[120] Additional clinical trials of sufficient size are clearly required in this very important area.

BREAST-CONSERVING THERAPY AFTER PREOPERATIVE CHEMOTHERAPY

Chemotherapy can also be administered in the preoperative setting (also known as neoadjuvant, primary or induction chemotherapy). There are several theoretical arguments for the use of preoperative chemotherapy. These include the ability to carry out in vivo assessment of tumor response, using the primary tumor to monitor and optimize treatment effects on micrometastases. Also, there is a theoretical advantage of decreasing drug resistance by early exposure to systemic therapy with the hope of improving disease-free and overall survival, as well as producing less favorable growth kinetics for micrometastases. Patients with a good response to neoadjuvant chemotherapy can become eligible for BCT even when their initial tumor was too large for this treatment.

In the NSABP-B27 study, 87% of patients had a clinical response and 26.1% had a pathological complete remission after a combination of AC and docetaxel neoadjuvant chemotherapy.[121] In the meta-analysis of neoadjuvant versus postsurgery adjuvant therapy clinical trials, there was a significant reduction in the number of mastectomies after neoadjuvant chemotherapy (16.6% absolute reduction; 95% confidence internal, (CI) 15.1–18.1%).[122] An as yet unanswered question is to what extent the choice for BCT in these patients that were treated after neoadjuvant chemotherapy has resulted in an increase in local recurrence rates. In four randomized controlled trials[123–126] long-term follow-up showed no difference in survival between the two treatment regimens, nor any significant difference in local tumor control. In the NSABP-18 trial,[125] for patients who underwent BCT, at 9 years an LR rate of 10.7% was found for the neoadjuvant chemotherapy group versus 7.6% in the adjuvant chemotherapy group. Because of the heterogeneity of the designs of these studies, firm conclusions cannot be drawn. In the meta-analysis[122] there was a 22% increase in the risk of local regional recurrence after neoadjuvant chemotherapy (relative risk (RR) 1.22; CI 1.04–1.43).[122] The risk of local recurrence was highest in studies where patients with a clinical complete remission,[124] or even with macroscopical remaining tumor, were treated with radiotherapy alone without surgery.[123,127,128] The relative risk increase of local recurrence in these three studies was 1.53 (CI 1.17–2.00). In the other studies combined, there was no increase in the risk of local recurrence (RR 1.10; CI 0.87–1.38). These results suggest that even after a complete remission, surgery remains an important component of BCT.

On the basis of a study in 340 patients after neoadjuvant chemotherapy, who all underwent BCT, investigators at the MD Anderson Cancer Center have developed a prognostic index.[129] Risk factors in this study were: clinical (c)N2 or cN3 nodal status; residual pathological tumor size >2 cm; lymphangio invasion; multifocal growth pattern of the remaining tumor. If two of these risk factors are present, the risk of local recurrence was considered too high for BCT (12% with two risk factors; 18% with three risk factors after 5 years).

This prognostic index based on three risk factors was validated in a dataset of 815 patients who underwent BCT after neoadjuvant chemotherapy.[130] In this study, patients with no risk factors or only one risk factor had very low local recurrence rates after 10 years; when more risk factors were present, 10-year local recurrence rates were as high as 61%. These findings highlight that good patient selection for BCT after neoadjuvant chemotherapy is extremely important.

In summary, mastectomy instead of BCT after neoadjuvant chemotherapy should be advised when: there are diffuse malignant microcalcifications throughout the breast; when the resection is not radical with more than focally involved resection margins; if there are contraindications for radiation therapy; if it is not possible to localize the tumor area after a complete remission (for this reason, leaving markers in the breast at the position of the tumor should be considered prior to neoadjuvant chemotherapy). Mastectomy should also be considered if two or more of the risk factors found in the MD Anderson study are present: cN2 or cN3 nodal status (before or after chemotherapy); remaining tumor size >2 cm; multifocal tumor (which is often observed in invasive lobular carcinoma); if there is lymphangio invasion.

If these guidelines are followed, neoadjuvant chemotherapy will help to enable selected patients with large tumors eligible for BCT. However, it should be kept in mind that the majority of patients are already eligible for BCT without neoadjuvant chemotherapy and only selected patients with large tumors will benefit in this way. Therefore, converting mastectomy to BCT is not a very important justification for the use of neoadjuvant chemotherapy.

CONCLUSIONS

BCT has become the first choice for the local treatment of primary invasive breast cancer for many patients. Risk factors for local recurrence play an important role in the decision-making processes on BCT. Based on the LR risk profile, the following questions need to be answered for an individual patient:

- Should mastectomy be advised instead of BCT?
- Should a re-excision be performed?
- Should a boost of radiotherapy be given; at what dose? What should be the target area?
- To what extent will systemic adjuvant treatment contribute to an acceptable LR risk?

To date, young age and a number of histopathological factors have been identified as risk factors for LR, and these factors are used to guide patient-tailored therapy. However, there still is much need for improvement and additional risk factors for LR will be of great clinical value. A risk of LR >1%/year is considered too high and may be an indication for converting BCT to mastectomy. It should,

however, be realized that even with an LR risk of 30% at 10 years, 70% of patients could be safely treated with BCT. Therefore, to identify risk factors that can be used *within* high-risk groups is greatly needed. Young patients, arbitrarily defined as those younger than 40 or 35 years of age, form one such risk group. Using the rapidly increasing knowledge on genetic alterations in breast cancer, and the emergence of high-throughput techniques such as gene expression profiling by microarray analysis, it should be possible to identify these greatly needed additional risk factors.

Optimal BCT should result in low LR rates. At the same time, every attempt should be made to obtain an optimal cosmetic result. Here, there is still need for improvement and standardization of surgical and radiotherapy techniques. Risk factors for LR should then be integrated into the process of optimizing both cosmesis and local control. BCT has become a recognized standard of care in the past decades; the coming years will hopefully provide us with more powerful tools to optimize patient-tailored therapy.

REFERENCES

1. Halsted WS. The results of radical operations for the cure of carcinoma of the breast. Annals Surgery 1907; 46(1): 1–19.
2. Fisher B, Anderson S, Bryant J et al. Twenty-year follow-up of a randomized trial comparing total mastectomy, lumpectomy, and lumpectomy plus irradiation for the treatment of invasive breast cancer. N Engl J Med 2002; 347(16): 1233–41.
3. Clark RM, Whelan T, Levine M et al. Randomized clinical trial of breast irradiation following lumpectomy and axillary dissection for node-negative breast cancer: an update. Ontario Clinical Oncology Group. J Natl Cancer Inst 1996; 88(22): 1659–64.
4. Liljegren G, Holmberg L, Bergh J et al. 10-Year results after sector resection with or without postoperative radiotherapy for stage I breast cancer: a randomized trial. J Clin Oncol 1999; 17(8): 2326–33.
5. Veronesi U, Marubini E, Mariani L et al. Radiotherapy after breast-conserving surgery in small breast carcinoma: long-term results of a randomized trial. Ann Oncol 2001; 12(7): 997–1003.
6. Blichert-Toft M, Rose C, Andersen JA et al. Danish randomized trial comparing breast conservation therapy with mastectomy: six years of life-table

analysis. Danish Breast Cancer Cooperative Group. J Natl Cancer Inst Monogr 1992; (11): 19–25.

7. Fisher B, Redmond C, Poisson R et al. Eight-year results of a randomized clinical trial comparing total mastectomy and lumpectomy with or without irradiation in the treatment of breast cancer. N Engl J Med 1989; 320(13): 822–8.

8. Lichter AS, Lippman ME, Danforth Jr DN et al. Mastectomy versus breast-conserving therapy in the treatment of stage I and II carcinoma of the breast: a randomized trial at the National Cancer Institute. J Clin Oncol 1992; 10(6): 976–83.

9. Sarrazin D, Le M, Rouesse J et al. Conservative treatment versus mastectomy in breast cancer tumors with macroscopic diameter of 20 millimeters or less. The experience of the Institut Gustave-Roussy. Cancer 1984; 53(5): 1209–13.

10. van Dongen JA, Bartelink H, Fentiman IS et al. Randomized clinical trial to assess the value of breast-conserving therapy in stage I and II breast cancer, EORTC 10801 trial. J Natl Cancer Inst Monogr 1992; (11): 15–18.

11. Veronesi U, Saccozzi R, del Vecchio M et al. Comparing radical mastectomy with quadrantectomy, axillary dissection, and radiotherapy in patients with small cancers of the breast. N Engl J Med 1981; 305(1): 6–11.

12. van Dongen JA, Voogd AC, Fentiman IS et al. Long-term results of a randomized trial comparing breast-conserving therapy with mastectomy: European Organization for Research and Treatment of Cancer 10801 trial. J Natl Cancer Inst 2000; 92(14): 1143–50.

13. Veronesi U, Cascinelli N, Mariani L et al. Twenty-year follow-up of a randomized study comparing breast-conserving surgery with radical mastectomy for early breast cancer. N Engl J Med 2002; 347(16): 1227–32.

14. Arriagada R, Le MG, Guinebretiere JM et al. Late local recurrences in a randomised trial comparing conservative treatment with total mastectomy in early breast cancer patients. Ann Oncol 2003; 14(11): 1617–22.

15. Poggi MM, Danforth DN, Sciuto LC et al. Eighteen-year results in the treatment of early breast carcinoma with mastectomy versus breast conservation therapy: the National Cancer Institute Randomized Trial. Cancer 2003; 98(4): 697–702.

16. NIH. NIH consensus conference. Treatment of early-stage breast cancer. JAMA 1991; 265(3): 391–5.

17. Holland R, Veling SH, Mravunac M, Hendriks JH. Histologic multifocality of Tis, T1–2 breast carcinomas. Implications for clinical trials of breast-conserving surgery. Cancer 1985; 56(5): 979–90.

18. Borger J, Kemperman H, Hart A et al. Risk factors in breast-conservation therapy. J Clin Oncol 1994; 12(4): 653–60.

19. Burke MF, Allison R, Tripcony L. Conservative therapy of breast cancer in Queensland. Int J Radiat Oncol Biol Phys 1995; 31(2): 295–303.

20. Dewar JA, Arriagada R, Benhamou S et al. Local relapse and contralateral tumor rates in patients with breast cancer treated with conservative surgery and radiotherapy (Institut Gustave Roussy 1970–1982). IGR Breast Cancer Group. Cancer 1995; 76(11): 2260–5.

21. Fourquet A, Campana F, Zafrani B et al. Prognostic factors of breast recurrence in the conservative management of early breast cancer: a 25-year follow-up. Int J Radiat Oncol Biol Phys 1989; 17(4): 719–25.

22. Gage I, Schnitt SJ, Nixon AJ et al. Pathologic margin involvement and the risk of recurrence in patients treated with breast-conserving therapy. Cancer 1996; 78(9): 1921–8.

23. Heimann R, Powers C, Halpem HJ et al. Breast preservation in stage I and II carcinoma of the breast. The University of Chicago experience. Cancer 1996; 78(8): 1722–30.

24. Mansfield CM, Komarnicky LT, Schwartz GF et al. Ten-year results in 1070 patients with stages I and II breast cancer treated by conservative surgery and radiation therapy. Cancer 1995; 75(9): 2328–36.

25. Park CC, Mitsumori M, Nixon A et al. Outcome at 8 years after breast-conserving surgery and radiation therapy for invasive breast cancer: influence of margin status and systemic therapy on local recurrence. J Clin Oncol 2000; 18(8): 1668–75.

26. Schnitt SJ, Abner A, Gelman R et al. The relationship between microscopic margins of resection and the risk of local recurrence in patients with breast cancer treated with breast-conserving surgery and radiation therapy. Cancer 1994; 74(6): 1746–51.

27. Spivack B, Khanna MM, Tafra L, Juillard G, Giuliano AE. Margin status and local recurrence after breast-conserving surgery. Arch Surg 1994; 129(9): 952–6.

28. Locker AP, Ellis IO, Morgan DA et al. Factors influencing local recurrence after excision and radiotherapy for primary breast cancer. Br J Surg 1989; 76(9): 890–4.

29. Veronesi U, Marubini E, del Vecchio M et al. Local recurrences and distant metastases after conservative breast cancer treatments: partly independent events. J Natl Cancer Inst 1995; 87(1): 19–27.

30. Veronesi U, Volterrani F, Luini A et al. Quadrantectomy versus lumpectomy for small size breast cancer. Eur J Cancer 1990; 26(6): 671–3.

31. Fisher ER, Anderson S, Redmond C, Fisher B. Ipsilateral breast tumor recurrence and survival following lumpectomy and irradiation: pathological findings from NSABP protocol B-06. Semin Surg Oncol 1992; 8(3): 161–6.

32. Clarke DH, Le MG, Sarrazin D et al. Analysis of local–regional relapses in patients with early breast cancers treated by excision and radiotherapy: experience of the Institut Gustave-Roussy. Int J Radiat Oncol Biol Phys 1985; 11(1): 137–45.

33. Kurtz JM, Jacquemier J, Torhorst J et al. Conservation therapy for breast cancers other than infiltrating ductal carcinoma. Cancer 1989; 63(8): 1630–5.

34. Mate TP, Carter D, Fischer DB et al. A clinical and histopathologic analysis of the results of conservation surgery and radiation therapy in stage I and II breast carcinoma. Cancer 1986; 58(9): 1995–2002.

35. du Toit RS, Locker AP, Ellis IO et al. Invasive lobular carcinomas of the breast – the prognosis of histopathological subtypes. Br J Cancer 1989; 60(4): 605–9.

36. Weiss MC, Fowble BL, Solin LJ, Yeh IT, Schultz DJ. Outcome of conservative therapy for invasive breast cancer by histologic subtype. Int J Radiat Oncol Biol Phys 1992; 23(5): 941–7.

37. Schnitt SJ, Connolly JL, Recht A, Silver B, Harris JR. Influence of infiltrating lobular histology on local tumor control in breast cancer patients treated with conservative surgery and radiotherapy. Cancer 1989; 64(2): 448–54.

38. Sastre-Garau X, Jouve M, Asselain B et al. Infiltrating lobular carcinoma of the breast. Clinicopathologic analysis of 975 cases with reference to data on conservative therapy and metastatic patterns. Cancer 1996; 77(1): 113–20.

39. Fisher B, Anderson S. Conservative surgery for the management of invasive and noninvasive carcinoma of the breast: NSABP trials. National Surgical Adjuvant Breast and Bowel Project. World J Surg 1994; 18(1): 63–9.

40. Elkhuizen PH, Voogd AC, van den Broek LC et al. Risk factors for local recurrence after breast-conserving therapy for invasive carcinomas: a case-control study of histological factors and alterations in oncogene expression. Int J Radiat Oncol Biol Phys 1999; 45(1): 73–83.

41. Elkhuizen PH, van de Vijver MJ, Hermans J et al. Local recurrence after breast-conserving therapy for invasive breast cancer: high incidence in young patients and association with poor survival. Int J Radiat Oncol Biol Phys 1998; 40(4): 859–67.

42. Fowble B, Gray R, Gilchrist K et al. Identification of a subgroup of patients with breast cancer and histologically positive axillary nodes receiving adjuvant chemotherapy who may benefit from postoperative radiotherapy. J Clin Oncol 1988; 6(7): 1107–17.

43. Recht A, Gray R, Davidson NE et al. Locoregional failure 10 years after mastectomy and adjuvant chemotherapy with or without tamoxifen without irradiation: experience of the Eastern Cooperative Oncology Group. J Clin Oncol 1999; 17(6): 1689–700.

44. Vicini FA, Recht A, Abner A et al. Recurrence in the breast following conservative surgery and radiation therapy for early-stage breast cancer. J Natl Cancer Inst Monogr 1992; (11): 33–9.

45. Boyages J, Recht A, Connolly JL et al. Early breast cancer: predictors of breast recurrence for patients treated with conservative surgery and radiation therapy. Radiother Oncol 1990; 19(1): 29–41.

46. Bartelink H, Borger JH, van Dongen JA, Peterse JL. The impact of tumor size and histology on local control after breast-conserving therapy. Radiother Oncol 1988; 11(4): 297–303.

47. Jacquemier J, Kurtz JM, Amalric R et al. An assessment of extensive intraductal component as a risk factor for local recurrence after breast-conserving therapy. Br J Cancer 1990; 61(6): 873–6.

48. Lindley R, Bulman A, Parsons P et al. Histologic features predictive of an increased risk of early local recurrence after treatment of breast cancer by local tumor excision and radical radiotherapy. Surgery 1989; 105(1): 13–20.

49. Delouche G, Bachelot F, Premont M, Kurtz JM. Conservation treatment of early breast cancer: long term results and complications. Int J Radiat Oncol Biol Phys 1987; 13(1): 29–34.

50. Spitalier JM, Gambarelli J, Brandone H et al. Breast-conserving surgery with radiation therapy for operable mammary carcinoma: a 25-year experience. World J Surg 1986; 10(6): 1014–20.

51. Fisher ER, Costantino J, Fisher B et al. Pathologic findings from the National Surgical Adjuvant Breast Project (NSABP) Protocol B-17. Intraductal carcinoma (ductal carcinoma in situ). The National Surgical Adjuvant Breast and Bowel Project Collaborating Investigators. Cancer 1995; 75(6): 1310–19.

52. Fisher ER, Dignam J, Tan-Chiu E et al. Pathologic findings from the National Surgical Adjuvant Breast Project (NSABP) eight-year update of Protocol B-17: intraductal carcinoma. Cancer 1999; 86(3): 429–38.

53. Vargas C, Kestin L, Go N et al. Factors associated with local recurrence and cause-specific survival in patients with ductal carcinoma in situ of the breast treated with breast-conserving therapy or mastectomy. Int J Radiat Oncol Biol Phys 2005; 63(5): 1514–21.

54. Silverstein MJ, Lagios MD, Groshen S et al. The influence of margin width on local control of ductal carcinoma in situ of the breast. N Engl J Med 1999; 340(19): 1455–61.

55. Cutuli B, Cohen-Solal-le Nir C, de Lafontan B et al. Breast-conserving therapy for ductal carcinoma in situ of the breast: the French Cancer Centers' experience. Int J Radiat Oncol Biol Phys 2002; 53(4): 868–79.

56. Elkhuizen PH, van Slooten HJ, Clahsen PC et al. High local recurrence risk after breast-conserving therapy in node-negative premenopausal breast cancer patients is greatly reduced by one course of perioperative chemotherapy. A European Organization for Research and Treatment of Cancer Breast Cancer Cooperative Group Study. J Clin Oncol 2000; 18(5): 1075–83.

57. Veronesi U, Salvadori B, Luini A et al. Breast conservation is a safe method in patients with small cancer of the breast. Long-term results of three randomised trials on 1,973 patients. Eur J Cancer 1995; 31A(10): 1574–9.

58. de la Rochefordiere A, Asselain B, Campana F et al. Age as prognostic factor in premenopausal breast carcinoma. Lancet 1993; 341(8852): 1039–43.

59. Voogd AC, Peterse JL, Crommelin MA et al. Histological determinants for different types of local recurrence after breast-conserving therapy of invasive breast cancer. Dutch Study Group on local Recurrence after Breast Conservation (BORST). Eur J Cancer 1999; 35(13): 1828–37.

60. Fowble BL, Schultz DJ, Overmoyer B et al. The influence of young age on outcome in early stage breast cancer. Int J Radiat Oncol Biol Phys 1994; 30(1): 23–33.

61. Kurtz JM, Spitalier JM, Amalric R et al. Mammary recurrences in women younger than forty. Int J Radiat Oncol Biol Phys 1988; 15(2): 271–6.

62. Pierce LJ, Strawderman MH, Douglas KR, Lichter AS. Conservative surgery and radiotherapy for early-stage breast cancer using a lung density correction: the University of Michigan experience. Int J Radiat Oncol Biol Phys 1997; 39(4): 921–8.

63. Matthews RH, McNeese MD, Montague ED, Oswald MJ. Prognostic implications of age in breast cancer patients treated with tumorectomy and irradiation or with mastectomy. Int J Radiat Oncol Biol Phys 1988; 14(4): 659–63.

64. Haffty BG, Fischer D, Rose M, Beinfield M, McKhann C. Prognostic factors for local recurrence in the conservatively treated breast cancer patient: a cautious interpretation of the data. J Clin Oncol 1991; 9(6): 997–1003.

65. Bartelink H, Horiot JC, Poortmans PM et al. Impact of a higher radiation dose on local control and survival in breast-conserving therapy of early breast cancer: 10-Year results of the Randomized Boost Versus No Boost EORTC 22881–10882 Trial. J Clin Oncol 2007 (in press).

66. Fisher ER, Anderson S, Tan-Chiu E et al. Fifteen-year prognostic discriminants for invasive breast carcinoma: National Surgical Adjuvant Breast and Bowel Project Protocol-06. Cancer 2001; 91(Suppl 8): 1679–87.

67. Kini VR, Vicini FA, Frazier R et al. Mammographic, pathologic, and treatment-related factors associated with local recurrence in patients with early-stage breast cancer treated with breast conserving therapy. Int J Radiat Oncol Biol Phys 1999; 43(2): 341–6.

68. Kurtz JM, Jacquemier J, Amalric R et al. Why are local recurrences after breast-conserving therapy more frequent in younger patients? J Clin Oncol 1990; 8(4): 591–8.

69. Brekelmans CT, Voogd AC, Botke G et al. Family history of breast cancer and local recurrence after breast-conserving therapy. The Dutch Study Group on Local Recurrence after Breast Conservation (BORST). Eur J Cancer 1999; 35(4): 620–6.

70. Haffty BG, Yang Q, Reiss M et al. Locoregional relapse and distant metastasis in conservatively managed triple negative early-stage breast cancer. J Clin Oncol 2006; 24(36): 5652–7.

71. Harrold EV, Turner BC, Matloff ET et al. Local recurrence in the conservatively treated breast cancer patient: a correlation with age and family history. Cancer J Sci Am 1998; 4(5): 302–7.

72. Jobsen JJ, Meerwaldt JH, van der Palen J. Family history in breast cancer is not a prognostic factor? Breast 2000; 9(2): 83–7.

73. Pierce LJ, Strawderman M, Narod SA et al. Effect of radiotherapy after breast-conserving treatment in women with breast cancer and germline BRCA1/2 mutations. J Clin Oncol 2000; 18(19): 3360–9.

74. Leopold KA, Recht A, Schnitt SJ et al. Results of conservative surgery and radiation therapy for multiple synchronous cancers of one breast. Int J Radiat Oncol Biol Phys 1989; 16(1): 11–16.

75. Ramachandra S, Machin L, Ashley S, Monaghan P, Gusterson BA. Immunohistochemical distribution of c-erbB-2 in in situ breast carcinoma – a detailed morphological analysis. J Pathol 1990; 161(1): 7–14.

76. van de Vijver MJ, Peterse JL, Mooi WJ et al. Neu-protein overexpression in breast cancer. Association with comedo-type ductal carcinoma in situ and limited prognostic value in stage II breast cancer. N Engl J Med 1988; 319(19): 1239–45.

77. Lowe SW, Bodis S, McClatchey A et al. p53 status and the efficacy of cancer therapy in vivo. Science 1994; 266(5186): 807–10.

78. O'Connor PM, Jackman J, Jondle D et al. Role of the p53 tumor suppressor gene in cell cycle arrest and radiosensitivity of Burkitt's lymphoma cell lines. Cancer Res 1993; 53(20): 4776–80.

79. Kreike B, Halfwerk H, Kristel P et al. Gene expression profiles of primary breast carcinomas from patients at high risk for local recurrence after breast-conserving therapy. Clin Cancer Res 2006; 12(19): 5705–12.

80. Nuyten DS, Kreike B, Hart AA et al. Predicting a local recurrence after breast-conserving therapy by gene expression profiling. Breast Cancer Res 2006; 8(5): R62.

81. Clarke M, Collins R, Darby S et al. Effects of radiotherapy and of differences in the extent of surgery for early breast cancer on local recurrence and 15-year survival: an overview of the randomised trials. Lancet 2005; 366(9503): 2087–106.

82. Forrest AP, Stewart HJ, Everington D et al. Randomised controlled trial of conservation therapy for breast cancer: 6-year analysis of the Scottish trial. Scottish Cancer Trials Breast Group. Lancet 1996; 348(9029): 708–13.

83. Pierquin B, Baillet F, Wilson JF. Radiation therapy in the management of primary breast cancer. AJR Am J Roentgenol 1976; 127(4): 645–8.

84. Arriagada R, Mouriesse H, Sarrazin D, Clark RM, Deboer G. Radiotherapy alone in breast cancer. I. Analysis of tumor parameters, tumor dose and local control: the experience of the Gustave-Roussy

Institute and the Princess Margaret Hospital. Int J Radiat Oncol Biol Phys 1985; 11(10): 1751–7.

85. Taylor ME, Perez CA, Halverson KJ et al. Factors influencing cosmetic results after conservation therapy for breast cancer. Int J Radiat Oncol Biol Phys 1995; 31(4): 753–64.

86. Kurtz JM, Amalric R, Brandone H, Ayme Y, Spitalier JM. How important is adequate radiotherapy for the long-term results of breast-conserving treatment? Radiother Oncol 1991; 20(2): 84–90.

87. Huang J, Barbera L, Brouwers M, Browman G, Mackillop WJ. Does delay in starting treatment affect the outcomes of radiotherapy? A systematic review. J Clin Oncol 2003; 21(3): 555–63.

88. Slotman BJ, Meyer OW, Njo KH, Karim AB. Importance of timing of radiotherapy in breast conserving treatment for early stage breast cancer. Radiother Oncol 1994; 30(3): 206–12.

89. Nixon AJ, Recht A, Neuberg D et al. The relation between the surgery–radiotherapy interval and treatment outcome in patients treated with breast-conserving surgery and radiation therapy without systemic therapy. Int J Radiat Oncol Biol Phys 1994; 30(1): 17–21.

90. Chauvet B, Reynaud-Bougnoux A, Calais G et al. Prognostic significance of breast relapse after conservative treatment in node-negative early breast cancer. Int J Radiat Oncol Biol Phys 1990; 19(5): 1125–30.

91. Mansfield CM, Komarnicky LT, Schwartz GF et al. Perioperative implantation of iridium-192 as the boost technique for stage I and II breast cancer: results of a 10-year study of 655 patients. Radiology 1994; 192(1): 33–6.

92. Perez CA, Taylor ME, Halverson K et al. Brachytherapy or electron beam boost in conservation therapy of carcinoma of the breast: a nonrandomized comparison. Int J Radiat Oncol Biol Phys 1996; 34(5): 995–1007.

93. Poortmans P, Bartelink H, Horiot JC et al. The influence of the boost technique on local control in breast conserving treatment in the EORTC 'boost versus no boost' randomised trial. Radiother Oncol 2004; 72(1): 25–33.

94. Galinsky DL, Sharma M, Hartsell WF, Griem KL, Murthy A. Primary radiation therapy to T1 and T2 breast cancer following conservative surgery. Which patients should be boosted? Am J Clin Oncol 1994; 17(1): 60–3.

95. Poortmans P, Collette L, Horiot JC et al. Impact of the boost dose on local control and survival in patients with early stage breast cancer after a microscopicaly incomplete lumpectomy: 10 years results of the randomised EORTC boost trial 22881/10882. Radiother Oncol 2006; 81 (Suppl 1): 19 [abstract].

96. Andry G, Suciu S, Vico P et al. Locoregional recurrences after 649 modified radical mastectomies: incidence and significance. Eur J Surg Oncol 1989; 15(6): 476–85.

97. Fentiman IS, Matthews PN, Davison OW, Millis RR, Hayward JL. Survival following local skin recurrence after mastectomy. Br J Surg 1985; 72(1): 14–16.

98. Fisher B, Anderson S, Fisher ER et al. Significance of ipsilateral breast tumour recurrence after lumpectomy. Lancet 1991; 338(8763): 327–31.

99. Haffty BG, Reiss M, Beinfield M et al. Ipsilateral breast tumor recurrence as a predictor of distant disease: implications for systemic therapy at the time of local relapse. J Clin Oncol 1996; 14(1): 52–7.

100. Whelan T, Clark R, Roberts R, Levine M, Foster G. Ipsilateral breast tumor recurrence postlumpectomy is predictive of subsequent mortality: results from a randomized trial. Investigators of the Ontario Clinical Oncology Group. Int J Radiat Oncol Biol Phys 1994; 30(1): 11–16.

101. Abner AL, Recht A, Eberlein T et al. Prognosis following salvage mastectomy for recurrence in the breast after conservative surgery and radiation therapy for early-stage breast cancer. J Clin Oncol 1993; 11(1): 44–8.

102. Fowble B, Solin LJ, Schultz DJ, Rubenstein J, Goodman RL. Breast recurrence following conservative surgery and radiation: patterns of failure, prognosis, and pathologic findings from mastectomy specimens with implications for treatment. Int J Radiat Oncol Biol Phys 1990; 19(4): 833–42.

103. Haffty BG, Fischer D, Beinfield M, McKhann C. Prognosis following local recurrence in the conservatively treated breast cancer patient. Int J Radiat Oncol Biol Phys 1991; 21(2): 293–8.

104. Kurtz JM, Amalric R, Brandone H et al. Local recurrence after breast-conserving surgery and radiotherapy. Frequency, time course, and prognosis. Cancer 1989; 63(10): 1912–17.

105. Kurtz JM, Spitalier JM, Amalric R et al. The prognostic significance of late local recurrence after breast-conserving therapy. Int J Radiat Oncol Biol Phys 1990; 18(1): 87–93.

106. Meijer-van Gelder ME, Look MP, Bolt-de Vries J et al. Breast-conserving therapy: proteases as risk factors in relation to survival after local relapse. J Clin Oncol 1999; 17(5): 1449–57.

107. Recht A, Schnitt SJ, Connolly JL et al. Prognosis following local or regional recurrence after conservative surgery and radiotherapy for early stage breast carcinoma. Int J Radiat Oncol Biol Phys 1989; 16(1): 3–9.

108. Voogd AC, van Tienhoven G, Peterse HL et al. Local recurrence after breast conservation therapy for early stage breast carcinoma: detection, treatment, and outcome in 266 patients. Dutch Study Group on Local Recurrence after Breast Conservation (BORST). Cancer 1999; 85(2): 437–46.

109. Fisher B, Dignam J, Mamounas EP et al. Sequential methotrexate and fluorouracil for the treatment of node-negative breast cancer patients with estrogen receptor-negative tumors: eight-year results from National Surgical Adjuvant Breast and Bowel Project

(NSABP) B-13 and first report of findings from NSABP B-19 comparing methotrexate and fluorouracil with conventional cyclophosphamide, methotrexate, and fluorouracil. J Clin Oncol 1996; 14(7): 1982–92.

110. Haffty BG, Wilmarth L, Wilson L et al. Adjuvant systemic chemotherapy and hormonal therapy. Effect on local recurrence in the conservatively treated breast cancer patient. Cancer 1994; 73(10): 2543–8.

111. Rose MA, Henderson IC, Gelman R et al. Premenopausal breast cancer patients treated with conservative surgery, radiotherapy and adjuvant chemotherapy have a low risk of local failure. Int J Radiat Oncol Biol Phys 1989; 17(4): 711–17.

112. Fisher B, Costantino J, Redmond C et al. A randomized clinical trial evaluating tamoxifen in the treatment of patients with node-negative breast cancer who have estrogen-receptor-positive tumors. N Engl J Med 1989; 320(8): 479–84.

113. Dalberg K, Johansson H, Johansson U, Rutqvist LE. A randomized trial of long term adjuvant tamoxifen plus postoperative radiation therapy versus radiation therapy alone for patients with early stage breast carcinoma treated with breast-conserving surgery. Stockholm Breast Cancer Study Group. Cancer 1998; 82(11): 2204–11.

114. Lingos TI, Recht A, Vicini F et al. Radiation pneumonitis in breast cancer patients treated with conservative surgery and radiation therapy. Int J Radiat Oncol Biol Phys 1991; 21(2): 355–60.

115. Markiewicz DA, Schultz DJ, Haas JA et al. The effects of sequence and type of chemotherapy and radiation therapy on cosmesis and complications after breast conservation therapy. Int J Radiat Oncol Biol Phys 1996; 35(4): 661–8.

116. Buchholz TA, Austin-Seymour MM, Moe RE et al. Effect of delay in radiation in the combined modality treatment of breast cancer. Int J Radiat Oncol Biol Phys 1993; 26(1): 23–35.

117. Hartsell WF, Recine DC, Griem KL, Murthy AK. Delaying the initiation of intact breast irradiation for patients with lymph node positive breast cancer increases the risk of local recurrence. Cancer 1995; 76(12): 2497–503.

118. Recht A, Come SE, Gelman RS et al. Integration of conservative surgery, radiotherapy, and chemotherapy for the treatment of early-stage, node-positive breast cancer: sequencing, timing, and outcome. J Clin Oncol 1991; 9(9): 1662–7.

119. Recht A, Come SE, Henderson IC et al. The sequencing of chemotherapy and radiation therapy after conservative surgery for early-stage breast cancer. N Engl J Med 1996; 334(21): 1356–61.

120. Bellon JR, Come SE, Gelman RS et al. Sequencing of chemotherapy and radiation therapy in early-stage breast cancer: updated results of a prospective randomized trial. J Clin Oncol 2005; 23(9): 1934–40.

121. Bear HD, Anderson S, Smith RE et al. Sequential preoperative or postoperative docetaxel added to preoperative doxorubicin plus cyclophosphamide for operable breast cancer: National Surgical Adjuvant Breast and Bowel Project Protocol B-27. J Clin Oncol 2006; 24(13): 2019–27.

122. Mieog JS, van der Hage JA, van de Velde CJ. Preoperative chemotherapy for women with operable breast cancer. Cochrane Database Syst Rev 2007; (2): CD005002.

123. Broet P, Scholl SM, de la Rochefordiere A et al. Short and long-term effects on survival in breast cancer patients treated by primary chemotherapy: an updated analysis of a randomized trial. Breast Cancer Res Treat 1999; 58(2): 151–6.

124. Mauriac L, MacGrogan G, Avril A et al. Neoadjuvant chemotherapy for operable breast carcinoma larger than 3 cm: a unicentre randomized trial with a 124-month median follow-up. Institut Bergonie Bordeaux Groupe Sein (IBBGS). Ann Oncol 1999; 10(1): 47–52.

125. Wolmark N, Wang J, Mamounas E, Bryant J, Fisher B. Preoperative chemotherapy in patients with operable breast cancer: nine-year results from National Surgical Adjuvant Breast and Bowel Project B-18. J Natl Cancer Inst Monogr 2001; (30): 96–102.

126. van der Hage JA, van de Velde CJ, Julien JP et al. Preoperative chemotherapy in primary operable breast cancer: results from the European Organization for Research and Treatment of Cancer trial 10902. J Clin Oncol 2001; 19(22): 4224–37.

127. Gazet JC, Ford HT, Gray R et al. Estrogen-receptor-directed neoadjuvant therapy for breast cancer: results of a randomised trial using formestane and methotrexate, mitozantrone and mitomycin C (MMM) chemotherapy. Ann Oncol 2001; 12(5): 685–91.

128. Scholl SM, Fourquet A, Asselain B et al. Neoadjuvant versus adjuvant chemotherapy in premenopausal patients with tumours considered too large for breast conserving surgery: preliminary results of a randomised trial: S6. Eur J Cancer 1994; 30A(5): 645–52.

129. Chen AM, Meric-Bernstam F, Hunt KK et al. Breast conservation after neoadjuvant chemotherapy. Cancer 2005; 103(4): 689–95.

130. Huang EH, Strom EA, Perkins GH et al. Comparison of risk of local–regional recurrence after mastectomy or breast conservation therapy for patients treated with neoadjuvant chemotherapy and radiation stratified according to a prognostic index score. Int J Radiat Oncol Biol Phys 2006; 66(2): 352–7.

The role of cell–cell and cell–stromal interactions in predicting breast cancer behavior

5

Deborah L Holliday and J Louise Jones

INTRODUCTION

There is a growing understanding of the importance of interactions between cells, and between cells and the surrounding stromal environment. Information may be transmitted to cells through chemokine and cytokine signaling, growth factor receptor binding or adhesive interactions. The integration of such signals controls tissue architecture, cellular differentiation and tissue-specific gene expression. In fact, it has been suggested that through such mechanisms, the microenvironment plays the dominant role in controlling tissue function, and restoration of appropriate interactions with the surrounding environment may revert features of the malignant phenotype even though genetic abnormalities persist.

Given the importance of these interactions in modulating cell behavior, it is not surprising that disruption of these normal signals can influence how tumors behave. Breast carcinomas frequently exhibit altered cell adhesion molecule expression, which influences how the tumor cells communicate with each other and with the surrounding matrix. Furthermore, there are changes in the composition of the environment, with altered matrix protein expression, changes in cellular components of the microenvironment, and extensive remodelling of the stroma. Such alterations have the capacity to generate novel signals between tumor cells and the environment, and this is likely to profoundly influence how tumors behave.

This chapter will focus on key changes in cell adhesion molecules and stromal components which have been shown to modulate breast cancer cell function, the potential for such features to act as predictive factors for breast cancer behavior, and the growing opportunity to use such alterations as therapeutic targets.

CELL ADHESION MOLECULES IN BREAST CANCER

Cell–cell adhesion

Epithelial cells mediate intercellular adhesion primarily through adherens junctions, desmosomes, and gap junctions. The molecules involved in these adhesive complexes – classical cadherins, desmosomal glycoproteins and connexins, respectively – have all been shown to exhibit altered expression in breast cancers.

The classical cadherins include E-cadherin, P-cadherin and N-cadherin, and of these the major focus in breast cancer has been E-cadherin. E-cadherin mediates homophilic Ca^{++}-dependent adhesion and, via interactions with cytoplasmic catenins and the actin cytoskeleton, it plays an important role in maintaining epithelial morphogenesis.[1] There is compelling evidence to indicate that E-cadherin acts as a tumor suppressor: in vitro studies have indicated an invasion-suppressor role for E-cadherin,[2,3] whilst loss of heterozygosity (LOH) at this site is frequently detected in breast carcinomas,[4] and hypermethylation of the E-cadherin promoter region, with reduced expression of the protein, is also common in breast cancer.[5,6] Numerous studies have examined the relationship between downregulated E-cadherin and breast cancer behavior. In infiltrating ductal carcinoma (IDC), reduced membrane E-cadherin has been associated with high tumor grade[7-9] and the presence of lymph node metastases,[9,10] though other studies show no relationship with conventional prognostic indices.[11,12] However, a recent meta-analysis confirmed interstudy heterogeneity, but an analysis of 10 retrospective studies found that reduced or absent E-cadherin significantly increased the risk of all-cause mortality, whilst a nonspecific association was identified for breast cancer-specific mortality.[13] In addition to reflecting differences in study design, the contradictory findings regarding the prognostic value of E-cadherin also likely reflects the complexity of its role in breast cancer spread. Thus, it has been suggested that downregulation of E-cadherin may be a transient event, with reexpression at a distant site;[14] and enhanced E-cadherin expression in nodal metastasis has been shown to be an independent marker of improved survival, whilst no such relationship was shown with E-cadherin levels in the primary tumor.[15]

In contrast to the tumor-suppressor function of E-cadherin, expression of P-cadherin in invasive breast carcinomas is consistently associated with features of more aggressive tumors, including high tumor grade and estrogen receptor negativity,[16,17] the presence of lymph node metastasis,[18] and reduced disease-free and overall survival.[17] Recent gene expression array studies cluster P-cadherin expression with the basal subtype of breast cancer,[19] which is also associated with poor patient outcome.[20] Furthermore, P-cadherin expression is strongly associated with BRCA-1-mutated breast carcinomas, and has been shown to be a predictor of poor prognosis, particularly in small node-negative tumors.[21] Expression of P-cadherin appears to be controlled primarily through methylation;[17,22] whilst the function of P-cadherin is poorly understood, one study demonstrated a pro-invasive effect of this cell adhesion molecule.[23]

Altered expression of other members of the cadherin family has also been reported in breast cancer, though little is known of their functional and prognostic impact. N-cadherin has been detected in up to 30% of invasive breast cancers,[24] and has been shown to promote tumor cell invasion[25] and enhance tumor metastasis in animal models.[26] However, limited studies to date suggest expression in primary breast carcinoma does not relate to tumor prognosis.[24]

Desmosomes are another major adhesive complex in epithelial cells, of which the desmosomal glycoprotein families of desmocollins (DSc) and desmogleins (DSg) are key components.[27,28] DSc and DSg exhibit a tissue-specific pattern of expression; in the breast DSc1 and -2 and DSg 1 and -2 proteins are expressed by all epithelial cells, whilst DSc3 and DSg3 are restricted to myoepithelial cells in the normal breast.[29] In the normal breast, desmosomal proteins mediate cell adhesion, induce polarity of mammary epithelium[29] and inhibit cell motility.[30] Despite a central role in maintaining tissue structure, little is understood about changes in desmosomes in cancer. Downregulation of DSc3 has been described as a common event in breast cancer,[31,32] which is frequently associated with promoter methylation.[32] Other desmosomal components are also downregulated in tumor compared to normal tissues, including desmoplakin and desmoglein 2,[33] though the functional importance of such changes remains to be established.

The connexin family of gap junction proteins are involved in regulation of cell growth, cell differentiation and tissue development, and they are widely regarded as having a tumor-suppressor role.[34,35] Connexin 26 (Cx26) and Cx43 are expressed in normal breast epithelium, and both reduced and enhanced levels of expression in breast carcinomas have been reported.[36,37] Experimental systems have indicated a dominant role for these proteins in control of breast differentiation, with overexpression of Cx26 and/or Cx43 leading to the reversion of the malignant phenotype through regulation of epithelial–mesenchymal transition and angiogenesis.[38] Once again, despite powerful experimental

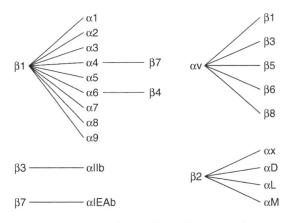

Figure 5.1 Integrin heterodiners. Each integrin comprises an α and β subchain which combine to form 23 integrins. Note that α4 combines with both β1 and β7, and α6 combines with β1 and β4.

evidence, the predictive value of assessing connexin expression in primary breast cancer has not been fully evaluated. It may not be as straightforward as anticipated, since there are suggestions that the functional impact of connexin expression may be context dependant, and there may be instances where they contribute to, rather than suppress, breast cancer progression.[39]

Cell–matrix adhesion

The integrin family of cell adhesion molecules is the major mediator of cellular interaction with the extracellular matrix. Integrins are cell surface receptors composed of noncovalently linked α and β subunits,[40] and at least 22 heterodimer receptors are now recognized (Figure 5.1). Cell–matrix interactions mediate many of the processes implicated in tumorigenesis, including proliferation, differentiation, migration and invasion,[41] thus, changes in expression on breast carcinoma cells may be expected to have an important impact on tumor cell behavior.

The integrin receptor profile for normal breast epithelium includes α2β1, α3β1, α6β1 and α6β4, with low level expression of α5β1 and αvβ3.[42,43] Strong expression of many of these receptors is localized, particularly within

the myoepithelial compartment, and α6β4 is largely confined to the junction with the basement membrane, consistent with its incorporation into hemidesmosomes. Evidence for the role of integrins in modulating tumor cell behavior comes both from in vitro functional studies, and tissue studies, though there are some discrepancies between these approaches. Thus, in three-dimensional culture models of breast cancer, blocking β1 integrin leads to increased apoptosis and decreased proliferation,[44] and induction of normal breast morphogenesis,[45] suggesting that β1 integrin promotes tumorigenesis. However, in apparent contradiction to this, a number of tissue studies report that reduced levels of β1 integrin are associated with higher tumor grade and with axillary lymph node metastases.[43,45–47] The simplest explanation for this discrepancy is that tissue studies do not measure levels of activated integrin, which is likely to be important. In support of this, activated (but not nonactivated) αvβ3 integrin has been implicated in promoting tumor metastasis.[48] However, a recent tissue study has found that high level β1 integrin staining on breast carcinomas is an independent predictor of disease-free and overall survival.[49] Whilst this appears more in keeping with the in vitro findings, it is difficult to reconcile with earlier studies, though it is notable that the latter study is the largest of all those reported, which is probably a result of successful antigen retrieval techniques allowing application to routinely fixed archival tissues. The possibility that β1 integrin could be targeted for therapy[49–51] means that further large-scale studies to determine the prognostic role of β1 integrin are imperative.

Another integrin heterodimer which plays a complex role in breast cancer is α6β4 integrin. In the normal breast, α6β4 is largely confined to the cell–basement membrane interface where it is incorporated into hemidesmosomes. Reduced or absent α6β4 has been a consistent finding in many studies of primary breast cancer,[46,48,52] though when detected it has been associated with poor patient prognosis in some series[53] but not in others.[54] Methodological differences between these studies may explain the discrepant findings. And both studies have limitations: the former is on a small sample cohort; the latter depends on in situ hybridization, which may not reflect the level of protein expression. Thus, the true prognostic significance of α6β4 in breast cancer is not fully established, though molecular subtyping using gene expression arrays has identified α6β4 integrin as one of the genes associated with the basal subtype of breast cancer,[19] and it may well contribute to the aggressive nature characteristic of this tumor group.[20] Certainly, experimental data indicate a role for α6β4 integrin in promoting tumor cell growth and invasion,[55–57] mediated at least in part through its collaboration with other signalling molecules such as c-met[58] and c-erbB2.[59] However, other data suggest an antitumor effect of α6β4 integrin: Weaver et al[60] found that upregulation of α6β4 in breast cancer cells reversed some features of the malignant phenotype and promoted glandular morphogenesis. Furthermore, upregulation of α6β4 has been shown to restore contact inhibition of growth[61] and reduce breast cancer cell invasion.[62] These apparent contradictions perhaps result from the different functions of α6β4 depending on its cytoskeletal attachments, as it mediates anchorage through intermediate filament-associated hemidesmosomes but migration in actin-associated adhesive structures.[63,64] Furthermore, the effect of α6β4 signalling may be dependent on coexpression of other molecules such as c-met. Such relationships require further investigation in primary tissues in order to fully understand the prognostic significance of α6β4 integrin.

The integrin αvβ6 is of interest in that it is epithelial specific; it is expressed weakly or is absent on normal adult epithelia, but is increased in injured or inflamed epithelium.[65,66] Importantly, high expression of αvβ6 integrin has been detected on many cancers[67] and correlates with reduced survival from colon cancer.[68] Work in our group has shown that upregulation of αvβ6 integrin is significantly associated with high tumor grade, though not lymph node status, but is an independent predictor of poor patient outcome (unpublished data). Since αvβ6 is rarely expressed in normal tissue, and has been shown to promote tumor cell invasion, it presents a plausible target for therapeutic attack.

STROMAL CHANGES IN BREAST CANCER

It has long been recognized that the stroma associated with breast carcinomas differs from normal;[69] however, it is only in the last decade that the critical role of the microenvironment in determining tumor behavior has been acknowledged. Indeed, a number of in vivo model studies suggest that stromal alterations alone can lead to induction of mammary carcinoma.[70,71] There are many components to the stromal microenvironment, each of which can contribute to the modulation of tumor behavior. Key features include cellular components, such as fibroblasts and inflammatory cells, and the extracellular matrix proteins. The tumor-associated vasculature clearly has an important influence on tumor behavior but is not covered here since this is a topic in its own right.

Cellular changes in the breast cancer microenvironment

One of the main cellular components of the stroma is the fibroblast population, which undergoes activation in the tumor environment to form myofibroblasts[72] which have a pleiotropic effect on tumor cells and the environment. Differences in the pattern of gene and protein expression have been identified between peri-tumoral and normal fibroblasts,[73,74] and a number of these gene families are implicated in promotion of tumor growth and invasion. For example, it has recently been shown that tumor-associated fibroblasts (TAFs) secrete high levels of the chemokine stromal cell-derived factor-1 (SDF-1), which binds to the CXCR4 receptor on breast cancer cells, promotes tumor growth and invasion,[75] and is critical for metastatic spread of breast cancer cells to bone and lung.[76] In keeping with this experimental data, it has been shown that elevated SDF-1 levels in human breast carcinomas correlate with the presence of lymph node metastases, and with reduced disease-free and overall survival.[77]

Fibroblasts are also the major source of extracellular matrix proteins and matrix-degrading proteolytic enzymes, both of which have important functions in tumor progression, and are discussed further below. However, as the contribution of TAFs to breast cancer progression becomes more widely accepted, attention has focused on determining the precise nature of these cells and how their altered function is generated. The changes in gene expression exhibited by TAFs are thought to arise largely as a response to tumor-derived signals; however, there is growing evidence to indicate that the peri-tumoral stromal population may undergo independent genetic and epigenetic modifications,[78–81] and such changes may influence the function of the stromal population and contribute to their tumor-promoter role. It has also been suggested that independently acquired genetic alterations in the stromal population may influence the diversity in clinical outcome observed in breast cancer.[78] This has recently been illustrated in an analysis of p53 mutations in tumor-associated stroma, whereby somatic p53 mutations in the stroma (but not in the epithelium) of breast cancer were associated with regional lymph node metastases,[82] and in the absence of p53 mutations, loss of heterozygosity and allelic imbalance at other loci in the stroma associated with metastases. This is one of the first studies to provide definitive evidence of the importance of stromal changes in breast cancer.

Changes in the extracellular matrix in breast cancer

The extracellular matrix (ECM) provides a scaffold for epithelial cells in tissues; through direct adhesive interactions, or via cross-talk with classical signalling cascades, the ECM has a central role in controlling epithelial cell growth, differentiation and migration.[83–85]

Basement membrane (BM) represents a specialized form of the ECM laid down at epithelial–stromal junctions and around blood vessels. In addition to a modulatory role, ECM and BM act as important physical barriers to invasion by tumor cells. It is clear then that changes in the composition and integrity of the ECM may profoundly influence tumor behavior.

The ECM around breast cancer differs from normal breast.[86] Fibronectin expression is increased in the stroma of many breast cancers, and changes in the isoform profile have been described with upregulation of protein containing the so-called ED-A and ED-B domains.[87,88] Whilst many in vitro studies indicate a role for fibronectin, particularly in promoting breast cancer cell motility or growth,[89,90] few tissue studies have established the prognostic value of enhanced fibronectin expression. Yao et al[49] recently demonstrated that high fibronectin expression was associated with reduced disease-free and overall survival in univariate, but not multivariate, analysis. This finding was in agreement with an earlier immunohistochemical study,[91] though this conclusion has not been universal.[92] Interestingly, most studies do not distinguish between the different fibronectin isoforms, which is likely to have an important influence on the results. A distinct form of truncated fibronectin, termed migration-stimulating factor (MSF), has been characterized; as the name implies, MSF stimulates cell migration but expression is confined to fetal and tumor tissues.[93] However, the prognostic significance of this isoform has not yet been established.

Another ECM protein shown to be consistently upregulated in breast cancer is Tenascin-C (TN-C). TN-C is a multifunctional protein which can influence cell behavior directly through interactions with cell surface receptors, and indirectly through binding to other matrix proteins such as fibronectin, and altering their interaction with cells.[94] High expression of TN-C has been related to the presence of lymph node metastases,[91] local and distant recurrence,[95] and reduced survival;[91] expression of TN-C in DCIS has been suggested to predict progression to invasion.[96] However, as with many of the ECM proteins, diversity is generated through expression of alternatively spliced isoforms, which introduces functionally relevant domains into the mature protein.[97] Several studies have indicated a switch towards larger molecular weight isoforms in tumor tissues compared to normal.[98–100] Work in our laboratory has detected very specific changes in TN-C isoform profile in breast cancers, with induction of two isoforms not usually found in normal breast tissue: one containing exon 16 (TN-C16) and one containing exons 14 plus 16 (TN-C14/16).[101] Whilst these isoforms appear to specifically promote breast cancer growth and invasion (unpublished data), their prognostic value is not yet established, partly due to lack of good reagents to these splice variants. A further member of the Tenascin family is TN-W, which has recently been shown to be upregulated in breast cancers though is undetectable in normal breast tissue.[102] Interestingly, TN-W appears to be particularly upregulated in low-grade breast cancers, and has been suggested to be an early marker of activated tumor stroma.[102] Extending the work on Tenascin members and their isoforms is likely to prove valuable since tumor-specific TN-C isoforms are already being successfully targeted in other malignancies.[103]

Further emphasizing the importance of tumor-specific splice variants, a recent report has shown that a switch in laminin isoform profile, from β2-containing to β1-containing laminins, occurs during progression of breast cancer.[104] These novel laminin isoforms are deposited in newly formed tumor blood vessels and again represent a potential therapeutic target.

From this discussion it is very apparent that the changes in ECM in tumors are complex. A recent study used gene expression microarray analysis to determine the patterns of ECM changes in breast cancer.[105] They showed that breast cancers could be classified according to their profile of ECM expression, and that this had clinical significance with tumors exhibiting overexpression of protease inhibitors

having a favorable outcome, whilst those with high expression of integrin and metallopeptidases having a poor prognosis.[105]

Matrix remodeling in breast cancer

In addition to changes in the extracellular matrix composition, the matrix is also altered through remodeling. This is generated through the action of proteolytic enzymes, of which there are many but those most commonly implicated in cancer include the matrix metalloproteinases (MMPs), the urokinase plasminogen activator system and the A disintegrin and metalloproteinases (ADAMs). Each of these protein families has been shown through, in vivo and in vitro model systems, to play a role in cancer progression, and parallel tissue studies are starting to identify their potential prognostic value. A large body of literature surrounds the MMP family and accordingly this discussion will focus on the role of the MMPs in breast cancer.

Matrix metalloproteinases

The human MMP family comprises 24 members which between them can degrade virtually all components of the extracellular matrix.[106–108] They are zinc-binding endopeptidases which share a number of functional domains including: (i) a signal peptide required for secretion; (ii) a propeptide domain which interacts with the zinc-binding site and maintains the enzyme in an inactive form; (iii) a catalytic domain which contains the zinc-binding site with the exception of the matrilysins; and (iv) a hemopexin/vitronectin-like domain connected to the catalytic domain via a hinge. Traditionally, MMPs have been classified according to their substrate specificity but with the growing complexity of the family, and their overlapping activity, they are increasingly classified on a structural basis (see Figure 5.2).

One of the defining characteristics of MMPs is the tight regulation of their activity. They are under the control of a variety of naturally occurring inhibitors including the

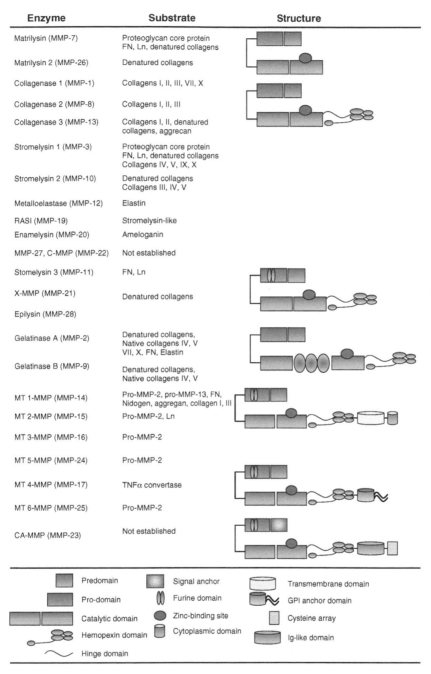

Enzyme	Substrate	Structure
Matrilysin (MMP-7)	Proteoglycan core protein FN, Ln, denatured collagens	
Matrilysin 2 (MMP-26)	Denatured collagens	
Collagenase 1 (MMP-1)	Collagens I, II, III, VII, X	
Collagenase 2 (MMP-8)	Collagens I, II, III	
Collagenase 3 (MMP-13)	Collagens I, II, denatured collagens, aggrecan	
Stromelysin 1 (MMP-3)	Proteoglycan core protein FN, Ln, denatured collagens Collagens IV, V, IX, X	
Stromelysin 2 (MMP-10)	Denatured collagens Collagens III, IV, V	
Metalloelastase (MMP-12)	Elastin	
RASI (MMP-19)	Stromelysin-like	
Enamelysin (MMP-20)	Ameloganin	
MMP-27, C-MMP (MMP-22)	Not established	
Stomelysin 3 (MMP-11)	FN, Ln	
X-MMP (MMP-21)	Denatured collagens	
Epilysin (MMP-28)		
Gelatinase A (MMP-2)	Denatured collagens, Native collagens IV, V VII, X, FN, Elastin	
Gelatinase B (MMP-9)	Denatured collagens, Native collagens IV, V	
MT 1-MMP (MMP-14)	Pro-MMP-2, pro-MMP-13, FN, Nidogen, aggrecan, collagen I, III	
MT 2-MMP (MMP-15)	Pro-MMP-2, Ln	
MT 3-MMP (MMP-16)	Pro-MMP-2	
MT 5-MMP (MMP-24)	Pro-MMP-2	
MT 4-MMP (MMP-17)	TNFα convertase	
MT 6-MMP (MMP-25)	Pro-MMP-2	
CA-MMP (MMP-23)	Not established	

Legend:
- Predomain
- Pro-domain
- Catalytic domain
- Hemopexin domain
- Hinge domain
- Signal anchor
- Furine domain
- Zinc-binding site
- Cytoplasmic domain
- Transmembrane domain
- GPI anchor domain
- Cysteine array
- Ig-like domain

Figure 5.2 Classification and structure of matrix metalloproteinases (MMPs). MMPs may be classified according to substrate specificity (collagenases, stromelysins, gelatinases) or according to structural similarity. The simplest MMP is the Matrilysin subgroup, comprising a signal prepeptide domain, a propeptide that maintains the enzyme in the inactive form, and the catalytic domain with the zinc-binding site. The collagenases, stromelysins, metalloelastase, enamelysin, MMP-19 and MMP-27 contain an additional hemopexin domain, which provides substrate specificity. The gelatinases also contain a series of fibronectin type II units, whilst stromelysin-3, epilysin and MMP-21 have a furin-like cleavage site which allows intracellular activation. The membrane type (MT)-MMPs form a distinct group and are linked to the cell membrane either via a transmembrane domain or with a glycosylophosphatidyl-inositol (GPI) anchor. CA-MMP contains a unique cystein array and immunoglobulin-like domain in the C-terminal, with an N-terminal signal anchor targeting it to the cell membrane. (Adapted from Chabottaux and Noel.[108])

tissue inhibitors of metalloproteinases (TIMPs) of which there are four,[109–112] as well as the plasma inhibitor α2-macroglobulin[113] and the so-called reversion-inducing cysteine-rich protein with Kazal motifs (RECK).[114] The majority of MMPs are secreted as inactive precursors or may be secreted in their active form following cleavage of the propeptide intracellularly by furin-like convertases.[115] A distinct group of MMPs are membrane associated, either via a transmembrane domain (MT1-, MT2-, MT3- and MT5-MMP), a glycosylphosphatidyl-inositol (GPI) anchor (MT4- and MT6-MMP) or an N-terminal signal anchor (SA) targeting it to the membrane (CA-MMP).[116]

In addition to their classical role in matrix degradation, MMPs are becoming recognized for a much broader range of activities. Thus, MMPs can control cell proliferation through release of matrix-bound growth factors, or activation of latent growth factors, such as MMP-3 release of insulin-like growth factor[117] or MMP-7 activation of heparin-binding epidermal growth factor (EGF)-like growth factor.[118] Both MMP-1 and MMP-3 have been shown to break down perlecan leading to the release of basic fibroblast growth factor (FGF), which is a potent mitogen for endothelial cells.[119] A number of other MMPs are involved in angiogenesis, including the gelatinases[120] or some of the MT-MMPs which can activate vascular endothelial growth factor (VEGF)[121] or directly enhance vascular tubulogenesis.[122] In contrast to the pro-angiogenic role of most MMPs, MMP-19 appears to be a negative regulator of tumor angiogenesis.[123] Many of the MMPs are also involved in mediating tumor cell invasion. The MT-MMPs have been implicated in directly breaching basement membrane barriers through the assembly of invasive pseudopodia.[124] MMP-3 and MMP-7 have been shown to enhance tumor invasion through cleavage of E-cadherin and induction of the epithelial–mesenchymal transition (EMT).[125,126] Having such multifaceted roles in the processes relevant to tumor progression, the relationship between MMP expression and prognosis has been much studied in breast cancer, and despite the complexity some clear patterns are beginning to emerge.

A number of studies have demonstrated a relationship between elevated gelatinase levels and unfavorable prognosis in breast cancer. Iwata et al[127] reported significantly higher levels of MMP-2 in lymph node-positive breast cancers compared to lymph node-negative ones, and elevated MMP-2 and MMP-9 relative to their inhibitors TIMP-2 and TIMP-1 have been associated with lymph node positivity and reduced survival.[128,129] In a separate study, MMP-2 positivity in breast cancer was identified as an independent predictor of reduced disease-free and overall survival,[130] and has also been shown to predict poor response to antiestrogen therapy.[131] The prognostic value of MMP-9 is less consistent, with some studies reporting a positive association with more aggressive disease,[132] others no association[133,134] and even an inverse relationship with outcome; Scorilas et al[135] found overexpression of MMP-9 to be an independent predictor of improved survival in node-negative patients. In contrast, two recent studies have shown MMP-9 to be related to reduced survival[136] and to act as an independent predictor of poor prognosis.[137]

The MT-MMPs are emerging as key enzymes in promoting breast cancer progression.[124,138] Several studies have demonstrated a relationship between MT1-MMP and the presence of lymph node and/or distant metastases:[133,139,140] and elevated MT1-MMP mRNA in breast carcinomas has been shown to predict significantly reduced survival even when adjusted for factors such as tumor size and lymph node status.[141] No such correlation has been shown with MT2-MMP, and MT3-MMP has not been detected in breast tissue.[139] Whereas MT4-MMP was identified in breast cancer cells, the role of this and MT5-MMP in breast cancer is not yet established,[142] and MT6-MMP appears to be expressed predominantly by leukocytes.[143]

Increased expression of MMP-1 has been associated with lymph node metastases[144] and poor prognosis[145] in breast cancer, and was also one of the genes in the 70-gene expression signature identified by Van't Veer et al[146] to predict distant metastases in lymph node-negative patients. MMP-1 is also implicated in mediating lung metastases in a mouse model of breast cancer.[147] And, interestingly, elevated mRNA levels have been identified as a marker for predicting the development of invasive carcinoma from atypical ductal hyperplasia.[148]

Stromelysin 3 (MMP-11) was initially cloned as a gene differentially expressed in malignant compared to benign breast tissue[149] and has been shown to be expressed exclusively by peri-tumoral fibroblasts.[150–152] Expression levels of MMP-11, either by in-situ hybridization (ISH) or by immunohistochemistry (IHC), are associated with the presence of lymph node metastases,[153] and both recurrence-free and overall survival;[153–156] and in node-positive patients, elevated MMP-11 provides a strong independent prognostic parameter for disease-free survival.[156]

Collagenase 3 (MMP-13) was also first identified in breast carcinomas and has been localized predominantly to stromal cells of invasive carcinomas.[157,158] In a recent study, including a series of ductal carcinoma in situ (DCIS) cases, MMP-13 was identified in the peri-ductal stroma of 7 of 8 cases exhibiting microinvasion, but not in 9 cases without microinvasion.[159] Although further studies are required to confirm this, it has been proposed that MMP-13 may play a pivotal role in the transition of DCIS to invasive disease, and may serve as a useful prognostic marker.

Finally, over recent years the impact of functional single nucleotide polymorphisms (SNPs) on modifying disease behavior has become evident. SNPs in the promoter region of several MMP genes influence levels of gene expression.[160–163] A study in our laboratory has shown that the 2G/2G genotype of MMP-1, which generates an increased level of gene expression, was more frequent in the lymph node-positive patients and conferred a 3.9-fold increased risk of lymph node metastasis, whilst the C/T genotype of MMP-9 was found to confer a 3.6-fold increased occurrence of lymph node metastasis.[164] Przybylowska et al[165] reported a similar association between the MMP-1 2G/2G genotype and lymph node metastasis – in patients with breast cancer they showed no such association with the MMP-9 T allele. Such studies underline the biological role of MMPs in breast cancer and these genetic variations may help explain some of the individual variation observed in breast cancer behavior.

CONCLUSIONS

There is considerable experimental evidence which indicates the importance of cell–cell and cell–stromal interactions in modulating tumor cell behavior, and some of these systems suggest that microenvironmental cues may have a dominant role in determining epithelial cell function. Given the profound impact of these interactions in model systems, it is perhaps somewhat surprising that many of the molecules involved such as cadherins, integrins, proteolytic enzymes and matrix proteins, do not have unequivocal prognostic value. This almost certainly relates, at least in part, to issues surrounding activity status and receptor functionality which are not easily resolved in tissue-based studies. However, despite these limitations, some consistent and interesting data are emerging. For example, the relationship between P-cadherin and the BRCA-1 phenotype, the interactions of α6β4 with signaling molecules frequently expressed in breast cancers, and the association of the αvβ6 integrin with aggressive tumor behavior, all contribute prognostic information, and also open therapeutic opportunities. Similarly, the identification of tumor-specific isoforms of extracellular matrix proteins is an exciting development, and whilst their prognostic value is not yet fully established they again may be exploited for therapy. Members of the MMP family continue to show prognostic value and functional relevance in breast cancer progression.

Finally, one of the most fascinating stories emerging is the concept that tumor-associated stroma may itself exhibit significant genetic abnormality: this challenges the widely held view of a 'reactive' stroma and really does suggest that the stroma is an intrinsic part of the tumor and could be just as important in predicting tumor behavior as the tumor cells themselves.

REFERENCES

1. Takeichi M. Morphogenetic role of classic cadherins. Curr Opin Cell Biol 1995; 7: 619–27.
2. Frixen UH, Behrens J, Sachs M et al. E-cadherin mediated cell–cell adhesion prevents invasiveness of human carcinoma cells. J Cell Biol 1991; 113: 173–85.
3. Vleminckx K, Vakaet L, Mareel M, Fiers W, Vanroy F. Genetic manipulation of E-cadherin expression by epithelial tumour cells reveal an invasion suppressor role. Cell 1991; 66: 107–19.
4. Chalmers J, Aubele M, Hartman E, Braungart E, Werner M. Mapping the chromosome 16 cadherin gene cluster to a minimal detected region in ductal breast cancer. Cancer Genet Cytogenet 2001; 126: 39–44.
5. Nass SJ, Herman JG, Gabrielson E et al. Aberrant methylation of the oestrogen receptor and E-cadherin 5′ CpG islands increases with malignant progression in breast cancer. Cancer Res 2000; 60: 4346–8.
6. Caldeira JRF, Prando EC, Quevedo FC et al. CDH1 promoter hypermethylation and E-cadherin protein expression in infiltrating breast cancer. BMC Cancer 2006; 6: 48–56.
7. Moll R, Mitze M, Frixen UH, Birchmeier W. Differential loss of E-cadherin expression in infiltrating ductal and lobular carcinomas. Am J Pathol 1993; 143: 1731–42.
8. Gonzalez HA, Pinder SE, Wencyk PM et al. An immunohistochemical examination of the expression of E-cadherin, alpha- and beta/gamma-catenins and alpha 2 and beta 1 integrins in invasive breast cancer. J Pathol 1999; 187: 523–9.
9. Oka H, Shiozaki H, Kobayashi K et al. Expression of E-cadherin cell adhesion molecule in human breast cancer tissues and its relationship to metastasis. Cancer Res 1993; 83(7): 1696–701.
10. Jones JL, Royall JE, Walker RA. E-cadherin relates to EGFR expression and lymph node metastasis in primary breast carcinomas. Br J Cancer 1996; 74: 1237–41.
11. Lipponen P, Saarelainen E, Ji H, Aaltomea S, Syrjanen K. Expression of E-cadherin as related to other prognostic factors and survival in breast cancer. J Pathol 1994; 174: 101–9.
12. Quereshi HS, Linden MD, Divine G, Raju UB. E-cadherin status in breast cancer correlates with histologic type but does not correlate with established prognostic parameters. Am J Clin Pathol 2006; 125: 377–85.
13. Gould Rothberg BE, Bracken MB. E-cadherin immunohistochemical expression as a prognostic factor in infiltrating ductal carcinoma of the breast: a systematic review and meta-analysis. Breast Cancer Res Treat 2006; 5: 139–48.
14. Kowalski PJ, Rubin MA, Kleer CG. E-cadherin expression in primary carcinomas of the breast and its distant metastases. Breast Cancer Res 2003; 5: R217–R222.
15. Harigopal M, Berger AJ, Camp RL, Rimm DL, Kluger HM. Automated quantitative analysis of E-cadherin expression in lymph node metastases is predictive of survival in invasive ductal breast cancer. Clin Cancer Res 2005; 11: 4083–89.
16. Palacios J, Benito N, Pizarro A et al. Anomalous expression of P-cadherin in breast carcinomas: correlation with E-cadherin and pathological features. Am J Pathol 1995; 146: 605–12.
17. Paredes J, Albergaria A, Oliveira JT et al. P-cadherin overexpression is an indictator of clinical outcome in invasive breast carcinomas and is associated with CDH3 promoter hypermethylation. Clin Cancer Res 2005; 11: 5869–77.
18. Gamallo C, Moreno-Bueno G, Sarrio D et al. The prognostic significance of P-cadherin in infiltrating breast carcinoma. Mod Pathol 2001; 14: 650–4.
19. Perou CM, Sorlie T, Eisen MB et al. Molecular portraits of human breast tumours. Nature 2000; 406: 747–52.
20. Sorlie T, Perou CM, Tibshirani R et al. Gene expression patterns of breast carcinomas distinguish tumour subclasses with clinical implications. Proc Natl Acad Sci USA 2001; 98: 10,869–74.
21. Arnes JB, Brunet JS, Stefansson I et al. Placemental cadherin and the basal epithelial phenotype of BRCA-1 related breast cancer. Clin Cancer Res 2005; 11: 4003–11.
22. Jarrard DF, Paul R, van Bokhoven A et al. P-cadherin is a basal cell specific epithelial marker that is not expressed in prostate cancer. Clin Cancer Res 1997; 3: 2121–8.
23. Paredes J, Stove C, Stove V et al. P-cadherin is upregulated by the anti-oestrogen ICI182, 780 and promotes invasion of human breast cancer cells. Cancer Res 2004; 64: 8309–17.
24. Kovacs A, Dhillon J, Walker RA. Expression of P-cadherin but not E-cadherin or N-cadherin relates to pathological and functional differentiation of breast carcinomas. Mol Pathol 2003; 56: 318–22.
25. Hazan RB, Phillips GR, Qiao RF, Norton L, Aaronson SA. Exogenous expression of N-cadherin in breast cancer cells induces cell migration, invasion and metastasis. J Cell Biol 2000; 148: 779–90.
26. Hulit J, Suvama K, Chung S et al. N-cadherin signalling potentiates mammary tumour metastasis via enhanced extracellular signal-regulated kinase activation. Cancer Res 2007; 67: 3106–16.
27. Koch PJ, Franke WW. Desmosomal cadherins: another growing multigene family of adhesion molecules. Curr Opin Cell Biol 1994; 6: 682–7.
28. Garrod DR, Merritt AJ, Nie Z. Desmosomal cadherins. Curr Opin Cell Biol 2002; 14: 537–45.

29. Runswick SK, O'Hare MJ, Jones JL, Streuli CH, Garrod DR. Desmosomal adhesion regulates epithelial morphogenesis and cell positioning. Nat Cell Biol 2001; 3: 823–30.

30. Tselepis C, Chidgey M, North A, Garrod DR. Desmosomal adhesion inhibits invasive behaviour. Proc Natl Acad Sci USA 1998; 95: 8064–9.

31. Klus GT, Rokaeus N, Bittner ML et al. Down-regulation of the desmosomal cadherin desmocollin 3 in human breast cancer. Int J Oncol 2001; 19: 169–74.

32. Oshiro MM, Kim KJ, Wozniack RJ et al. Epigenetic silencing of DSC3 is a common event in human breast cancer. Breast Cancer Res 2005; 7: R669–R680.

33. Davies EL, Gee JM, Cochrane RA et al. The immunohistochemical expression of desmoplakin and its role in vivo in the progression and metastasis of breast cancer. Eur J Cancer 1991; 35: 902–7.

34. Saez JC, Berthoud VM, Branes MC, Martinez AD, Beyer EC. Plasma membrane channels formed by connexins: their regulation and functions. Physiol Rev 2003; 83: 1359–400.

35. Hirschi KK, Xu CE, Tsukamoto T, Sager R. Gap junction genes CX26 and CX43 individually suppress the cancer phenotype of human mammary carcinoma cells and restore differentiation potential. Cell Growth Differ 1996; 7: 861–70.

36. Kanczuga-Koda L, Sulkowski S, Lenczewski A et al. Increased expression of connexins 26 and 43 in lymph node metastases of breast cancer. J Clin Pathol 2006; 59: 429–33.

37. Jamieson S, Going JJ, D'Arcy R, George WD. Expression of gap junction proteins connexin 26 and connexin 43 in normal human breast and in breast tumours. J Pathol 1998; 184: 37–43.

38. McLachlan E, Shao Q, Wang HL, Langlois S, Laird DW. Connexins act as tumour suppressors in three-dimensional mammary cell organoids by regulating differentiation and angiogenesis. Cancer Res 2006; 66: 9886–94.

39. McLachlan E, Shao Q, Laird DW. Connexins and gap junctions in mammary gland development and breast cancer progression. J Membr Biol 2007; 218: 107–21.

40. Hynes RO. Integrins – a family of cell surface receptors. Cell 1987; 48: 549–54.

41. Roskelley CD, Srebrow A, Bissell MJ. A hierarchy of ECM-mediated signalling regulates tissue-specific gene expression. Curr Opin Cell Biol 1995; 7: 736–47.

42. Koukoulis GK, Virtanen I, Korhonen M et al. Immunohistochemical localisation of integrins in the normal, hyperplastic and neoplastic breast – correlations with their functions as receptors and cell adhesion molecules. Am J Pathol 1991; 139: 787–99.

43. Jones JL, Critchley DR, Walker RA. Alterations of stromal protein and integrin expression in breast – a marker of premalignant change. J Pathol 1992; 167: 399–406.

44. Park CC, Zhang H, Pallavicini M et al. β1 integrin inhibiting antibody induces apoptosis of breast cancer cells, inhibits growth, and distinguishes malignant from normal phenotype in three dimensional cultures and in vivo. Cancer Res 2006; 66: 1526–35.

45. Pignatelli M, Hanby AM, Stamp GWH. Low expression of beta 1, alpha 2 and alpha 3 subunits of VLA integrins in malignant mammary tumours. J Pathol 1991; 165: 25–32.

46. Zutter MM, Mazou Jian G, Santoro SA. Decreased expression of integrin adhesive protein receptors in adenocarcinoma of the breast. Am J Pathol 1990; 137: 863–70.

47. Gui GP, Wells CA, Browne PD et al. Integrin expression in primary breast cancer and its relation to axillary node status. Surgery 1995; 117: 102–8.

48. Felding-Habermann B, O'Toole TE, Smith JW et al. Integrin activation controls metastasis in human breast cancer. Proc Natl Acad Sci USA 2001; 98: 1853–8.

49. Yao ES, Zhang H, Chen Y-Y et al. Increased β1-integrin is associated with decreased survival in invasive breast cancer. Cancer Res 2007; 67: 659–64.

50. Shannon KE, Keene JL, Settle SL et al. Anti-metastatic properties of RGD-peptidomimetic agents 5137–5247. Clin Exp Metastasis 2004; 21: 129–38.

51. Stoeltzing O, Liu W, Reinmuth N et al. Inhibition of integrin α5β1 function with a small peptide (ATN-161) plus continuous 5-FU infusion reduces colorectal liver metastases and improves survival in mice. Int J Cancer 2003; 104: 496–503.

52. Natali PG, Nicotra MR, Botti C et al. Changes in expression of alpha 6 beta 4 integrin heterodimer in primary and metastatic breast cancer. Br J Cancer 1992; 66: 318–22.

53. Tagliabue E, Ghirelli C, Squicciarini P et al. Prognostic value of alpha6beta4 integrin expression is affected by laminin production from tumour cells. Cancer Res 1998; 4: 407–10.

54. Diaz LK, Cristofanilli M, Zhou X et al. β4 integrin subunit gene expression correlates with tumour size and nuclear grade in early breast cancer. Mod Pathol 2005; 18: 1165–75.

55. Rabinovitz I, Mercurio AM. The integrin alpha 6 beta 4 functions in carcinoma cell migration on laminin-1 by mediating the formation and stabilization of actin-containing motility structures. Mol Biol Cell 1997; 8: 1533.

56. Shaw LM, Rabinovitz I, Wang HH et al. Activation of phosphoinositide 3-OH kinase by the alpha6beta4 integrin promoted carcinoma invasion. Cell 1997; 91: 949–60.

57. Chung J, Bachelder RE, Lipscomb EA et al. Integrin alpha6beta4 regulation of eIF-4E activity and VEGF translation: a survival mechanism for carcinoma cells. J Cell Biol 2002; 158: 165–74.

58. Bertollti A, Comoglio PM, Trussolino L. Beta 4 integrin is a transforming molecule that unleashes Met tyrosine kinase tumourigenesis. Cancer Res 2005; 65: 10,674–9.

59. Guo W, Pylayeva Y, Pepe A et al. Beta 4 integrin amplifies erbB2 signalling to promote mammary tumourigenesis. Cell 2006; 126: 489–502.

60. Weaver VM, Petersen OW, Wang F et al. Reversion of the malignant phenotype of human breast cells in three-dimensional culture and in-vivo by integrin blocking antibodies. J Cell Biol 1997; 137: 231–45.

61. Sun H, Santoro SA, Zutter MM. Downstream events in mammary gland morphogenesis mediated by re-expression of the alpha(2)beta(1) integrin: the role of the alpha(6) and beta(4) integrin subunits. Cancer Res 1998; 58: 2224–33.

62. Jones LJ, Royall JE, Critchley DR, Walker RA. Modulation of the myoepithelial associated alpha 6 beta 4 integrin in a breast cancer cell line alters invasive potential. Exp Cell Res 1997; 235: 325–33.

63. Carter WG, Kaur P, Gil SG, Gahr PJ, Wayner EA. Distinct functions for integrins alpha-3-beta-1 in focal adhesions and alpha-6-beta-4 and bullous pemphigoid antigen in a new stable anchoring contact (sac) of keratinocytes – relation to hemidesmosomes. J Cell Biol 1990; 111: 3141–54.

64. Rabinovitz I, Toker A, Mercurio AM. Protein kinase C dependent mobilization of the alpha6beta4 integrin from hemidesmosomes and its association with actin-rich cell protrusions drive the chemotactic migration of carcinoma cells. J Cell Biol 1999; 146: 1147–60.

65. Breuss JM, Gillett N, Lu L, Sheppard D, Pytela R. Restricted distribution of integrin beta-6 messenger RNA in primate epithelial tissues J Histochem Cytochem 1993; 41: 1521–7.

66. Breuss JM, Gallo J, DeLisser HM et al. Expression of the β6 integrin subunit in development, neoplasia and tissue repair suggests a role in epithelial remodelling. J Cell Sci 1995; 108: 2241–51.

67. Thomas GJ, Nystrom ML, Marshall JF. αvβ6 integrin in wound healing and cancer of the oral cavity. J Oral Pathol Med 2006; 35: 1–10.

68. Bates RC, Bellovin DI, Brown C et al. Transcriptional activation of integrin β6 during the epithelial–mesenchymal transition defines a novel prognostic indicator of aggressive colon carcinoma. J Clin Invest 2005; 115: 339–47.

69. Jackson JG, Orr JW. The ducts of carcinomatous breasts with particular reference to connective tissue changes. J Pathol Bacteriol 1957; 74: 265–73.

70. Barcellos-Hoff MH, Ravani SA. Irradiated mammary gland stroma promotes the expression of tumourigenic potentially unirradiated epithelial cells. Cancer Res 2000; 60: 1254–60.

71. Kuperwasser C, Chavarria T, Wu M et al. Reconstruction of functionally normal and malignant human breast tissues in mice. Proc Natl Acad Sci USA 2004; 100: 4966–71.

72. Desmouliere A, Guyot C, Gabbiani G. The stroma reaction myofibroblast: a key player in the control of tumour cell behaviour. Int J Dev Biol 2004; 48: 509–17.

73. Chang HY, Sneddon JB, Alizadeh AA et al. Gene expression signature of fibroblast serum response predicts human cancer progression: similarities between tumours and wounds. PLoS Biology 2004; 2: 206–13.

74. Singer CF, Gschwantler-Kaulich D, Fink-Retter A et al. Differential gene expression profile in breast cancer derived stromal fibroblasts. Breast Cancer Res Treat 2007 (e-pub ahead of print).

75. Kang H, Watkins G, Parr C et al. Stromal cell derived factor-1: its influence of invasiveness and migration of breast cancer cells in vitro and its association with prognosis and survival in human breast cancer. Breast Cancer Res Treat 2005; 7: R402–R410.

76. Orimo A, Gupta PD, Sgroi DC et al. Stromal fibroblasts present in invasive human breast carcinomas promote tumour growth and angiogenesis through elevated SDF-1/CXCL12 secretion. Cell 2005; 121: 335–48.

77. Kato M, Kitayama J, Kazama S, Nagawa H. Expression pattern of CXC chemokine receptor-4 is correlated with lymph node metastasis in human invasive ductal carcinoma. Breast Cancer Res 2003; 5: R144–R150.

78. Moinfar F, Man YG, Arnould L et al. Concurrent and independent genetic alterations in the stromal and epithelial cells of mammary carcinoma: implications for tumorigenesis. Cancer Res 2000; 60: 2562–6.

79. Fukino K, Shen L, Matsumoto S et al. Combined total genome loss of heterozygosity scan of breast cancer stroma and epithelium reveals multiplicity of stromal targets. Cancer Res 2004; 64: 7231–6.

80. Hu M, Yao J, Cai L et al. Distinct epigenetic changes in the stromal cells of breast cancers. Nat Genet 2005; 37: 899–905.

81. Hanson JA, Gillespie JW, Grover A et al. Gene promoter methylation in prostate tumor-associated stromal cells. J Natl Cancer Inst 2006; 98: 255–61.

82. Patocs A, Zhang L, Xu Y et al. Breast cancer stromal cells with TP53 mutations and nodal metastases. New Eng J Med 2007; 357: 2543–51.

83. Howe A, Aplin AE, Alahari SK, Juliano RL. Integrin signaling and cell growth control. Curr Opin Cell Biol 1998; 10: 220–31.

84. Farrelly N, Lee Y-J, Oliver J, Dive C, Streuli CH. Extracellular matrix regulates apoptosis in mammary epithelium through a control on insulin signaling. J Cell Biol 1999; 144: 1337–48.

85. Lee Y-J, Streuli CH. Extracellular matrix selectively modulates the response of mammary epithelial cells to different soluble signaling ligands. J Cell Biol 1999; 274: 22401–8.

86. Ronnov-Jenson L, Petersen OW, Bissell MB. Cellular changes in the conversion of normal to malignant breast: the importance of the stromal reaction. Physiol Rev 1996; 76: 69–125.

87. Kaczmarek J, Castellani P, Nicolo G et al. Distribution of oncofetal fibronectin isforms in normal, hyperplastic and neoplastic human breast tissues. Int J Cancer 1994; 59: 11–16.

88. Castellani P, Viale G, Dorcaratto A et al. The fibronectin isoform containing the ED-B oncofetal domain: a marker of angiogenesis. Int J Cancer 1994; 59: 612–18.

89. Hu M, Carles-Kinch KL, Zelinski DP, Kinch MS. EphA2 induction of fibronectin creates a permissive microenvironment for malignant cells. Mol Cancer Res 2004; 2: 533–40.

90. Sisci D, Aquila S, Middea E et al. Fibronectin and type IV collagen activate ER alpha AF-1 by c-src pathway: effect on breast cancer cell motility. Oncogene 2004; 23: 8920–30.

91. Ioachim E, Charchanti A, Briasoulis E et al. Immunohistochemical expression of extracellular matrix components tenascin, fibronectin, collagen type IV and laminin in breast cancer: their prognostic value and role in tumour invasion and progression. Eur J Cancer 2002; 38: 2362–70.

92. Swiatoniowski G, Mathowski R, Suder E et al. E-cadherin and fibronectin expression have no prognostic role in stage II ductal breast cancer. Anticancer Res 2005; 25: 2879–83.

93. Schor SL, Ellis IR, Jones SJ et al. Migration-stimulating factor: a genetically truncated oncofetal fibronectin isoform expressed by carcinoma and tumour-associated stromal cells. Cancer Res 2003; 63: 8827–36.

94. Chiquet-Ehrismann R, Matsuoka Y, Hofer U et al. Tenascin variants: differential binding to fibronectin and distinct distribution in cell cultures and tissues. Cell Reg 1991; 2: 927–38.

95. Jahkola T, Toivonen T, Virtanen I et al. Tenascin-C expression in the invasive border of early breast cancer: a predicator of local and distant recurrence. Br J Cancer 1998; 78: 1507–13.

96. Jahkola T, Toivonen T, Virtanen I et al. Expression of tenascin-C in intraductal carcinoma of human breast: relationship to invasion. Eur J Cancer 1998; 34: 1687–92.

97. Jones PL, Jones FS. Tenascin-C in development and disease: gene regulation and cell function. Matrix Biol 2000; 19: 581–96.

98. Borsi L, Carnemolla B, Nicolo G et al. Expression of different tenascin isoforms in normal, hyperplastic and neoplastic human breast tissues. Int J Cancer 1992; 52: 688–92.

99. Hindermann W, Berndt A, Borsi L et al. Synthesis and protein distribution of the unspliced large tenascin-C isoform in oral squamous cell carcinoma. J Pathol 1999; 189: 475–80.

100. Dueck M, Riedl S, Hinz U et al. Detection of tenascin-C isoforms in colorectal mucosa, ulcerative colitis, carcinomas and liver metastases. Int J Cancer 1999; 82: 477–83.

101. Adams M, Jones JL, Walker RA et al. Changes in tenascin-C isoform expression in invasive and pre-invasive breast disease. Cancer Res 2002; 62: 3289–97.

102. Degen M, Brellier F, Kain R et al. Tenascin-W is a novel marker for activated tumor stroma in low-grade human breast cancer and influences cell behavior. Cancer Res 2007; 67: 9169–79.

103. Reardon DA, Zalutsky MR, Bigner DD. Anti-tenascin-C monoclonal antibody radioimmunotherapy for malignant glioma patients. Expert Rev Anticancer Ther 2007; 7: 675–87.

104. Fujita M, Khazenzon NM, Bose S et al. Overexpression of beta1-chain-containing laminins in capillary basement membranes of human breast cancer and its metastases. Breast Cancer Res 2005; 7: R411–R421.

105. Bergamaschi A, Tagliabue E, Sørlie T et al. Extracellular matrix signature identifies breast cancer subgroups with different clinical outcome. J Pathol 2008; 214: 357–67.

106. Page-McCaw A, Ewald AJ, Werb Z. Matrix metalloproteinases and the regulation of tissue remodelling. Nat Rev Mol Cell Biol 2007; 8: 221–3.

107. Cauwe B, Van den Steen PE, Opdenakker G. The biochemical, biological and pathological kaleidoscope of cell surface substrates processed by matrix metalloproteinses. Crit Rev Biochem Mol Biol 2007; 42: 113–85.

108. Chabottaux V, Noel A. Breast cancer progression: insights into multifaceted matrix metalloproteinases. Clin Exp Metastasis 2007; 24: 647–56.

109. Docherty AJP, Lyons A, Smith BJ et al. Sequence of human-tissue inhibitor of metalloproteinases and its identity to erythroid-potentiating activity. Nature 1985; 318: 66–9.

110. Stetler-Stevenson WG, Krutzsch HC, Liotta LA. Tissue inhibitor of metalloproteinase (TIMP-2) – a new member of the metalloproteinase inhibitor family. J Biol Chem 1989; 264: 17,374–8.

111. Apte SS, Hayashi K, Seldin MF et al. Gene encoding a novel murine tissue inhibitor of metalloproteinases (TIMP), TIMP-3, is expressed in developing mouse epithelia, cartilage and muscle, and is located on chromosome 10. Development Dyn 1994; 200: 177–97.

112. Greene J, Wang MS, Liu YLE et al. Molecular cloning and characterization of human tissue inhibitor of metalloproteinase 4. J Biol Chem 1996; 271: 30,375–80.

113. Visse R, Nagase H. Matrix metalloproteinases and tissue inhibitors of metalloproteinases: structure function and biochemistry. Circ Res 2003; 92: 827–39.

114. Oh J, Takahashi R, Kondo S et al. The membrane anchored MMP inhibitor RECK is a key regulator of extracellular matrix integrity and angiogenesis. Cell 2001; 107: 789–800.

115. Folgueras AR, Pendas AM, Sanchez LM, Lopez-Otin C. Matrix metalloproteinases in cancer: from new functions to improved inhibition strategies. Int J Dev Biol 2004; 48: 411–24.

116. Zucker S, Pei D, Cao J, Lopex-Otin C. Membrane type-matrix metalloproteinases (MT-MMP). Curr Top Dev Biol 2003; 54: 1–74.

117. Manes S, Mira E, Barnacid MD et al. Identification of insulin-like growth factor binding protein-1 as a

potential physiological substrate for stromelysin-3. J Biol Chem 1997; 272: 25,706–12.

118. Miyamato S, Nakamura M, Yano K et al. Matrix metalloproteinase-7 triggers the matricrine action of insulin-like growth factor-II via proteinase activity on insulin-like growth factor binding protein 2 in the extracellular matrix. Cancer Sci 2007; 98: 685–91.

119. Forough R, Weylie B, Collins C et al. Transcription factor Ets-1 regulates fibroblast growth factor-1-mediated angiogenesis in vivo: role of Ets-1 in the regulation of the PI3K/AKT/MMP-1 pathway. J Vasc Res 2006; 43: 327–37.

120. Masson V, de la Ballina LR, Munaut C et al. Contribution of host MMP-2 and MMP-9 to promote tumour vascularisation and invasion of malignant keratinocytes. FASEB J 2005; 18: 234–6.

121. Sounni NE, Devy L, Hajitou A et al. MT1-MMP expression promotes tumour growth and angiogenesis through up-regulation of vascular endothelial growth factor receptor expression. FASEB J 2002; 16: 555–64.

122. Lafleur MA, Handsley MM, Knauper V, Murphy G, Edwards DR. Endothelial tubulogenesis within fibrin gels specifically requires the activity of membrane type matrix metalloproteinases (MT-MMPs). J Cell Sci 2002; 115: 3427–8.

123. Jost M, Folgueras AR, Frerast F et al. Earlier onset of tumoural angiogenesis in matrix metalloproteinase-19 deficient mice. Cancer Res 2006; 66: 5234–41.

124. Hotary K, Li XY, Allen E, Stevens SL, Weiss SJ. A cancer cell metalloproteinase triad regulates the basement membrane transmigration program. Genes Dev 2006; 20: 2673–86.

125. Noe V, Fingleton B, Jacobs K et al. Release of an invasion-promoter E-cadherin fragment by matrilysin and stromelysin-1. J Cell Sci 2001; 114: 111–18.

126. Orlichenko LS, Radisky DC. Matrix metalloproteinases stimulate epithelial to mesenchymal transition during tumour development. Clin Exp Metastasis 2008 (e-pub ahead of print).

127. Iwata H, Kobayashi S, Iwase H et al. Production of matrix metalloproteinases and tissue inhibitors of metalloproteinases in human breast carcinomas. Jpn J Cancer Res 1996; 87: 602–11.

128. Onisto M, Riccio MP, Scannapieco P et al. Gelatinase A/TIMP-2 imbalance in lymph node positive breast carcinomas, as measured by RT-PCR. Int J Cancer 1995; 63: 621–6.

129. Jinga DC, Blidaru A, Condreas I et al. MMP-9 and MMP-2 gelatinases and TIMP-1 and TIMP-2 inhibitors in breast cancer: correlations with prognostic factors. J Cell Mol Med 2006; 10: 499–510.

130. Talvensaari-Mattila A, Paakko P, Hoyhtya M, Blanco-Sequeiros G, Turpeenniemi-Hujanen T. MMP-2 immunoreactive protein: a mark of aggressiveness in breast carcinoma. Cancer 1998; 183: 1153–62.

131. Talvensaari-Mattila A, Paakko P, Hoyhtya M, Blanco-Sequeiros G, Turpeenniemi-Hujanen T. Matrix metalloproteinase 2 (MMP-2) is associated with the risk for a relapse in postmenopausal patients with node-positive breast carcinoma treated with antiestrogen adjuvant therapy. Breast Cancer Res Treat 2001; 65: 55–61.

132. Davies B, Miles DW, Happerfield LC et al. Activity of type-IV collagenases in benign and malignant breast disease. Br J Cancer 1993; 67: 1126–31.

133. Jones JL, Glynn P, Walker RA. Expression of MMP-2 and MMP-9, their inhibitors and the activator MT1-MMP in primary breast carcinomas. J Pathol 1999; 189: 161–8.

134. Remacle AG, Noel A, Duggan C et al. Assay of matrix metalloproteinases types 1, 2, 3 and 9 in breast cancer. Br J Cancer 1998; 77: 926–31.

135. Scorilas A, Karameris A, Arnogiannaki N et al. Overexpression of matrix metalloproteinase 9 in human breast cancer: a potential favourable indicator in node negative patients. Br J Cancer 2001; 84: 1488–96.

136. Wu ZS, Wu Q, Yang JH et al. Prognostic significance of MMP-9 and TIMP-1 serum and tissue expression in breast cancer. Int J Cancer 2008; 122: 2050–6.

137. Mylona E, Nomikos A, Magkou C et al. The clinicopathological and prognostic significance of membrane type MMP and MMP-9 according to the localisation in invasive breast carcinoma. Histopathology 2007; 50: 338–47.

138. Wolf C, Wu YI, Liu Y et al. Multi-step pericellular proteolysis controls the transition from individual to collective cancer cell invasion. Nat Cell Biol 2007; 9: 893–904.

139. Ueno H, Nakamura H, Inoue M et al. Expression and tissue localisation of membrane types 1, 2, and 3 matrix metalloproteinases in human invasive breast carcinomas. Cancer Res 1997; 57: 3159–67.

140. Mimori K, Ueo H, Shirasaka C, Mori M. Clinical significance of MT1-MMP mRNA expression in breast cancer. Oncol Rep 2001; 8: 401–3.

141. Tetu B, Brisson J, Wang CS et al. The influence of MMP-14, TIMP-2 and MMP-2 expression on breast cancer prognosis. Breast Cancer Res 2006; 8: R28–R37.

142. Pei DQ. Identification and characterization of the fifth membrane-type matrix metalloproteinase MT5-MMP. J Biol Chem 1999; 274: 8925–32.

143. Pei D. Leukolysin/MMP-25/MT6-MMP: a novel matrix metalloproteinase specifically expressed in the leukocyte lineage. Cell Res 1999; 9: 291–303.

144. Nakopoulou L, Giannopoulou I, Gakiopoulou H et al. Matrix metalloproteinase-1 and -3 in breast cancer: correlation with progesterone receptors and other clinicopathologic features. Hum Pathol 1999; 30: 436–42.

145. Vizoso FJ, Gonzalez LO, Corte MD et al. Study of matrix metalloproteinases and their inhibitors in breast cancer. Br J Cancer 2007; 96: 903–11.

146. van't Veer LJ, Dai HY, van de Vijver MJ et al. Gene expression profiling predicts clinical outcome of breast cancer. Nature 2002; 415: 530–6.

147. Minn AJ, Gupta GP, Siegel PM et al. Genes that mediate breast cancer metastasis to lung. Nature 2005; 436: 518–24.

148. Poola I, DeWitty RL, Marshalleck JJ et al. Identification of MMP-1 as a putative breast cancer predictive marker by global gene expression analysis. Nat Med 2005; 11: 481–3.

149. Basset P, Bellocq JP, Wolf C et al. A novel metalloproteinase gene specifically expressed in stromal cells of breast carcinomas. Nature 1990; 348: 699–704.

150. Kossakowska AE, Huchcroft SA, Urbanski SJ, Edwards DR. Comparative analysis of the expression patterns of metalloproteinases and their inhibitors in breast neoplasia, sporadic colorectal neoplasia, pulmonary carcinomas and malignant non-Hodgkins lymphoma in humans. Br J Cancer 1996; 73: 1401–8.

151. Hahnel E, Harvey JM, Joyce R et al. Stromelysin-3 expression in breast cancer biopsies: clinicopathological correlations. Int J Cancer 1993; 55: 771–4.

152. Heppner KJ, Matrisian LM, Jensen RA, Rodgers WH. Expression of most matrix metalloproteinase family members in breast cancer represents a tumor-induced host response. Am J Pathol 1996; 149: 273–82.

153. Tetu B, Brisson J, Lapointe H, Bernard P. Prognostic significance of stromelysin 3, gelatinase A, and urokinase expression in breast cancer. Hum Pathology 1998; 29: 979–85.

154. Ahmed A, Marshall JF, Bassett P, Anglard P, Hart IR. Modulation of human stromelysin 3 promoter activity and gene expression by human breast cancer cells. Int J Cancer 1997; 73: 290–6.

155. Chenard MP, O'Siorain L, Shering S et al. High levels of stromelysin 3 correlate with poor prognosis in patients with breast carcinoma. Int J Cancer 1996; 69: 448–51.

156. Engel G, Heselmeyer K, Auer G et al. Correlation between stromelysin 3 mRNA level and outcome of human breast cancer. Int J Cancer 1994; 58: 830–5.

157. Uria JA, Stahl-Backdahl M, Seiki M, Fueyo A, Lopez-Otin C. Regulation of collagenase 3 expression in breast carcinomas is mediated by stromal–epithelial cell interactions. Cancer Res 1997; 57: 4882–8.

158. Pendas AM, Uria JA, Jimenez MG et al. An overview of collagenase-3 expression in malignant tumours and analysis of its potential value as a target in antitumour therapies. Clin Chim Acta 2000; 291: 137–55.

159. Nielsen BS, Rank F, Lopez JM et al. Collagenase-3 expression in breast myofibroblasts as a molecular marker of transition of ductal carcinoma in situ lesions to invasive ductal carcinomas. Cancer Res 2001; 61: 7091–100.

160. Rutter JL, Mitchell TI, Buttice G et al. A single nucleotide polymorphism in the matrix metalloproteinase-1 promoter creates an Ets binding site and augments transcription. Cancer Res 1998; 58: 5321–5.

161. Ye S, Eriksson P, Hamsten A et al. Progression of coronary atherosclerosis is associated with a common genetic variant of the human stromelysin-1 promoter which results in reduced gene expression. J Biol Chem 1996; 271: 13055–60.

162. Zhang B, Ye S, Herrmann SM et al. Functional polymorphism in the regulatory region of gelatinase B gene in relation to severity of coronary atherosclerosis. Circulation 1999; 99: 1788–94.

163. Zhang J, Jin X, Fang S et al. The functional polymorphism in the matrix metalloproteinase-7 promoter increases susceptibility to esophageal squamous cell carcinoma, gastric cardiac adenocarcinoma and non-small cell lung carcinoma. Carcinogenesis 2005; 26: 1748–53.

164. Hughes S, Agbaje O, Bowen RL et al. Matrix metalloproteinase single nucleotide polymorphisms and haplotypes predict breast cancer progression. Clin Cancer Res 2007; 13: 6673–80.

165. Przybylowska K, Kluczna A, Zadrozny M et al. Polymorphisms of the promoter regions of matrix metalloproteinases genes MMP-1 and MMP-9 in breast cancer. Breast Cancer Res Treat 2006; 95: 65–72.

Color Plates

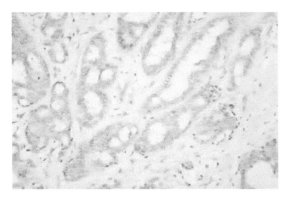

Figure 2.2 Hematoxylin and eosin section showing tubule formation.

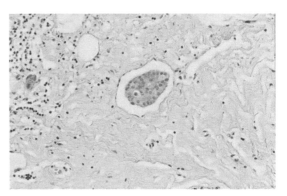

Figure 2.3 Hematoxylin and eosin section showing lymphovascular invasion.

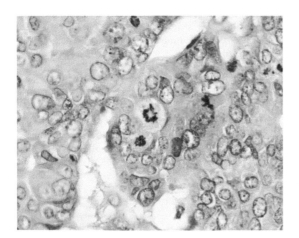

Figure 3.1 Mitotic figure as seen in hematoxylin and eosin (H&E)-stained section.

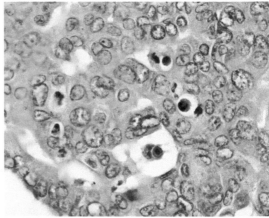

Figure 3.3 Apoptotic cells as they can be recognized in hematoxylin and eosin (H&E)-stained sections of a breast cancer.

ITC   MICROMETASTASIS

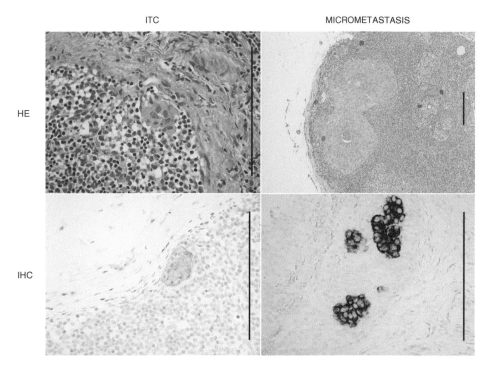

Figure 6.1 Isolated tumor cells (ITC; left side images) and micrometastases (right side images) can be detected by both hematoxylin and eosin staining (HE; top images) and cytokeratin immunohistochemistry (IHC; bottom images). Note that ITC are generally visualized by IHC but larger clusters close to 0.2 mm can also be first seen on HE slides. Likewise small micrometastases may escape HE detection and may require IHC for identification. Bars, 0.2 mm; all images at 400× magnification, except top right at 100×.

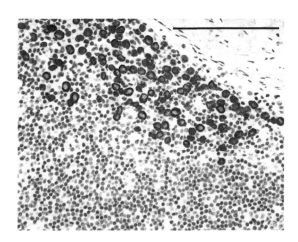

Figure 6.2 Discohesive pattern of a micrometastasis from lobular carcinoma. Note that some pathologists would consider this as multiple "isolated tumor cells" (requiring a comment about overall nodal tumor volume) because none of the cells or touching cell clusters are >0.2 mm. Bar, approximately 0.2 mm; 400× magnification, cytokeratin. Courtesy of Professor Simonetta Bianchi, Florence, Italy.

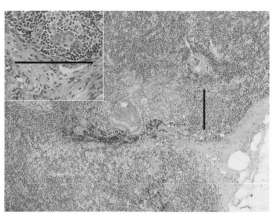

Figure 6.3 The "tip of the iceberg" phenomenon. The sentinel lymph node containing the 90 mm large cluster of cells (classified as "isolated tumor cells") shown in the inset was further sectioned at 250 mm, and turned out to be involved by a micrometastasis measuring 390 mm shown on the main field. Due to the fact of sampling, the lesion might have been somewhat larger in one of the unsampled levels. It should be accepted that size measurements are generally not perfect and despite objective measures they represent only the best approximation we can make. Similarly, micrometastases may be upstaged to macrometastases. Bars, 0.2 mm; inset 400×; main picture ×100.

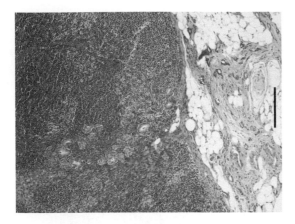

Figure 6.4   Extracapsular extension of a nodal micrometastasis from a tubulolobular carcinoma.

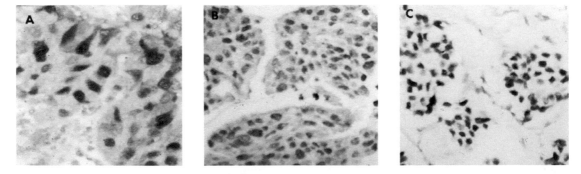

Figure 10.3   Activation of mitogen-activated protein kinase family members in clinical breast cancer: (a) phosphorylated extracellular signal regulated kinases 1 and 2; (b) phosphorylated c-jun N-terminal kinases; (c) phosphorylated p38.

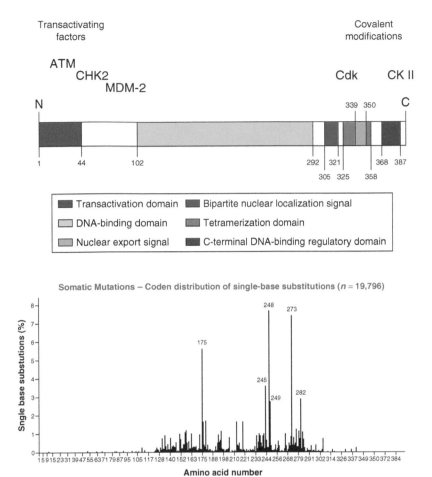

Figure 12.2   p53 comprises a 393 amino acid protein including transactivation, DNA binding, oligomerization, and negative regulatory domains. At the N-terminal end of the molecule, ATM, CHK2 and (MDM)-2 are amongst the many proteins that interact with p53; at the C-terminus, covalent modification (phosphorylation, acetylation) and interactions with cyclin-dependent kinases (Cdk) and casein kinase II (CK II) affect the function of p53.

The mutations detected in p53 predominantly occur in the DNA-binding domain (lower panel) with specific sites being more common in human cancer (numbered amino acids, e.g. 175, versus frequency).

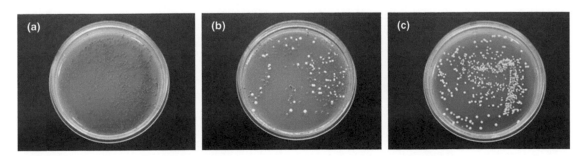

Figure 12.3   Methods used to detect p53 aberrations include: (a) the yeast functional assay where mutation in p53 appears as red colonies on the agar plate, yeast colonies with wild-type p53 as white colonies and a tumor sample demonstrates a mix of red colonies from cancer cells with mutant p53 and white colonies from the normal tissue in the biopsy specimen (after Duddy et al 2000).

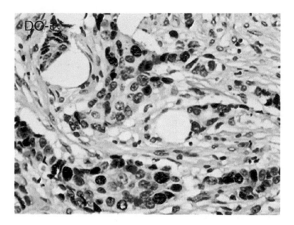
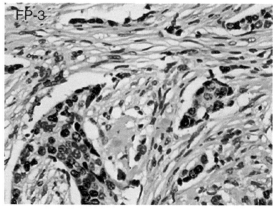

Figure 12.5 Immunohistochemical staining of a cancer for p53 using the antibodies DO-1 (binds to the N-terminal end of p53) and FP3 (binds to the phosphorylated serine 392 residue at the C-terminus. Nuclear p53 staining of most cells for p53 (DO-1) and many cells for activated, phosphorylated p53 (FP3) is demonstrated.

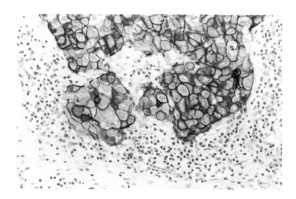
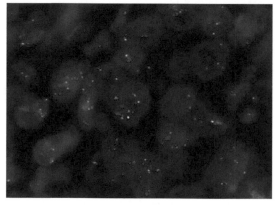

Figure 13.1 Overexpression of the HER2 protein by immunohistochemistry.

Figure 13.2 Amplification of the HER2 gene detected by fluorescence in situ hybridization (FISH) using a Vysis Kit with an inbuilt control (chromosome 17 probe).

Sentinel nodes, micrometastases and isolated tumor cells

6

Gábor Cserni

"… there are truths but there is not truth"

A Camus: Le mythe de Sisyphe

INTRODUCTION

This chapter will summarize several aspects of nodal micrometastases in breast cancer. It will briefly deal with the term itself, the methods used for the detection of these low-volume metastases, and some interpretation issues. Finally, it will discuss the prognostic and predictive implications of micrometastases: whether they have a prognostic impact on survival, and whether they are predictive of nonsentinel node involvement when found within a sentinel lymph node. Obviously, predictive, in this sense is different from the general use of this term, but is nevertheless justified.

MICROMETASTASES, OCCULT METASTASES, ISOLATED TUMOR CELLS, AND THEIR DEFINITIONS

Metastases (from Greek: changing state/change of state) are tumor deposits away from the primary neoplasm. Although instances of metastasis are known in benign conditions, this is generally the most important hallmark of malignant behavior. The prefix micro- (from Greek: small) suggests that micrometastases are indeed small metastases, and in this context the term reflects that they cannot be identified clinically or by naked-eye observation.

If one delves in the fields of medical history, it may happen that who was the first to make a statement in some area is challenged by others. To my knowledge, micrometastases were originally named so by Huvos et al,[1] because they had been supposed to be detectable only by microscopy instead of being picked up at gross examination. A noninclusive size limit of 2 mm was suggested by these authors, who found no survival disadvantage for breast cancer patients with only micrometastases as compared to those with no metastasis at all, after a minimum follow-up of 8 years. Although this study suffers from low patient numbers (only 18 patients with micrometastasis) and lack of detail on the pathologic assessment of the lymph nodes (probably meaning that a single hematoxylin and eosin (H&E)-stained slide was assessed for each), it can be credited for a definition of micrometastases. It also suggested that not only the number of metastatic nodes but also the tumor burden in the lymph nodes may be an important aspect of nodal involvement.

Occult metastases have been well known by pathologists for more than 50 years[2,3] and were often reported to be of no real prognostic value. However, the fact of being occult, i.e. not disclosed by first microscopic inspection but identified later by a more thorough or more sensitive work-up (this definition of "occult metastasis" will be used), does not reflect a size or tumor burden adequately. Such metastases may be smaller or larger than 2 mm, depending on what size the lymph node investigated is and what the "standard" or original pathologic examination consisted of.[4] Because the size of a metastasis influences its chances of being detected by limited sampling, micrometastases are linked to occult metastases since many of them would remain occult if a single H&E section were to be assessed per lymph node; both terms reflect low-volume metastatic involvement.

The definitions of micrometastasis are not uniform. Most investigators use the 2 mm inclusive upper cut-off limit, as suggested by the tumor node metastasis (TNM) classification of malignant tumors,[5,6] whereas others use a 1 mm cut-off size,[7,8] a larger 0.2 cm² or a <1 mm² cut-off area.[9,10] The European Working Group for Breast Screening Pathology recently assessed the pathology practice relating to sentinel lymph nodes (SLNs) by means of a questionnaire and found that the term micrometastasis was used by 93% of the responders; the definitions given for this category included 17 somewhat different entities.[11] For uniformity of use, adherence to the TNM definition of micrometastasis, last updated in 2002, which includes a lower cut-off value of 0.2 mm, is strongly recommended. However, it must be noted that this definition is not unanimously reflected in current and earlier publications, and one should always check definitions before interpreting retrospective data.

According to the current definition, the former group of micrometastasis was split into two diagnostic categories: the micrometastases per se and a disputed category labeled with the misnomer of "isolated tumor cells" (ITCs).[5,6,12] The latter is also called submicrometastasis by some,[13] but the name of nanometastasis has also been suggested.[14]

Although the Union Internationale Contre le Cancer (UICC) and the American Joint Committee on Cancer (AJCC) are supposed to use the same TNM system for the determination of the anatomic extent of malignant disease, the wording in the two main relevant publications of these bodies differ in a minimal extent, and this may be the source of some differences in interpretation and hence classification. The sixth edition of the UICC TNM Classification of MalignantTumours[5] defines ITC as "single tumor cells or small clusters not more than 0.2 mm in greatest dimension, that are usually detected by immunohistochemistry or molecular methods; they do not typically show evidence of metastatic activity or penetration of vascular or lymphatic sinus walls." The AJCC Cancer Staging Manual[6] and its abridged variant used a somewhat different wording, and defined ITC as "single cells or small clusters of cells not greater than 0.2 mm in largest dimension, usually with no histological evidence of malignant activity (such as proliferation or stromal reaction)." The relation to sinus walls is not mentioned in the latter description.[6] The use of the pN0(i+) symbol to denote ITC was also different in the AJCC publications[6] from the one suggested in the UICC publications.[5,12] However, in a revision it was made clear that the "(i+)" denoted the presence of ITC and not immunohistochemistry (IHC) as the method of its detection (Figure 6.1).[15,16] Although it may seem that size is a major criterion to distinguish between ITC and micrometastases, and therefore a node-negative and a node-positive stage (from staging and management aspects), both major publications[5,6] cite a UICC paper where the tumor cell location within the lymph node, and the so-called metastatic activity, were also listed as distinguishing features.[12]

The present TNM categories were also endorsed by the United Kingdom National Health Service Breast Screening Programme[17] and their respective labels are given below:

- pN1mi: micrometastasis;
- pN0(i+): isolated tumor cells, identified by microscopy, i.e. morphological methods, including H&E staining and/or IHC;
- pN0(mol+): evidence of ITCs by molecular methods, most commonly reverse transcription polymerase chain reaction (RT-PCR) only;
- whenever ITCs are looked for by morphologic or molecular studies, but these yield negative results, the pN0(i–) and pN0(mol–) symbols are to be used;
- pN0 is to be used when no metastases are found, but no special methods are used for the search of "occult" metastases.

ITC   MICROMETASTASIS

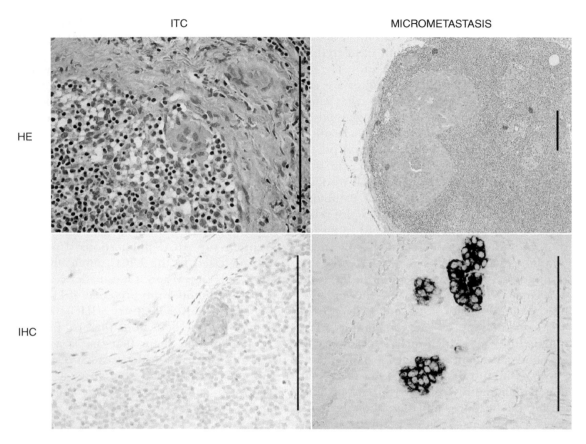

Figure 6.1   Isolated tumor cells (ITC; left side images) and micrometastases (right side images) can be detected by both hematoxylin and eosin staining (HE; top images) and cytokeratin immunohistochemistry (IHC; bottom images). Note that ITC are generally visualized by IHC but larger clusters close to 0.2 mm can also be first seen on HE slides. Likewise small micrometastases may escape HE detection and may require IHC for identification. Bars, 0.2 mm; all images at 400× magnification, except top right at 100×.

The TNM classification also suggests that whenever there are multiple distinct foci of metastatic involvement, only the largest should be considered for classification.

With all this in mind, it must be mentioned that the reproducibility of these staging categories is less than optimal. A group of European pathologists with expertise in breast pathology examined and interpreted 50 cases represented by digital images, all approaching the differential diagnosis of micrometastases and ITCs. The kappa value for the consistency of categorizing low-volume nodal load into micrometastasis, ITCs or none of these was 0.39 (reflecting fair reproducibility) when each participant used his/her interpretation of the TNM definitions. This figure changed to 0.49 (still reflecting only moderate reproducibility) in a second circulation of the same set of images performed after a discussion aimed at making the interpretation of the definitions more uniform.[18] The kappa value was ≤0.57 even on a single institutional level.[19] One source of interpretative trouble stems from the classification of nodal metastases of invasive lobular carcinomas, which often infiltrate the lymph nodes by a noncohesive single cell pattern (Figure 6.2). A group of pathologists could achieve a very good consistency in diagnosing such lesions following the partly

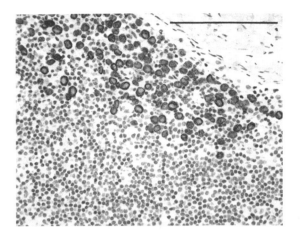

Figure 6.2 Discohesive pattern of a micrometastasis from lobular carcinoma. Note that some pathologists would consider this as multiple "isolated tumor cells" (requiring a comment about overall nodal tumor volume) because none of the cells or touching cell clusters are >0.2 mm. Bar, approximately 0.2 mm; 400× magnification, cytokeratin. Courtesy of Professor Simonetta Bianchi, Florence, Italy.

image-guided interpretative guidelines agreed on before testing, but several pathologists within that study, including the present author, raised concerns about diagnosing a relatively high total metastatic nodal volume as ITCs on the basis of the infiltrative pattern (Roderick Turner, personal communication, June 2007). Another source of confusion comes from the localization of low volume (≤0.2 mm in greatest dimension) nodal involvement; some would not consider this a matter of diagnostic distinction between micrometastases and ITCs, and would make the distinction simply on the basis of size criteria, whereas others would consider extrasinusoidal and intraparenchymal lesions of this size as micrometastases.[18,20] Such interpretative issues may seriously affect prognostic, prediction and consequently therapy-related conclusions of most studies lacking a uniform pathology review of SLN slides. These problems in interpretation also highlight the need for a more precise definition of ITCs and micrometastasis categories, preferably with visual aid and examples on how to classify challenging cases.

THE USE OF MULTILEVEL ASSESSMENT, IMMUNOHISTOCHEMISTRY AND MOLECULAR TECHNIQUES FOR THE DETECTION OF LYMPH NODE/SENTINEL LYMPH NODE INVOLVEMENT

The presence of occult metastases can be confirmed by a more detailed sampling of the lymph nodes and/or the use of a more sensitive method to detect them. As a consequence, examining several slices or step sections from a lymph node and/or introducing immunostains in their investigation leads to an increase in occult nodal involvement and an upstaging from node-negative to node-positive status when compared to a methodology which does not use these tools.

It has been known for a long time that IHC aimed at highlighting the presence of epithelial markers (mainly cytokeratins) in lymph nodes may increase the detection rate of small metastases.[21] However, it must be remembered that not everything that is cytokeratin-positive represents metastatic nodal deposits; cytokeratin-positive dendritic cells are normal constituents of the lymph nodes,[22,23] and benign epithelial inclusions[24] or dislodged papillary fragments[25] are also positive. Rarely, macrophages and plasma cells may also stain nonspecifically, and different contaminants and carry-over may hinder interpretation of cytokeratin immunostaining.[26] In cases of uncertainty, the TNM general rules suggest that the lower category (less advanced disease stage) should be opted for. Therefore, a node-negative status should be the conclusion if one is in doubt about the nature of the cytokeratin positivity.[27]

SLNs can be defined as lymph nodes with direct lymph drainage from the primary tumor site.[26] Sentinel lymph node biopsy (SLNB) seems an ideal surgical method for selecting the most likely sites of regional nodal metastases, and therefore selecting the few or only lymph nodes which should be subjected to more scrutiny in order to identify otherwise occult metastases. According to the first relevant report on this issue, the addition (per half

SLN) of two extra H&E stained levels and one stained with cytokeratin IHC resulted in a 13% nodal upstaging as compared to a previous series of comparable breast cancer patients staged by axillary dissection with a standard pathological assessment of the lymph nodes.[28] The upstaging was mainly due to the higher detection rate of micrometastases (38% in the SLNB group vs 10% in the axillary clearance group). Many other studies have confirmed these observations, and the upstaging rates vary between 9 and 47%.[29]

The use of cytokeratin IHC is one of the most controversial issues in the examination of axillary lymph nodes. SLNs are often subjected to this method when negative by H&E. Although several guidelines do not recommend the routine use of IHC for the evaluation of SLNs,[30] a questionnaire based survey by the European Working Group for Breast Screening Pathology suggested that 71% of the 240 pathology laboratories assessed used IHC regularly for SLNs negative by H&E.[11] This rate may be even higher in the United States (Roderick Turner, personal communication, at Sentinel Node 2004, Santa Monica, December 2004).

The value of cytokeratin staining in highlighting occult nodal involvement depends on several factors. When step sectioning is done, the smaller the steps, the lower is the extra yield in nodal positivity detected by adding IHC to the standard histological stains.[31–33] The size of the metastatic involvement is also important, since most of the cases identified by IHC belong to the micrometastasis or ITC categories. The pattern of nodal involvement of lobular carcinomas is often prone to escape traditional detection by light microscopy: therefore, the addition of cytokeratin IHC increases the rate of nodal positivity more than in cases of ductal carcinomas.[34–36] IHC of SLNs also suggests a higher upstaging rate if the primary tumor is of the lobular type, and with this histological type immunostaining may highlight not only ITCs and micrometastases but also some smaller macrometastases.[37]

Although cytokeratin IHC may increase the detection rate of nodal involvement, it disproportionally increases the detection rate of ITCs, many of which may escape detection even if visible. The results of automated analysis of SLNs immunostained with cytokeratin antibodies suggest that very small volumes may remain unnoticed by conventional microscopic examination.[38,39]

Once it is established that the cytokeratin-positive cells are from the tumor, histopathology cannot differentiate between cells which got to the lymph node by an active metastatic process and those which were dislodged by prior manipulation of the tumor. Indeed, diagnostic and localization procedures (needle biopsies, wire or radioisotopic localizations) and massage, sometimes used in order to promote the migration of the tracers during SLNB, have been reported as, or supposed to be, possible ways of tumoral seeding.[25,40,41] If noticed, such seeding would most likely be labeled as ITC, giving further support for including these in the pN0 category.

The combination of multilevel assessment and IHC yields the highest rate of upstaging when compared to a single H&E level assessment.[29] Most macrometastases are discovered on the first or first few levels of sectioning SLN tissue blocks. Micrometastases may need a more intensive search, whereas ITCs are rather randomly distributed in the lymph nodes.[31–33,42] Targeting the search for nodal involvement and concentrating it to the area around the junction of the tumor-draining afferent lymphatic channel, visualized by either the blue coloration or the highest intranodal radioactivity count, may help in finding most nodal involvement with less effort,[43,44] but this needs further prospective investigation. It seems obvious that no histology protocol can aim at detecting all ITCs in a lymph node, and histology protocols should be devised in a way to be able to exclude a given size metastasis with a reasonable accuracy.[45] Whether micrometastases should be the category to exclude is a matter of debate, and this will be discussed further at the end of this chapter.

Molecular methods to highlight nodal involvement of very low volume include flow cytometry[46] and RT-PCR assays.[29] These are very sensitive but lack sufficient specificity: a challenge which mandates the use of several markers. Most reports on RT-PCR in lymph nodes report false-negative cases, i.e. lymph nodes with histologically proven metastatic involvement but negative molecular testing. Whereas such nodes are obviously positive, those which test positive with the RT-PCR assay but are negative by histology may either represent false-positive testing or histologically occult nodal involvement.[47] This may also justify labeling them as pN0(mol+). Real-time quantitative RT-PCR assays are more promising, as manipulations of the cut-off levels may make the tests more specific.[48,49] However, it must be remembered that molecular staging may also be biased by sampling errors[43,44,50] and nontumoral epithelial tissue presence,[24] and this strengthens the need for histological verification of molecular results.

Histopathology will therefore remain the standard diagnostic approach to SLNs and nodal staging. The differences in histology protocols may however cause differences in treatment options,[51] and perhaps even outcome. Such differences may be overcome by devising regional, national or international guidelines on the minimum requirements in SLN histopathology. Without such standardization, outcome data will not be consistently comparable.

THE PROGNOSTIC IMPACT OF NODAL MICROMETASTASES

Nodal status is generally considered an important prognostic factor. Several studies have highlighted that the volume of metastatic nodal load also represents a prognostic parameter beyond the node-positive versus node-negative status. At one end of the spectrum, metastasis in a large number of lymph nodes is associated with a worse prognosis than the involvement of a few lymph nodes,[52,53] or the involvement of a larger proportion of the examined lymph nodes is worse than a lower ratio of metastatic lymph nodes.[54,55] When only a few lymph nodes are involved, small metastases lumped into the category of micrometastasis may also represent a smaller prognostic disadvantage than larger metastases.[56]

The prognostic impact of micrometastases in breast cancer is largely disputed. Some authors found no survival disadvantage for micrometastatic nodal involvement; others have reported a worse associated outcome, but only for disease-free survival and not for overall survival; and still others described a definite disadvantage (Table 6.1). Occult metastases are often admixed with micrometastases in the quoted studies, especially in the earlier ones. The methods of pathological evaluation are also different from study to study and many would be considered less than optimal with our current knowledge; most studies were aimed at detecting some occult metastases and were not devised to exclude all occult metastases of a given size. It is likely that no attempt was ever made to exclude the possibility of the identified micrometastases being the tip of a larger metastasis "iceberg" (Figure 6.3). As shown in Table 6.1, the micrometastatic group often comprised only a few cases and the follow-up was also limited. Therefore, many of the series have insufficient power to demonstrate a minor benefit.

After reviewing many of the series published, it was concluded that micrometastases are of prognostic impact, but only large series with long follow-up can demonstrate this.[78,79] The need for a long follow-up, especially for better differentiated tumors, was also stressed by the analysis of the Survival Epidemiology and End Results database.[80] With the advent of SLNB, nodal micrometastases are not only found more frequently[28] but smaller micrometastases and ITCs are also increasingly discovered. Theoretically, this may suggest an even lesser survival disadvantage, which would be backed up by most studies on the predictive role of these small metastases, but some recent studies report a worse disease-free survival even with ITCs (Table 6.1).[14,74,75] These later studies are in keeping with the hypothesis that metastases may develop early in the neoplastic process as determined by the molecular signature of the tumor.[81,82]

Table 6.1 Studies on the survival effect (prognostic significance) of low-volume metastases

First author	Method of detection	Number of patients/details	Type of metastasis	Prognostic significance
Pickren[3]	Single HE vs SS	40 pN0 vs 11 pN0 upstaged to pN+ by SS	Occult	No (minimum 5-year follow-up)
Huvos[1]	NI	164 pN0 vs 18 pN1mi (<2mm)	Micrometastasis	No (minimum 8-year follow-up)
Fisher[57]	Single HE vs SS	59 pN0 vs 19 pN0 upstaged to pN+ by SS	Occult	No (mean follow-up: 61 months)
Fisher[58]	Single HE	287 pN0 vs 21 pN1mi (<2mm)	Micrometastasis	No (mean follow-up: 49 months)
Rosen[59]	NI	77 macrometastatic vs 70 pN1mi	Micrometastasis	Yes for DFS of T1 tumors (minimum 10 year follow-up)
Wilkinson[60]	HE vs SS	441 pN0 vs 84 pN0 upstaged to pN+ by SS	Occult	No (minimum follow-up: 5 years)
Trojani[61]	HE vs IHC of same sections	129 pN0 vs 21 pN0 upstaged to pN+ by IHC	Occult	Yes for DFS and OS (mean follow-up: 10 years)
Friedman[62]	Serial HE	637 pN0 vs 41 with sinusoidal low-volume metastases in a single lymph node	"Occult", sinusoidal	Yes (relative risk of distant metastasis at least 1.7 for occult metastases)
Sedmak[63]	HE vs new HE+IHC	36 pN0 vs 9 pN0 upstaged to pN+ by IHC	Occult	Yes for OS (minimum follow-up 10 years)
IBCSG[64]	Single level vs SS	838 pN0 vs 83 pN0 upstaged to pN+ by SS	Occult	Yes for DFS and OS (median follow-up: 5 years)
Galea[65]	HE vs IHC	89 pN0 vs 9 pN0 upstaged to pN+ by IHC (8 micrometastasis and 1macrometastasis)	Occult	No (follow-up out to 14 years)
De Mascarel[66]	HE vs IHC of same sections	168 pN0 vs 50 pN0 upstaged to pN+ by IHC; same series as Trojani et al[61] but longer follow-up	Occult	Yes – for DFS and ductal cancers (median follow up: 15.6 for ductal cancers)
Hainsworth[67]	1 HE vs 1 IHC	302 pN0 vs 41 pN0 upstaged to pN+ by IHC (31 micrometastasis and 10 macrometastasis)	Occult	Yes – only for DFS, but not for OS (follow-up: median 79 months)
Nasser[68]	HE vs SS+IHC	151pN0 vs 50 pN0 upstaged to pN+ by SS+IHC	Occult	No for all. Yes for both DFS and OS for occult metastases >0.2 mm (mean follow-up: 11 years)
McGuckin[69]	HE vs SS (4 levels) + IHC	155 pN0 vs 53 pN0 upstaged to pN+ by SS+IHC	Occult	Yes – only for DFS, but not for OS (median follow-up: 92 months)
Clare[70]	HE+IHC (5 levels each)	75 pN0 vs 11 pN0 upstaged to pN+ by SS+IHC	Occult	Yes – for disease-specific 5-year survival (median follow-up: 80 months)

(Continued)

Table 6.1 (Continued)

First author	Method of detection	Number of patients/details	Type of metastasis	Prognostic significance
Cote[71]	HE vs 6 levels HE and 1 level IHC	588 pN0 vs 148 pN0 upstaged to pN+ by IHC; same series as IBCSG,[64] but IHC added and longer follow-up	Occult	Yes – for both DFS and OS in postmenopausal women (median follow-up: 12 years)
Colpaert[72]	HE vs 2 further levels IHC	80 pN0 vs 24 pN0 upstaged to pN+ by IHC (17 ITC and 7 pN1mi)	Occult (ITC and micrometastasis)	No (median follow-up for patients with and without relapse: 25 months and 91.5 months, respectively)
Millis[73]	HE vs IHC	417pN0 vs 60 pN0 upstaged to pN+ by IHC	Occult	No (median follow-up: 18.9 years)
Kuijt[56]	No data (registry data)	4377 pN0 vs 179 pN1mi	Micrometastasis	Yes for 10 year OS (minimum follow-up: 52 months)
Mullenix[74]	HE + IHC	175 pN0(i–)(sn) vs 8 pN0(i+)(sn) or pN1mi(sn)	ITC and micrometastasis	Yes for DFS, but insufficient data (median follow-up: 25 months)
Colleoni[75]	No data, but step FS and IHC of suspicious cases on the basis of other reports from the same institution[31,48]	1400 pN0 (i–)(sn) vs 232 pN0(i+)(sn) or pN1mi(sn)	ITC and micrometastasis	Yes for DFS, but not for OS (median follow-up: 50 months)
Imoto[76]	HE+IHC	147 pN0(i–)(sn) vs 17 pN0(sn) upstaged to pN0(i+)(sn)	ITC	No (minimum follow-up: 5 years)
Nagashima[77]	HE/2 mm slice (+IHC in suspicious cases)	241 pN0(sn) vs 19 pN1mi(sn)	Micrometastasis	No (median follow-up: 30 months)
Querzoli[14]	(HE+IHC) + (HE+IHC) pairs being separated by 100 μm/both half	328 pN0(i–) vs 49 pN0 upstaged to pN+ (24 pN0(i+) and 25 pN1mi)	Occult (ITC and micrometastasis)	Yes for DFS (median follow-up: 8 years)

DFS, Disease-free survival; HE, hematoxylin and eosin; IBCSG, International Breast Cancer Study Group; IHC, immunohistochemistry; ITC, isolated tumor cells; NI, no information available; OS, overall survival; pN0(i+), isolated tumor cells (as defined in the articles in question); pN0(i–), no nodal involvement identified with multilevel assessment or immunostains; pN1mi, micrometastasis (≤2 mm, unless otherwise stated); pN+, any nodal involvement identified; (sn), symbol for nodal status established on the basis of sentinel lymph node biopsy without axillary clearance; SS, multiple level assessment by serial sectioning or step sectioning.

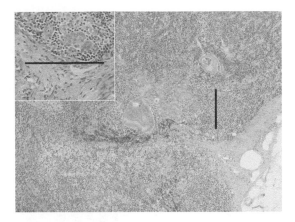

Figure 6.3 The "tip of the iceberg" phenomenon. The sentinel lymph node containing the 90 μm large cluster of cells (classified as "isolated tumor cells") shown in the inset was further sectioned at 250 μm, and turned out to be involved by a micrometastasis measuring 390 μm shown on the main field. Due to the fact of sampling, the lesion might have been somewhat larger in one of the unsampled levels. It should be accepted that size measurements are generally not perfect and despite objective measures they represent only the best approximation we can make. Similarly, micrometastases may be upstaged to macrometastases. Bars, 0.2 mm; inset 400×; main picture 100×.

On the whole, the data relating to the prognostic significance of micrometastases and ITCs are nonconclusive, and partly due to the lack of similar pathology methods (including sampling of all lymph nodes, sectioning them, using IHC, interpreting the findings, etc) they are also incomparable. It can be expected that the search for low-volume metastases in the SLNs will result in a stage migration[83] by diluting the traditional node-positive group with the "better prognosis" micrometastatic cases, and by concentrating the traditional node-negative group by taking out of it some cases with occult nodal involvement, resulting in a virtual improvement of prognosis in both new groups of node-positive and node-negative cases. This phenomenon makes the new results even less comparable with the historical reports listed in Table 6.1. The clinical trials on SLNB have not yet had sufficient long-term follow-up for definite conclusions about survival with micrometastases, although

they support SLNB as a low morbidity staging procedure. It may however be hypothesized that patients with nodal micrometastases receiving adjuvant systemic treatment would derive some benefit from this treatment.[56,77]

One should not forget that when systemic treatment decisions are based on nodal status, this is considered as a marker of metastatic dissemination – albeit a rather imperfect marker. Indeed, node-negative patients may die of disease and a subset of node-positive cases may survive with locoregional treatment alone. Therefore, it is not surprising that the role of nodal status in influencing adjuvant treatment decisions has lost some weight, or that other prognostic factors have gained significance in outcome prediction and therapeutic planning. Although lymph node involvement is still considered an important prognosticator, according to the newer St Gallen consensus statements, it does not automatically define high risk and should be considered with other risk factors.[84,85] Interestingly enough, these guidelines suggest that both ITCs and micrometastases should be ignored in risk allocation and treatment decisions.[84] The latter recommendation is made despite the contradictory evidences outlined in Table 6.1, with greater favor being given to the significance of micrometastases than to their lack. This is also in opposition with the arbitrary TNM segregation of ITCs and micrometastases into the pN0 and pN1 categories, respectively.

SENTINEL LYMPH NODE MICROMETASTASES AND THE PREDICTION OF NONSENTINEL NODE INVOLVEMENT

When SLNB is performed, the finding of a metastasis is generally perceived as an indication for axillary dissection or radiotherapy. The detailed histological or molecular analysis of the SLN and non-SLN status has led to the recognition that many breast cancer patients have metastases limited to the SLNs, in keeping with the theory that the SLNs are the most likely sites of regional nodal metastasis.[86–91] It has also been a common finding that the frequency of non-SLN metastases is dependent on SLN metastasis size[92] and some other factors. In this context, micrometastases are often reported to be associated with such a low rate, and therefore risk of non-SLN involvement, that several reports have concluded that no further axillary treatment is necessary in case of micrometastatic SLN positivity. In contrast, other studies have concluded that even ITCs in the SLNs are associated with a rate of non-SLN positivity which justifies axillary clearance as a general treatment option for any SLN involvement, and such findings also support the use of cytokeratin IHC in the evaluation of SLNs (Table 6.2).

The relevant studies are rather heterogeneous from several aspects, and therefore their meta-analysis may give more idea about the risk of non-SLN metastases than any of the individual reports.[117] Until the relevant clinical trials reach a reasonable follow-up time for relevant conclusions, a 10–15% overall risk may be the best estimation of non-SLN involvement for cases with SLN micrometastases.[117] This risk is very similar to the 5–10% false-negative rate of SLNB itself.

It must also be considered that micrometastases, as currently defined, are heterogeneous and this also relates to their size: they form a continuum. Larger ones at the macrometastasis edge probably reflect more harm than the smaller ones at the ITC edge. Likewise, some authors found that the rate of non-SLN involvement is significantly higher in patients with SLN micrometastases >1 mm than in those with smaller SLN micrometastases.[111,114] Another study identified 1.3 mm as a possible cut-off for higher (>10%) and smaller non-SLN metastasis risk,[118] whereas an Austrian paper suggested that micrometastases <0.5 mm were those in which the rate of non-SLN positivity could be considered negligible.[115] It must also be remembered that studies which found it sufficient to identify ITCs in a single IHC-stained slide of a 3 mm thick slice of an SLN, and failed to exclude a larger metastasis underlying this, must be considered with caution as regards the size of the

SLN involvement and the associated rate of non-SLN positivity. On the other hand, studies using an enhanced method of metastasis detection for SLNs, but a standard one to a few H&E levels approach to non-SLNs (a very rational, acceptable and practical approach to nodal staging), are likely to underestimate the risks of overall non-SLN involvement, but not of macrometastatic non-SLN involvement. (Pathological methods used are briefly summarized in Table 6.2.)

Another consideration which should be taken into account is the contribution of other factors in models assessing the risk of non-SLN involvement. Tumor size and lymphovascular invasion (LVI) are often reported as parameters influencing this risk, along with the number of SLNs involved, the number of SLNs found, or alternately the ratio of SLNs involved.

Therefore, despite the fact that the overall risk of non-SLN positivity associated with SLN micrometastases and ITCs found in different publications is generally low, and the estimate of 10–15% quoted previously[117] may generally work well, there may be combinations of other factors increasing or lowering this risk. For example, patients with in situ carcinomas,[119,120] small pT1a and pT1b (up to 1 cm large) tumors without demonstrable LVI[116,119] or with some special type tumors of good prognosis (like tubular or cribriform carcinomas)[116,121] would most certainly not benefit from axillary dissection after the finding of a micrometastatic SLN.

The interaction of different parameters has generated the search for predictive tools such as: the nomograms created at the Memorial Sloan-Kettering Cancer Center (MSKCC)[122] and at the Mayo Clinic;[123] the scoring systems generated by the MD Anderson Cancer Center,[97] the Tenon Hospital[124] and the Louisville sentinel lymph node study;[125] or the decision table stemming from an Australian study.[126] Some of these tools have been validated on independent datasets, but it seems that the group with the lowest risk of non-SLN involvement is very small, and this is where the predictive tools may perform more

Table 6.2 Studies on SLNB-based prediction of non-SLN metastasis including a minimum of 25 relevant cases

First author	Number of patients with small metastases (non-SLN+; %)	Findings	Pathology of SLNs; comments
Reynolds[93]	27 N1mi or ITC (6; 22%)	• T and SLN metastasis size (micro vs macro) are independent predictors of non-SLN+ • T1 and pN1mi(sn) have low risk of non-SLN+	4 HE + IHC; N1mi and ITC considered as one category
Wong[94]	28 only IHC-positive (3; 11%)	• pT category and number of positive SLNs are independent factors predicting non-SLN+ • A small subset of patients with only IHC-positive SLNs have obvious non-SLN metastases	HE/2 mm + IHC performed on only 49% of the cases The influence of SLN metastasis size could not be assessed reliably; probably mainly ITC identified
Marin[95]	29 N1mi or ITC (8; 28%); 18 only IHC-positive (4; 22%)	• Patients with micrometastatic SLN have a risk of non-SLN involvement, that might be minimal for ductal-type T1 tumors without LVI	1–7 HE + IHC (whole thickness at 0.5 mm steps); N1mi and ITC considered as one category
Rutledge[96]	29 N1mi (1; 3%)	• Non-SLN positivity differs significantly between cases with SLN micrometastasis and macrometastasis • Risk-benefit assessment is needed for decisions on ALND	3 level HE (+IHC not specified); N1mi and ITC considered as separate categories
Rahusen[10]	30 N1mi (<1 mm²) (8; 27%)*	• Patients with T1a tumors or SLN micrometastases <1 mm² still have a risk of non-SLN+	5HE + IHC; N1mi and ITC considered as one category; micrometastasis definition: <1 mm²
Hwang[97]	30 (5; 17%)	• SLN metastasis size (micro/ITC vs macro), pT (pT1 vs >2 cm) and LVI are the independent factors influencing non-SLN+	1 HE/2–3 mm slice – subset: 3 serial HE and 1 IHC; N1mi and ITC probably considered as one category
den Bakker[98]	32 (11 of which 4 ITC; 34%)*	• T (T1 vs >2 cm) and histological grade are associated with non-SLN+ • ALND is supported for low-volume SLN involvement	4 HE + 4 IHC at 250 μm/slice – non-SLNs also 3–10 IHC; N1mi and ITC considered as separate categories; ITC limited to 3 cells
Abdessalam[99]	35 N1mi or ITC (7; 20%); 5 only IHC-positive (1; 20%)	• SLN involvement, macrometastatic SLNs, LVI, extracapsular nodal involvement all increase the likelihood of non-SLN+	6FS + SS (HE) +IHC; N1mi and ITC considered as one category
Fréneaux[100]	35 only IHC-positive (1; 3%)	• IHC detected occult metastases are rarely associated with non-SLN+	1–4HE + (1–4)×6IHC; N1mi and ITC considered as one category; overlap with Houvenaeghel et al[116]

(Continued)

Table 6.2   (Continued)

First author	Number of patients with small metastases (non-SLN+; %)	Findings	Pathology of SLNs; comments
Zgajnar[101]	31 N1mi and 5 ITC (4; 11% for all, 13% for N1mi, 0% for ITC)	• No non-SLN macrometastases are likely if the ultrasound examination of the axilla is negative and the SLN contains only micrometastases or ITC	HE SS+IHC; N1mi and ITC considered as separate categories
Csermi[102]	43 N1mi or ITC (5; 12% for all, 4/39 for N1mi, 1/4 for ITC)	• Tumor size, SLN metastasis size, SLN+ ratio, extracapsular spread are predictors of non-SLN+	HE SS at 50–100 or 250 μm+multiple IHC; N1mi and ITC considered as separate categories
Kamath[103]	46 N1mi or ITC (7; 15%); 26 only IHC-positive (2; 8%)	• SLN micrometastases detected by IHC only are associated with a low risk of non-SLN+	SS(HE)+IHC; N1mi and ITC considered as one category; divided by method of detection; overlap with Jakub et al[107]
Carcoforo[104]	58 N1mi (8; 14%)	• pT (T1 vs >2 cm), LVI, and MIB-1 proliferation index (>10% vs <10%) are factors influencing non-SLN+ • Patients with micrometastatic SLNs but without LVI, MIB1 index <10%, and T1 tumors can probably avoid ALND	HE SS+IHC; ITCs not included in the SLN-positive group
Calhoun[105]	61 only IHC/ITC-positive (3; 5%)	• ALND is not supported for ITC involved SLNs	4–6 HE+2IHC; overlap with Turner et al[112]
Menes[106]	61 (12; 20% for all, 20% for N1mi, 19% for ITC)	• SLN metastasis size (micro/ITC vs macro), positive SLN ratio are the only factors associated with non-SLN+ • High risk of residual disease if ALND is not done for micrometastatic or ITC involved SLNs	5HE and 2IHC/SLN; N1mi and ITC considered as separate categories
Jakub[107]	62 only IHC-positive (9; 15%)	• Both IHC of SLNs and ALND for SLNs positive with IHC only are justified	HE+IHC/2–3 mm slice; N1mi and ITC not distinguished, probably mainly ITCs considered; overlap with Kamath et al[103]
Krauth[108]	62 (14; 23% for all, 21% for N1mi, 26% for ITC)	• Only LVI associated with non-SLN+ • ALND is indicated for minimal SLN involvement too	HE+IHC/1–2 mm slice (later cases also step sectioned at 0.5 or 0.2 mm); N1mi and ITC considered as separate categories
Di Tommaso[109]	62 N1mi or ITC (10; 16% for all; 7/25 (28%) for N1mi >1 mm, 3/37 (8%) for N1mi ≤1 mm; 9/31 (29%) for intraparenchymal N1mi and 1/31 (3%) for intrasinusoidal N1mi	• Micrometastases are less likely to be associated with non-SLN involvement than macrometastases.	HE SS on FS, no IHC; N1mi and ITC considered as one category

(Continued)

Table 6.2 (Continued)

First author	Number of patients with small metastases (non-SLN+; %)	Findings	Pathology of SLNs; comments
Mignotte[110]	68 N1mi or ITC (15; 22%); 44 only IHC-positive (7; 16%)	• No subset with very low risk of non-SLN+ could be identified	SS at 1–2 mm (HE) + 6 IHC; N1mi and ITC considered as one category, divided by method of detection; overlap with Houvenaeghel et al [116]
Leidenius[111]	84 N1mi (22; 26% for all, 37% for N1mi>1 mm, 21% for both N1mi<1 mm and ITC)	• Ratio of positive SLNs ≤0.2 makes the risk of non-SLN+ negligible • High overall risk of residual disease in the axilla if no completion ALND is done for micrometastatic SLNs	FS + 2HE + IHC/1–1.5 mm slice; ITC not mentioned, N1mi and ITC probably considered as one category
Turner[112]	89 N1mi or ITC (9; 10%); {20; 22%};* 39 only IHC-positive (5; 13%); {10; 26%}*	• SLN metastasis size (micro/ITC vs macro), pT (pT1a–b vs >1 cm) and LVI are the independent factors influencing non-SLN+ • Micrometastatic T1–2 tumors without LVI, hilar extracapsular nodal spread have low risk of non-SLN+	4–6HE + 2IHC; * overalp with Calhoun et al[105]
Weiser[113]	93 N1mi or ITC (17; 18%)	• SLN metastasis size (micro/ITC vs macro), pT (pT1a–b vs >1 cm) and LVI are the independent factors influencing non-SLN+ • Micrometastatic T1a–b tumors without LVI, have low risk of non-SLN+	FS + SS + IHC; N1mi and ITC considered as one category
Viale[114]	109 N1mi (24; 22% for all; 12/33 (36%) for pN1mi >1 mm, 12/77 (16%) or pN1mi ≤1 mm)	• Omission of ALND may be considered for micrometastases ≤1 mm	HE SS on FS + IHC; N1mi and ITC considered as one category
Schrenk[115]	122 N1mi or ITC (22; 18% for all; 18/78 (23%) for pN1mi, 4/44 (9%) for pN0(i+)	• Size of pN1mi and LVI significantly associated with non-SLN+	SS at 250 μm + IHC; N1mi and ITC considered as separate categories
Houvenaeghel[116]	700 N1mi or ITC (94; 13%)	• pT, detection method (IHC vs HE), LVI are factors influencing non-SLN+ • pT1a–b and some special type pT1a–b–c cancers have low risk of non-SLN+	HE + IHC; N1mi and ITC considered as separate categories

ALND, Axillary lymph node dissection; FS, frozen sections; HE, hematoxylin and eosin; IHC, immunohistochemistry; ITC, isolated tumor cells; LVI, lymphovascular invasion; non-SLN+, positive nonsentinel lymph node(s); pN1mi: micrometastasis (≤2 mm, unless otherwise stated); (p)T, tumor size as reflected by the T or pT categories of the TNM classification; SLN, sentinel lymph node; SLNB, sentinel lymph node biopsy; (sn), symbol for nodal status established on the basis of SLNB without axillary clearance; SS, multiple level assessment by serial sectioning or step sectioning; *, (results gained when) non-SLN also assessed with enhanced histopathology; TNM, tumor node metastasis classification of malignant tumors.

*Results gained when nonsentinel lymph nodes were also assessed with enhanced histopathology.

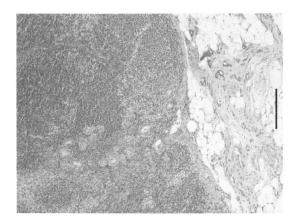

Figure 6.4 Extracapsular extension of a nodal micrometastasis from a tubulolobular carcinoma.

poorly.[127–129] It has also been found that the MSKCC nomogram is unreliable when SLNs are only micrometastatic.[130] Interestingly, several of the mentioned predictive tools do not include the size of the SLN metastasis as a variable.[122,125] The Louisville clinical prediction rule uses only factors which can be available during the SLNB procedure itself, to allow an intraoperative decision,[125] whereas the MSKCC nomogram reflects metastasis size only by its detection method (frozen section vs serial HE vs IHC).[122]

Many publications have documented that extracapsular spread of the SLN metastasis is a factor associated with increased risk of non-SLN involvement.[99,102,112,131,132] Although this phenomenon is perceived as a sign of nodal obliteration,[133] and therefore massive involvement, some micrometastases also show this feature,[134] especially in tumors with tubular histology (Figure 6.4). In such instances, the presence of extracapsular extension may be less associated with non-SLN metastases than in general.[121,134]

CONCLUSIONS

Nodal micrometastases represent low-volume lymph node involvement, which using the most common current definitions are arbitrarily separated from even lesser nodal involvement termed ITCs. Reports are contradictory on the prognostic impact of micrometastases, but it seems that larger series and longer follow-up are likely to document some prognostic disadvantage for patients with micrometastatic breast cancers as compared to their node-negative counterparts. It is also likely that the volume of the nodal metastatic load is important and that larger micrometastases convey a somewhat worse prognosis than smaller ones. With the introduction of SLNB in the axillary staging of breast carcinoma, micrometastases are more commonly found and this gives an opportunity to study their prognostic impact. Some recent studies have already documented survival disadvantages even with ITCs. SLNB also offers a tool for the selective treatment of the axilla. While it is largely accepted that SLN-negative patients do not require further axillary treatment, the therapeutic consequences of finding ITCs and micrometastases in the axillary SLNs are controversial and under intensive investigation. It is likely that the presence of ITCs does not mandate further axillary intervention and a large majority of patients with micrometastatic SLNs will also fall into this category. At least a number of them may be predictable with reasonable accuracy on the basis of clinical and pathological findings. However, care should be taken when interpreting results relating to micrometastases and ITC. The methods of lymph node evaluation are different from institution to institution,[11] and a less detailed histological assessment may not only result in more metastases remaining occult but may also underestimate the size of a metastasis by labeling larger metastases as micrometastasis. The distinction between micrometastases and ITCs is also suboptimal[18–20] (R Turner, personal communication) and this may also somewhat bias the results.

Whether one should look for micrometastases or ITCs is dependent on several factors, including the resources available. Although it was previously acknowledged that micrometastases might be of prognostic value, it has been suggested that their impact is not a major one. Also the importance of nodal status in determining systemic treatment has changed.[84,85] These factors could be taken as being against the need to search for micrometastases. On the other hand, there is evidence that micrometastases are associated with an overall risk of non-SLN metastasis in the range of 10–15%, and therefore further axillary treatment may be indicated in every seventh to tenth patient harboring micrometastasis in her/his axillary SLN. This may be interpreted as an argument in favor of looking for micrometastases. Taking into account other factors that bear on the risk of non-SLN positivity, such as a low ratio of involved/removed SLNs, small tumor size and the lack of LVI, the risk of having non-SLN involvement may be so minimal that looking for micrometastases is not worthwhile. Removing a micrometastatic SLN and not identifying the micrometastasis in it is probably acceptable in most cases where the predictive profile of non-SLN involvement is otherwise favorable.[135] In contrast, with an unfavorable predictive profile, the risk of non-SLN involvement associated with micrometastases may be >15%, and this is an important point to make.

Therefore, searching for micrometastases should be weighed against several factors, such as the patient perception of an acceptable risk of having axillary residual disease, other factors influencing the risk of non-SLN positivity, and available resources. The European guidelines relating to the histopathological assessment of SLNs require all macrometastases to be identified in SLNs, and suggest that the identification of all micrometastases would be optimal.[136] The first approach would be met by assessing levels separated by 1 mm, whereas the other would require step sectioning at 150–250 μm.[136,137] According to these guidelines, IHC is not mandatory in the evaluation of SLNs, but it is also not discouraged as it can make the recognition of micrometastases easier.[136] The guidelines of the German Senologic Society seem a reasonable compromise between these two options of nodal examination by advocating the examination of the whole SLN at levels separated by 500 μm.[138] Adherence to guidelines recommending a consistent and systematic examination of the SLNs can make the accuracy of nodal staging

(and the rate of missed occult metastases) comparable between laboratories and the therapy-related recommendations more uniform. In contrast, lack of a systematic sampling will fail to give similar levels of accuracy as it will allow metastases of different sizes (depending on the thickness of the tissue block left unsampled) to remain occult.

Concerning the identification of ITCs, no histopathological protocol, other than the IHC-aided investigation of the whole SLN at steps not larger than the smallest dimension of the actual tumor cell, would be able to exclude nodal involvement by such a low tumor volume, and this is well over the acceptable compromise any laboratory can make.[139,140] As a consequence, it should be remembered that the pN0(i+) symbol reflects the identification of ITCs within a lymph node, but the failure to identify, i.e. the pN0(i−), does not necessarily mean that the lymph node does not harbor such a small volume of secondary tumor.[47,140] Depending on the size of the metastasis which the histological protocol targets, and the protocol itself, a similar statement can also be made for micrometastases. Since no histopathological protocol can aim at identifying all ITCs, it may be envisaged that molecular methods would be a better approach. However, RT-PCR assays, although very sensitive, fail to be specific enough[20,29] and are not recommended for routine practice.[30,136] It can therefore be concluded that the prognostic and predictive impact of ITCs is at most controversial and obscured by interpretation problems. As a consequence, it is not recommended to search for ITCs, but it is recommended to report them whenever they are found. Although not supported by all publications (see Tables 6.1 and 6.2), at present, ignoring ITCs for therapeutic planning is a reasonable approach, and reflects published guidelines and consensus statements.[5,6,13,30,136]

To avoid confusion of the data for prospective analysis (and also for decisions stemming from the pathological findings), whenever micrometastases or ITCs are found in a lymph node, care should be taken to exclude larger size nodal involvement by examining deeper layers of the tissue block. Reporting the greatest dimension of the largest metastasis is an advisable, reasonable and practical approach to estimate the metastatic volume. Such an approach will hopefully help in clarifying the predictive and prognostic impact of low-volume nodal involvement, which is somewhat obscured by the diversity of the available data.

REFERENCES

1. Huvos AG, Hutter RVP, Berg JW. Significance of axillary macrometastases and micrometastases in mammary cancer. Ann Surg 1971; 173: 44–6.

2. Saphir O, Amromin GD. Obscure axillary lymph node metastasis in carcinoma of the breast. Cancer 1948; 1: 238–41.

3. Pickren JW. Significance of occult metastases. A study of breast cancer. Cancer 1961; 14: 1266–71.

4. Cserni G. Surgical pathological staging of breast cancer by sentinel lymph node biopsy with special emphasis on the histological work-up of axillary sentinel lymph nodes. Breast Cancer 2004; 11: 242–9.

5. Sobin LH, Wittekind Ch, eds. UICC TNM Classification of Malignant Tumours, 6th edn. New York: John Wiley and Sons, 2002.

6. Greene FL, Page DL, Morrow M et al, eds. AJCC Cancer Staging Manual, 6th edn. New York: Springer, 2002.

7. Sachdev U, Murphy K, Derzie A et al. Predictors of nonsentinel lymph node metastasis in breast cancer patients. Am J Surg 2002; 183: 213–17.

8. Chua B, Ung O, Taylor R et al. Frequency and predictors of axillary lymph node metastases in invasive breast cancer. ANZ J Surg 2001; 71: 723–8.

9. Hartveit F, Lilleng PK. Breast cancer: two micrometastatic variants in the axilla that differ in prognosis. Histopathology 1996; 28: 241–6.

10. Rahusen FD, Torrenga H, van Diest PJ et al. Predictive factors for metastatic involvement of nonsentinel nodes in patients with breast cancer. Arch Surg 2001; 136: 1059–63.

11. Cserni G, Amendoeira I, Apostolikas N et al. Discrepancies in current practice of pathological evaluation of sentinel lymph nodes in breast cancer. Results of a questionnaire based survey by the European Working Group for Breast Screening Pathology. J Clin Pathol 2004; 57: 695–701.

12. Hermanek P, Hutter RV, Sobin LH et al. International Union Against Cancer. Classification of isolated tumor cells and micrometastasis. Cancer 1999; 86: 2668–73.

13. Schwartz GF, Giuliano AE, Veronesi U et al. Proceedings of the consensus conference on the role of sentinel lymph node biopsy in carcinoma of the breast, April 19–22, 2001, Philadelphia, Pennsylvania. Cancer 2002; 94: 2542–51.

14. Querzoli P, Pedriali M, Rinaldi R et al. Axillary lymph node nanometastases are prognostic factors for disease-free survival and metastatic relapse in breast cancer patients. Clin Cancer Res 2006; 12: 6696–701.

15. Singletary SE, Greene FL, Sobin LH. Classification of isolated tumor cells: clarification of the 6th edition of the American Joint Committee on Cancer Staging Manual. Cancer 2003; 98: 2740–1.

16. Singletary SE, Connolly JL. Breast cancer staging: working with the sixth edition of the AJCC Cancer Staging Manual. CA Cancer J Clin 2006; 56: 37–47.

17. Ellis IO, Pinder SE, Bobrow L et al. Pathology reporting of breast disease. NHS Publication No 58. Sheffield: NHS Cancer Screening Programmes and the Royal College of Pathologists, 2005. http:// www. cancerscreening.nhs.uk/breastscreen/publications/ nhsbsp58-low-resolution.pdf (last viewed 12 July 2007).

18. Cserni G, Bianchi S, Boecker W et al. Improving the reproducibility of diagnosing micrometastases and isolated tumor cells. Cancer 2005; 103: 358–67.

19. Cserni G, Sapino A, Decker T. Discriminating between micrometastases and isolated tumor cells in a regional and institutional setting. Breast 2006; 15: 347–54.

20. Lebeau A, Cserni G, Dietel M et al. Pathological examination of sentinel lymph nodes: Work-up – Interpretation-Clinical implications. Breast Care 2007; 2: 102–8.

21. Giuliano AE, Kelemen PR. Sophisticated techniques detect obscure lymph node metastases in carcinoma of the breast. Cancer 1998; 83: 391–3.

22. Linden MD, Zarbo RJ. Cytokeratin immunostaining patterns of benign, reactive lymph nodes: applications for the evaluation of sentinel lymph node specimen. Appl Immunohistochem Mol Morphol 2001; 9: 297–301.

23. Xu X, Roberts SA, Pasha TL et al. Undesirable cytokeratin immunoreactivity of native nonepithelial cells in sentinel lymph nodes from patients with breast carcinoma. Arch Pathol Lab Med 2000; 124: 1310–13.

24. Maiorano E, Mazzarol GM, Pruneri G et al. Ectopic breast tissue as a possible cause of false-positive axillary sentinel lymph node biopsies. Am J Surg Pathol 2003; 27: 513–18.

25. Bleiweiss IJ, Nagi CS, Jaffer S. Axillary sentinel lymph nodes can be falsely positive due to iatrogenic displacement and transport of benign epithelial cells in patients with breast carcinoma. J Clin Oncol 2006; 24: 2013–18.

26. Cserni G. Pathological evaluation of sentinel lymph nodes. Surg Oncol Clin North Am 2007; 16: 17–34.

27. Wittekind C, Greene FL, Henson DE et al, eds. TNM Supplement: A Commentary on Uniform Use, 3rd edn. New York: John Wiley and Sons, Inc., 2003: 7.

28. Giuliano AE, Dale PS, Turner RR et al. Improved axillary staging of breast cancer with sentinel lymphadenectomy. Ann Surg 1995; 180: 700–4.

29. Cserni G, Amendoeira I, Apostolikas N et al. Pathological work-up of sentinel lymph nodes in breast cancer. Review of current data to be considered for the formulation of guidelines. Eur J Cancer 2003; 39: 1654–67.

30. Cserni G. Histopathologic examination of the sentinel lymph nodes. Breast J 2006; 12 (Suppl 2): S152–S156.

31. Viale G, Bosari S, Mazzarol G et al. Intraoperative examination of axillary sentinel lymph nodes in breast carcinoma patients. Cancer 1999; 85: 2433–8.

32. Farshid G, Pradhan M, Kollias J et al. Computer simulations of lymph node metastasis for optimizing the pathologic examination of sentinel lymph nodes in patients with breast carcinoma. Cancer 2000; 89: 2527–37.

33. Cserni G. Complete step sectioning of axillary sentinel lymph nodes in patients with breast cancer. Analysis of two different step sectioning and immunohistochemistry protocols in 246 patients. J Clin Pathol 2002; 55: 926–31.

34. Wells CA, Heryet A, Brochier J et al. The immunocytochemical detection of axillary micrometastases in breast cancer. Br J Cancer 1984; 50: 193–7.

35. Bussolati G, Gugliotta P, Morra I et al. The immunohistochemical detection of lymph node metastases from infiltrating lobular carcinoma of the breast. Br J Cancer 1986; 54: 631–6.

36. Trojani M, de Mascarel I, Bonichon F et al. Micrometastases to axillary lymph nodes from carcinoma of breast: detection by immunohistochemistry and prognostic significance. Br J Cancer 1987; 55: 303–6.

37. Cserni G, Bianchi S, Vezzosi V et al. The value of cytokeratin immunohistochemistry in the evaluation of axillary sentinel lymph nodes in patients with lobular breast carcinoma. J Clin Pathol 2006; 59: 518–22.

38. Mesker WE, Torrenga H, Sloos WC et al. Supervised automated microscopy increases sensitivity and efficiency of detection of sentinel node micrometastases in patients with breast cancer. J Clin Pathol 2004; 57: 960–4.

39. Weaver DL, Krag DN, Manna EA et al. Detection of occult sentinel lymph node micrometastases by immunohistochemistry in breast cancer. An NSABP protocol B-32 quality assurance study. Cancer 2006; 107: 661–7.

40. Diaz LK, Wiley EL, Venta LA. Are malignant cells displaced by large-gauge needle core biopsy of the breast? Am J Roentgenol 1999; 173: 1303–13.

41. Hansen NM, Ye X, Grube BJ et al. Manipulation of the primary breast tumor and the incidence of sentinel node metastases from breast cancer. Arch Surg 2004; 139: 634–40.

42. Cserni G. Metastases in axillary sentinel lymph nodes in breast cancer as detected by intensive histopathological work-up. J Clin Pathol 1999; 52: 922–4.

43. Cserni G. Mapping metastases in sentinel lymph nodes of breast cancer. Am J Clin Pathol 2000; 113: 351–4.

44. Diaz LK, Hunt K, Ames F et al. Histologic localization of sentinel lymph node metastases in breast cancer. Am J Surg Pathol 2003; 27: 385–9.

45. Weaver DL. Pathological evaluation of sentinel lymph nodes in breast cancer: a practical academic perspective from America. Histopathology 2005; 46: 702–6.

46. Leers MP, Schoffelen RH, Hoop JG et al. Multiparameter flow cytometry as a tool for the detection of micrometastatic tumour cells in the sentinel lymph node procedure of patients with breast cancer. J Clin Pathol 2002; 55: 359–66.

47. Cserni G. What is a positive sentinel lymph node in a breast cancer patient? A practical approach. Breast 2007; 16: 152–60.

48. Viale G, Mastropasqua MG, Maiorano E et al. Pathologic examination of the axillary sentinel lymph nodes in patients with early-stage breast carcinoma: current and resolving controversies on the basis of the European Institute of Oncology experience. Virchows Arch 2006; 448: 241–7.

49. Weigelt B, Verduijn P, Bosma AJ et al. Detection of metastases in sentinel lymph nodes of breast cancer patients by multiple mRNA markers. Br J Cancer 2004; 90: 531–7.

50. Smith PA, Harlow SP, Krag DN et al. Submission of lymph node tissue for ancillary studies decreases the accuracy of conventional breast cancer axillary node staging. Mod Pathol 1999; 12: 781–5.

51. Bolster MJ, Bult P, Schapers RF et al. Differences in sentinel lymph node pathology protocols lead to differences in surgical strategy in breast cancer patients. Ann Surg Oncol 2006; 13: 1466–73.

52. Nemoto T, Vana J, Bedwani RN et al. Management and survival of female breast cancer: results of a national survey by the American College of Surgeons. Cancer 1980; 45: 2917–24.

53. Vinh-Hung V, Burzykowski T, Cserni G et al. Functional form of the effect of the numbers of axillary nodes on survival in early breast cancer. Int J Oncol 2003; 22: 697–704.

54. Vinh-Hung V, Verschraegen C, Promish DI et al. Ratios of involved nodes in early breast cancer. Breast Cancer Res 2004; 6: R680–R688.

55. Woodward WA, Vinh-Hung V, Ueno NT et al. Prognostic value of nodal ratios in node-positive breast cancer. J Clin Oncol 2006; 24: 2910–16.

56. Kuijt GP, Voogd AC, van de Poll-Franse LV et al. The prognostic significance of axillary lymph-node micrometastases in breast cancer patients. Eur J Surg Oncol 2005; 31: 500–5.

57. Fisher ER, Swamidoss S, Lee CH et al. Detection and significance of occult axillary node metastases in patients with invasive breast cancer. Cancer 1978; 42: 2025–31.

58. Fisher ER, Palekar A, Rockette H et al. Pathologic findings from the National Surgical Adjuvant Breast

Project (protocol No. 4). V. Significance of axillary nodal micro- and macrometastases. Cancer 1978; 42: 2032–8.

59. Rosen PP, Saigo P, Weathers E et al. Axillary micro- and macrometastases in breast cancer: prognostic significance of tumor size. Ann Surg 1981; 194: 585–91.

60. Wilkinson EJ, Hause LL, Hoffman RG et al. Occult axillary lymph node metastases in invasive breast carcinoma: characteristics of the primary tumor and significance of the metastases. Pathol Ann 1982; 17: 67–91.

61. Trojani M, Mascarel ID, Bonichon F et al. Micrometastases to axillary lymph nodes from carcinoma of breast: detection by immunohistochemistry and prognostic significance. Br J Cancer 1987; 55: 303–6.

62. Friedman S, Bertin F, Mouriesse H et al. Importance of tumor cells in axillary node sinus margins ('clandestine' metastases) discovered by serial sectioning in operable breast carcinoma. Acta Oncol 1988; 27: 483–7.

63. Sedmak D, Meineke T, Knechtges D et al. Prognostic significance of cytokeratin-positive breast cancer metastases. Mod Pathol 1989; 2: 516–20.

64. International Breast Cancer Study Group. Prognostic importance of occult axillary lymph node micrometastases from breast cancers. Lancet 1990; 335: 1565–8.

65. Galea M, Athanassiou E, Bell J et al. Occult regional lymph node metastases from breast carcinoma: immunohistochemical detection with antibodies CAM 5.2 and NCRC-11. J Pathol 1991; 165: 221–7.

66. De Mascarel I, Bonichon F, Coindre J et al. Prognostic significance of breast cancer axillary lymph node micrometastases assessed by two special techniques: reevaluation with longer follow-up. Br J Cancer 1992; 66: 523–7.

67. Hainsworth PJ, Tjandra JJ, Stillwell RG et al. Detection and significance of occult metastases in node-negative breast cancer. Br J Surg 1993; 80: 459–63.

68. Nasser IA, Lee AKC, Bosari S et al. Occult axillary lymph node metastases in 'node-negative' breast carcinoma. Hum Pathol 1993; 24: 950–7.

69. McGuckin MA, Cummings MC, Walsh MD et al. Occult axillary node metastases in breast cancer: their detection and prognostic significance. Br J Cancer 1996; 73: 88–95.

70. Clare SE, Sener SF, Wilkens W et al. Prognostic significance of occult lymph node metastases in node-negative breast cancer. Ann Surg Oncol 1997; 4: 447–51.

71. Cote RJ, Peterson HF, Chaiwun B et al. Role of immunohistochemical detection of lymph-node metastases in management of breast cancer. Lancet 1999; 354: 896–900.

72. Colpaert C, Vermeulen P, Jeuris W et al. Early distant relapse in 'node-negative' breast cancer patients is not predicted by occult axillary lymph node metastases, but by features of the primary tumour. J Pathol 2001; 193: 442–9.

73. Millis RR, Springall R, Lee AHS et al. Occult axillary lymph node metastases are of no prognostic significance in breast cancer. Br J Cancer 2002; 86: 396–401.

74. Mullenix PS, Brown TA, Meyers MO et al. The association of cytokeratin-only-positive sentinel lymph nodes and subsequent metastases in breast cancer. Am J Surg 2005; 189: 606–9.

75. Colleoni M, Rotmensz N, Peruzzotti G et al. Size of breast cancer metastases in axillary lymph nodes: clinical relevance of minimal lymph node involvement. J Clin Oncol 2005; 23: 1379–89.

76. Imoto S, Ochiai A, Okumura C et al. Impact of isolated tumor cells in sentinel lymph nodes detected by immunohistochemical staining. Eur J Surg Oncol 2006; 32: 1175–9.

77. Nagashima T, Sakakibara M, Nakano S et al. Sentinel node micrometastasis and distant failure in breast cancer patients. Breast Cancer 2006; 13: 186–91.

78. Dowlatshahi K, Fan M, Snider HC, Habib FA. Lymph node micrometastases from breast carcinoma. Reviewing the dilemma. Cancer 1997; 80: 1188–97.

79. Sakorafas GH, Geraghty J, Pavlakis G. The clinical significance of axillary lymph node micrometastases in breast cancer. Eur J Surg Oncol 2004; 30: 807–16.

80. Tai P, Yu E, Cserni G et al. Minimum follow-up time required for the estimation of statistical cure of cancer patients: verification using data from 42 cancer sites in the SEER database. BMC Cancer 2005; 5(1): 48.

81. Ramaswamy S, Ross KN, Lander ES et al. A molecular signature of metastasis in primary solid tumors. Nat Genet 2003; 33: 49–54.

82. Weigelt B, Hu Z, He X et al. Molecular portraits and 70-gene prognosis signature are preserved throughout the metastatic process of breast cancer. Cancer Res 2005; 65: 9155–8.

83. Feinstein AR, Sosin DM, Wells CK. The Will Rogers phenomenon. Stage migration and new diagnostic techniques as a source of misleading statistics for survival in cancer. N Engl J Med 1985; 312: 1604–8.

84. Goldhirsch A, Glick JH, Gelber RD et al. Meeting highlights: international expert consensus on the primary therapy of early breast cancer 2005. Ann Oncol 2005; 16: 1569–83.

85. Costa SD, Bischoff J. ...and the winner is: the individualized therapy. Breast Care 2007; 2: 126–9.

86. Turner RR, Ollila DW, Krasne DL et al. Histopathologic validation of the sentinel lymph node hypothesis for breast carcinoma. Ann Surg 1997; 226: 271–6.

87. Czerniecki BJ, Scheff AM, Callans LS et al. Immunohistochemistry with pancytokeratins improves the sensitivity of sentinel lymph node biopsy in patients with breast carcinoma. Cancer 1999; 85: 1098–103.

88. Weaver DL, Krag DN, Ashikaga T et al. Pathologic analysis of sentinel and nonsentinel lymph nodes in breast carcinoma. Cancer 2000; 88: 1099–107.

89. Sabel MS, Zhang P, Barnwell JM et al. Accuracy of sentinel node biopsy in predicting nodal status in patients with breast carcinoma. J Surg Oncol 2001; 77: 243–6.

90. Stitzenberg KB, Calvo BF, Iacocca MV et al. Cytokeratin immunohistochemical validation of the sentinel node hypothesis in patients with breast cancer. Am J Clin Pathol 2002; 117: 729–37.

91. Mikhitarian K, Martin RH, Mitas M et al. Molecular analysis improves sensitivity of breast sentinel lymph node biopsy: results of a multi-institutional prospective cohort study. Surgery 2005; 138: 474–81.

92. Degnim AC, Griffith KA, Sabel MS et al. Clinicopathologic features of metastasis in nonsentinel lymph nodes of breast carcinoma patients. Cancer 2003; 98: 2307–15.

93. Reynolds C, Mick R, Donohue JH et al. Sentinel lymph node biopsy with metastasis: can axillary dissection be avoided in some patients with breast cancer? J Clin Oncol 1999; 17: 1720–6.

94. Wong SL, Edwards MJ, Chao C et al. Predicting the status of the nonsentinel axillary nodes. A multicenter study. Arch Surg 2001; 136: 563–8.

95. Marin C, Mathelin C, Neuville A et al. Sentinel lymph node biopsy with micrometastases in breast cancer. Histological data and surgical implications. Bull Cancer 2003; 90: 459–65.

96. Rutledge H, Davis J, Chiu R et al. Sentinel node micrometastasis in breast carcinoma may not be an indication for complete axillary dissection. Mod Pathol 2005; 18: 762–8.

97. Hwang RF, Krishnamurthy S, Hunt KK et al. Clinicopathologic factors predicting involvement of nonsentinel axillary nodes in women with breast cancer. Ann Surg Oncol 2003; 10: 248–54.

98. den Bakker MA, van Weeszenberg A, de Kantep AY et al. Non-sentinel lymph node involvement in patients with breast cancer and sentinel node micrometastasis; too early to abandon axillary clearance. J Clin Pathol 2002; 55: 932–5.

99. Abdessalam SF, Zervos EE, Prasad M et al. Predictors of positive axillary lymph nodes after sentinel lymph node biopsy in breast cancer. Am J Surg 2001; 182: 316–20.

100. Fréneaux P, Nos C, Vincent-Salomon A et al. Histological detection of minimal metastatic involvement in axillary sentinel nodes: a rational basis for a sensitive methodology usable in daily practice. Mod Pathol 2002; 15: 641–6.

101. Zgajnar J, Besic N, Podkrajsek M et al. Minimal risk of macrometastases in the non-sentinel axillary lymph nodes in breast cancer patients with micrometastatic sentinel lymph nodes and preoperatively ultrasonically uninvolved axillary lymph nodes. Eur J Cancer 2005; 41: 244–8.

102. Cserni G, Burzykowski T, Vinh-Hung V et al. Axillary sentinel node and tumour-related factors associated with non-sentinel node involvement in breast cancer. Jpn J Clin Oncol 2004; 34: 519–24.

103. Kamath VJ, Giuliano R, Dauway E et al. Characteristics of the sentinel lymph node in breast cancer predict further involvement of higher-echelon nodes in the axilla. Arch Surg 2001; 136: 688–92.

104. Carcoforo P, Maestroni U, Querzoli P et al. Primary breast cancer features can predict additional lymph node involvement in patients with sentinel node micrometastases. World J Surg 2006; 30: 1653–7.

105. Calhoun KE, Hansen NM, Turner RR et al. Nonsentinel node metastases in breast cancer patients with isolated tumor cells in the sentinel node: implications for completion axillary node dissection. Am J Surg 2005; 190: 588–91.

106. Menes TS, Tartter PI, Mizrachi H et al. Breast cancer patients with pN0(i+) and pN1(mi) sentinel nodes have high rate of nonsentinel node metastases. J Am Coll Surg 2005; 200: 323–7.

107. Jakub JW, Diaz NM, Ebert MD et al. Completion axillary lymph node dissection minimizes the likelihood of false negatives for patients with invasive breast carcinoma and cytokeratin positive only sentinel lymph nodes. Am J Surg 2002; 184: 302–6.

108. Krauth JS, Charitansky H, Isaac S et al. Clinical implications of axillary sentinel lymph node 'micrometastases' in breast cancer. Eur J Surg Oncol 2006; 32: 400–4.

109. Di Tommaso L, Arizzi C, Rahal D et al. Anatomic location of breast cancer micrometastasis in sentinel lymph node predicts axillary status. Ann Surg 2006; 243: 706–7.

110. Mignotte H, Treilleux I, Faure C et al. Axillary lymph-node dissection for positive sentinel nodes in breast cancer patients. Eur J Surg Oncol 2002; 28: 623–6.

111. Leidenius MH, Vironen JH, Riihela MS et al. The prevalence of non-sentinel node metastases in breast cancer patients with sentinel node micrometastases. Eur J Surg Oncol 2005; 31: 13–18.

112. Turner RR, Chu KU, Qi K et al. Pathologic features associated with nonsentinel lymph node metastases in patients with breast carcinoma in a sentinel lymph node. Cancer 2000; 89: 574–81.

113. Weiser MR, Montgomery LL, Tan LK et al. Lymphovascular invasion enhances the prediction of non-sentinel node metastases in breast cancer patients with positive sentinel nodes. Ann Surg Oncol 2001; 8: 145–9.

114. Viale G, Maiorano E, Mazzarol G et al. Histologic detection and clinical implications of micrometastases in axillary sentinel lymph nodes for patients with breast carcinoma. Cancer 2001; 92: 1378–84.

115. Schrenk P, Konstantiniuk P, Wolfl S et al. Prediction of non-sentinel lymph node status in breast cancer with a micrometastatic sentinel node. Br J Surg 2005; 92: 707–13.

116. Houvenaeghel G, Nos C, Mignotte H et al. Micrometastases in sentinel lymph node in a multicentric study: predictive factors of nonsentinel lymph node involvement. J Clin Oncol 2006; 24: 1814–22.

117. Cserni G, Gregori D, Merletti F et al. Meta-analysis of non-sentinel node metastases associated with micrometastatic sentinel nodes in breast cancer. Br J Surg 2004; 91: 1245–52.

118. Cserni G. Sentinel lymph-node biopsy-based prediction of further breast cancer metastases in the axilla. Eur J Surg Oncol 2001; 27: 532–8.

119. Cserni G, Bianchi S, Vezzosi V et al. Sentinel lymph node biopsy in staging small (up to 15 mm) breast carcinomas. Results from a European multi-institutional study. Pathol Oncol Res 2007; 13: 5–14.

120. Van Deurzen CH, Hobbelink MG, van Hillegersberg R et al. Is there an indication for sentinel node biopsy in patients with ductal carcinoma in situ of the breast? A review. Eur J Cancer 2007; 43: 993–1001.

121. Cserni G, Bianchi S, Vezzosi V et al. Sentinel lymph node biopsy and non-sentinel node involvement in special type breast carcinomas with a good prognosis. Eur J Cancer 2007; 43: 1407–14.

122. Van Zee KJ, Manasseh DM, Bevilacqua JL et al. A nomogram for predicting the likelihood of additional nodal metastases in breast cancer patients with a positive sentinel node biopsy. Ann Surg Oncol 2003; 10: 1140–51.

123. Degnim AC, Reynolds C, Pantvaidya G et al. Nonsentinel node metastasis in breast cancer patients: assessment of an existing and a new predictive nomogram. Am J Surg 2005; 190: 543–50.

124. Barranger E, Coutant C, Flahault A et al. An axilla scoring system to predict non-sentinel lymph node status in breast cancer patients with sentinel lymph node involvement. Breast Cancer Res Treat 2005; 91: 113–19.

125. Chagpar AB, Scoggins CR, Martin RC 2nd et al. Prediction of sentinel lymph node-only disease in women with invasive breast cancer. Am J Surg 2006; 192: 882–7.

126. Farshid G, Pradhan M, Kollias J et al. A decision aid for predicting non-sentinel node involvement in women with breast cancer and at least one positive sentinel node. Breast 2004; 13: 494–501.

127. Dauphine CE, Haukoos JS, Vargas MP et al. Evaluation of three scoring systems predicting nonsentinel node metastasis in breast cancer patients with a positive sentinel node biopsy. Ann Surg Oncol 2007; 14: 1014–19.

128. Cserni G. Comparison of different validation studies on the use of the Memorial-Sloan Kettering Cancer Center nomogram predicting nonsentinel node involvement in sentinel node positive breast cancer patients. Am J Surg 2007; 194: 699–700.

129. Cserni G, Bianchi S, Vezzosi V et al. Validation of clinical prediction rules for a low probability of nonsentinel and extensive lymph node involvement in breast cancer patients. Am J Surg 2007; 194: 288–93.

130. Alran S, De Rycke Y, Fourchotte V et al. Validation and limitations of use of a breast cancer nomogram predicting the likelihood of non-sentinel node involvement after positive sentinel node biopsy. Ann Surg Oncol 2007 Feb 9 (e-pub ahead of print).

131. Palamba HW, Rombouts MC, Ruers TJ et al. Extranodal extension of axillary metastasis of invasive breast carcinoma as a possible predictor for the total number of positive lymph nodes. Eur J Surg Oncol 2001; 27: 719–22.

132. Stitzenberg KB, Meyer AA, Stern SL et al. Extracapsular extension of the sentinel lymph node metastasis: a predictor of nonsentinel node tumor burden. Ann Surg 2003; 237: 607–13.

133. Goyal A, Douglas-Jones AG, Newcombe RG et al. Effect of lymphatic tumor burden on sentinel lymph node biopsy in breast cancer. Breast J 2005; 11: 188–94.

134. Cserni G. Axillary sentinel lymph node micrometastases with extracapsular extension: a distinct pattern of breast cancer metastasis? J Clin Pathol 2007 Apr 27 (e-pub ahead of print).

135. Cserni G. The potential therapeutic effect of sentinel lymphadenectomy. Eur J Surg Oncol 2002; 28: 689–91.

136. Perry N, Broeders M, de Wolf C et al, eds. European Guidelines for Breast Screening and Diagnosis, 4th edn. Luxemburg: European Communities, 2006.

137. Cserni G. A model for determining the optimum histology of sentinel lymph nodes in breast cancer. J Clin Pathol 2004; 57: 467–71.

138. Kuehn T, Bembenek A, Decker T et al. A concept for the clinical implementation of sentinel lymph node biopsy in patients with breast carcinoma with special regard to quality assurance. Cancer 2005; 103: 451–61.

139. Van Diest PJ. Histopathological workup of sentinel lymph nodes: how much is enough? J Clin Pathol 1999; 52: 871–3.

140. Weaver DL. Sentinel lymph nodes and breast carcinoma: which micrometastases are clinically significant? Am J Surg Pathol 2003; 27: 842–5.

7

Detection of minimal residual disease in predicting outcome

Volkmar Müller, Catherine Alix-Panabières and Klaus Pantel

INTRODUCTION

Metastasis is the main cause of breast cancer-related death. Early tumor cell dissemination occurs even in patients with early breast cancer, and bone marrow (BM) is a common homing organ for blood-borne disseminated tumor cells (DTC) derived from primary breast carcinomas. However, this early spread usually remains undetected even by high-resolution imaging technologies. Sensitive immunocytochemical and molecular assays allow specific detection of "occult" metastatic tumor cells at the single-cell stage, and the detection of systemic tumor cell dissemination in the peripheral blood and BM before the occurrence of incurable overt metastases. Evidence has emerged that the detection of DTC and circulating tumor cells (CTC) may provide important prognostic information, and in addition might help to monitor efficacy of therapy. Many studies have been also published on the detection of DTC in lymph nodes (see Chapter 6).[1–3] This chapter will focus on the detection, biology and clinical relevance of hematogeneous tumor cell spread, since this seems to be the most crucial step in breast cancer progression.

METHODS FOR THE DETECTION OF DISSEMINATED TUMOR CELLS

Immunocytochemical staining

Several different assays have been developed to detect DTC in breast cancer and other types of carcinomas. One major approach to identify DTC is immunocytochemical staining with monoclonal antibodies against epithelial or tumor-associated antigens.[4–7] To date, cytokeratins have become the most widely accepted protein markers for the detection of epithelial tumor cells in mesenchymal tissues such as BM, blood or lymph nodes.[8–10] However, different staining techniques can result in specificity variations.[11,12] Several international organizations have therefore recognized the need for standardization of the immunocytochemical assay and for its evaluation in prospective studies (see www.dismal-project.eu).[13,14]

Immunocytochemical analysis is usually used in combination with density gradient centrifugation, immunomagnetic procedures or size filtration methods to enrich tumor cells prior to their detection.[15–18] One way to improve current detection assays for single tumor cells is to develop better tumor cell enrichment procedures using improved density gradients[19] and antibody-coupled magnetic particles.[20–22] At present, it is unclear whether these new enrichment techniques provide more clinically relevant information than the standard density gradient procedure used to isolate the mononuclear cell fraction (Figure 7.1).

The use of new automated devices for microscopic screening of immunostained slides may help slides to be read more rapidly and increase reproducibility of the read-out (Figure 7.1).[20,23–27] Among the commercially available automated systems, the CellSearch™ system has gained considerable attention because it allows an automated immunomagnetic enrichment and cytokeratin staining of blood samples.[28] A recent validation study demonstrated the reproducibility indicating

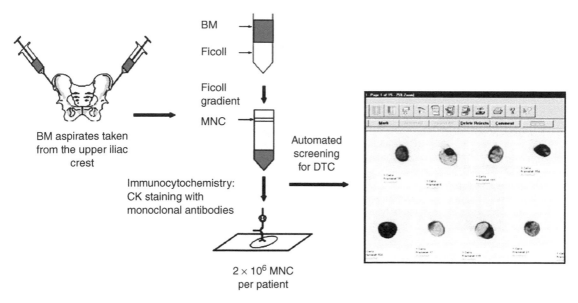

Figure 7.1   Immunocytochemical detection of disseminated tumor cells (DTC) in the bone marrow (BM) of patients with epithelial tumors. The detection process begins with Ficoll density gradient centrifugation to isolate mononuclear cells (MNC) and uses cytokeratin (CK) antibodies. The detection of the stained DTC can be performed automatically and suspect cells are displayed in an image gallery.

that multicenter studies with shipment of samples are possible.[29]

Polymerase chain reaction approach for the detection of disseminated tumor cells

A widely used alternative to immunocytochemical assays for the detection of DTC became molecular detection procedures. In principle, the nucleic acid in a sample can be amplified by polymerase chain reaction (PCR) so that very small numbers of tumor cells can be detected in a heterogeneous population of cells. However, the tumor cells must have changes in DNA or mRNA expression patterns which distinguish them from the surrounding hematopoetic cells. At the DNA level, breast carcinomas are genetically quite heterogeneous, so that there is no universally applicable DNA marker available. Therefore, the main approach to develop molecular diagnostic assays for breast carcinomas has focused on RNA markers. A multimarker approach with a panel of tumor-specific mRNA markers may improve the sensitivity

for the detection of DTC over single marker assays.[30,31]

Up to date, many transcripts have been evaluated as "tumor-specific" markers such as cytokeratins (CK) CK18, CK19 and CK20, mucin-1 (MUC1), and carcinoembryonic antigen.[32] However, many of these transcripts can also be identified by reverse transcription (RT)-PCR in normal BM, blood, and lymph node tissue.[33–35] Preanalytical depletion of the interfering normal cell fraction (e.g. granulocytes which express CK20) and/or quantitative RT-PCR determinations with well-defined cut-off values might solve this problem. In addition, expression of the mRNA marker might be downregulated, which argues in favor of the use of a multimarker RT-PCR approach.[36]

Enzyme-linked immunospot technology

A drawback of both immunocytochemistry and RT-PCR is the fact that these technologies are usually unable to distinguish between viable and apoptotic cells. Recently, a new technique which allows this important

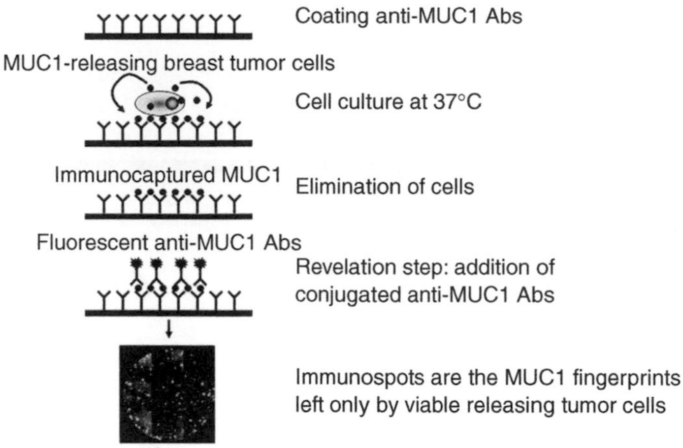

 Coating anti-MUC1 Abs

MUC1-releasing breast tumor cells

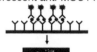 Cell culture at 37°C

Immunocaptured MUC1 Elimination of cells

Fluorescent anti-MUC1 Abs

Revelation step: addition of conjugated anti-MUC1 Abs

Immunospots are the MUC1 fingerprints left only by viable releasing tumor cells

Figure 7.2 Description of the mucin-I (MUC1)-epithelial immunospot (EPISPOT) assay. Plates are coated with anti-MUC1 antibodies (Abs). Next, the cells are seeded in each well and cultured for 48 hours. During this incubation period, the released MUC1 molecules are directly immunocaptured by the Abs on the bottom of the well. The cells are then eliminated and the presence of the released MUC1 protein is revealed by the addition of a second anti-MUC1 antibody conjugated to a fluorochrome.

discrimination was introduced for DTC/CTC analyses.[37] This technique was designated epithelial immunospot (EPISPOT) and is based on the secretion or active release of specific marker proteins using an adaptation of the enzyme-linked immunospot (ELISPOT) technology (Figure 7.2). The EPISPOT assay offers the advantage that only viable tumor cells will be detected and that protein secretion can be detected at an individual cell level.[38] For the detection of breast cancer-derived DTC/CTC, MUC1 and CK19 were used as marker proteins.[39] MUC1-secreting CTC were detected in all metastatic breast cancer patients analyzed, whereas such cells were not observed in healthy controls. Moreover, the enumeration of both MUC1- and CK19-secreting cells allowed the detection of viable DTC in BM of 90% and 54% of breast cancer patients, with and without overt distant metastasis, respectively.[39]

These data demonstrate the high specificity and sensitivity of the new EPISPOT technology, which reveals a unique fingerprint of single viable tumor cells and therefore opens a new avenue in the understanding of the biology of early metastatic spread.

MOLECULAR AND FUNCTIONAL CHARACTERIZATION OF DISSEMINATED TUMOR CELLS

DTC in BM of breast cancer patients have been characterized with immunological double staining to identify biological features which might favor early dissemination. Multiple characterization approaches of DTC in BM show a considerable phenotypic heterogeneity; in particular, the human epidermal growth factor receptor 2 (HER2) proto-oncogene appears to define a very aggressive subset of DTC with an increased invasive capability[40,41] and has gained substantial importance as a biological target for systemic therapy in breast cancer.[42]

It can be demonstrated that the presence of HER2 expressing DTC is also associated with impaired prognosis.[43] Furthermore, there is also some evidence of a prognostic effect of HER2-positive CTCs in stage I–III breast cancer.[44] In addition, most DTC and CTC do not express the proliferation antigen Ki67 and may therefore be resistant to chemotherapy.[45,46]

A detailed molecular description of DTC in BM of breast cancer patients without clinical signs of overt metastases demonstrated that these cells are genetically heterogeneous[47] and lack genomic aberrations observed in arbitrary selected areas of the primary tumors.[48] Thus, DTC may be derived from small subclones within the primary tumor which can be easily missed and/or they may undergo genetic changes after their homing in the BM.

By applying gene expression analysis of primary breast cancers in relation to the presence or absence of DTC in BM, specific gene signatures in primary tumors of patients with DTC in BM were observed.[49] These findings challenge the traditional concept that tumor cells acquire

Table 7.1 Examples of studies examining prognostic relevance of disseminated tumor cells identified by immuno-cytochemistry in bone marrow of breast cancer patients without overt distant metastases (stage M0)

First author (year)	Detection rate (%)	Prognostic value (number of patients)
Schlimok[85] (1987)	18	DDFS (155)
Cote[86] (1991)	37	DFS, OS* (49)
Harbeck[87] (1994)	38	DFS, OS* (100)
Diel[88] (1996)	31	DFS,* OS (727)
Molino[89] (1997)	31	None (109)
Mansi[90] (1999)	25	DFS, OS (350)
Braun[10] (2000)	36	DFS,* OS* (552)
Gebauer[4] (2001)	42	DFS,* OS* (393)
Gerber[6] (2001)	31	DFS,* OS* (484)
Wiedswang[21] (2003)	13	DDFS,* BCSS* (817)
Braun[56] (2005): pooled analysis	31	DDFS,* OS* (4703)

*Confirmed by multivariate analysis.
BCSS, breast cancer-specific survival; DDFS, distant-DFS; DFS, disease-free survival; OS, overall survival.

their metastatic genotype and phenotype late during tumor development, but rather support the alternative concept that tumor cells acquire the genetic changes relevant to their metastatic capacity early in tumorigenesis,[50] so that the metastatic potential of human tumors is encoded in the bulk of a primary tumor.[50,51] This concept could also explain the presence of DTC in BM at early stages of breast cancer.

Numerous studies have shown that BM is a common homing organ for disseminating tumor cells derived from various epithelial tumors, including breast, prostate, lung and colon cancer.[15,52] The properties of primary tumor cells to disseminate to BM are still under investigation and some mechanisms like adhesion molecules or hypoxia have been suggested.[49,53–55]

BIOLOGY OF MINIMAL RESIDUAL DISEASE

Only half of the breast cancer patients with DTC relapse, whereas the other half remain free of overt metastasis over a 10-year follow-up period (Table 7.1).[56] This finding is in line with data from animal models and suggests that a significant fraction of DTC might never develop into overt metastases but might remain in a "dormant" state. However, the persistence of DTC in BM even years after primary treatment is linked to an increased risk of late metastatic relapses in breast cancer.[57] Thus far, little is known about the conditions required for the escape from the dormant or quiescent phase into the dynamic phase of metastasis formation. The steady-state regulating dormancy might be disturbed by both changes in the DTC (e.g. additional mutations) and the surrounding microenvironment (e.g. decrease in immune surveillance or increased angiogenetic potential).[58–60] Among the protein characteristics, expression of the tyrosine kinase receptor HER2 on DTC and CTC appears to be linked to metastatic relapse.[44,61] Thus, HER2-mediated signaling might be important for the transition of DTC from a dormant to an active growth stage.

Recently, the search for breast cancer stem cells has gained increasing attention with the discovery of new stem cell markers and signatures.[39,62–64] It is assumed that breast cancer stem cells especially can disseminate from the primary tumor to distant sites. The significant correlation between the presence of DTC in BM and metastatic relapse[64] suggests that the founder cells of overt metastases might be among those DTC as metastatic stem cells. Furthermore, most DTC/CTC are nonproliferating (i.e. Ki-67-negative) and resistant to chemotherapy,[46,65,66] as postulated for cancer stem cells. Moreover, many DTC have a

CD44[+]CD24[−/low] breast cancer stem cell phenotype,[67,68] and a subpopulation of viable DTC are CK19[+]MUC1[−], also previously suggested as a breast stem cell phenotype.[39] More recently, EpCAM has been identified as a new breast cancer stem cell marker,[64] and this adhesion molecule is expressed on more than 60% of DTC in BM of breast cancer patients.[52]

CLINICAL RELEVANCE OF DISSEMINATED TUMOR CELLS AND CIRCULATING TUMOR CELLS FOR PREDICTING OUTCOME AND MONITORING THERAPY

The prognostic impact of DTC analysis performed at the time of primary surgery was confirmed in a large recent pooled analysis including 4703 patients with a 10-year follow-up.[56] In addition to their use as prognostic factor in breast cancer, monitoring of BM postsurgery (i.e. during and after systemic adjuvant therapy) might be able to provide a unique information for the clinical management of the individual cancer patient (Table 7.1).[57,65,66,69,70] The identification of patients at increased risk for recurrence after completion of adjuvant chemotherapy is an application of high clinical relevance, since these patients might benefit from an additional "second-line" treatment, e.g. bisphosphonates or targeted therapies like anti-HER2 approaches or antiangiogenetic drugs.

Sequential peripheral blood analyses should be more acceptable than BM aspirations and many research groups are currently assessing CTC in clinical studies. Depending on the detection technique used, CTC were revealed in 50–100% of patients with metastatic breast cancer.[15] However, even in patients with no clinical signs of overt metastases, detection rates range from 10% to 60%.[71] In contrast to one report that suggested that CTC are mostly apoptotic,[72] we have recently shown that viable CTC were frequently present both in patients with early and late stage breast cancer.[39]

The clinical relevance of CTC measurements is still under investigation. Detection of CTC with the CellSearch™ system provided significant prognostic information before and also early (4 weeks) after initiation of chemotherapy in patients with measurable metastatic breast cancer,[28] and the prognostic impact of increased CTC numbers was also maintained when repeated examinations during follow-up were performed.[73] Interestingly, CTC determinations seem to be superior over conventional imaging methods for response evaluation.[74] In contrast to patients with metastatic disease, the prognostic relevance of CTC in the blood of patients with early-stage disease without overt metastasis is still under investigation and needs to be demonstrated in prospective multicenter studies.[75] In patients with primary breast cancer, several studies have used RT-PCR based methods and showed a prognostic impact.[76–78]

To date, it is not clear if CTC measurements could replace the examination of BM. Previously, two immunocytochemical studies demonstrated statistically significant correlations between DTC detection in BM and blood, but BM was more frequently positive than blood.[46,79] One possible explanation is that BM is a homing organ for DTC, whereas blood analyses allow only a "snapshot" of tumor cell dissemination. Recently, it was also described that detection of DTC in BM had superior prognostic significance in comparison with CTC measurements in blood, analyzing patients with metastatic and nonmetastatic breast cancer by a quantitative RT-PCR assay for CK19 and mammaglobin mRNAs.[80] In line with this, another report using immunocytochemistry showed that only BM but not blood analyses provided prognostic information.[81] Currently, these findings do not support an exchange of DTC in BM with CTC from blood, but future studies with improved detection technologies may help to clarify this issue.

IDENTIFICATION OF THERAPEUTIC TARGETS ON DISSEMINATED TUMOR CELLS AND CIRCULATING TUMOR CELLS

A striking potential of DTC/CTC could also be to identify therapeutic targets on these cells, which might enable a more individual antimetastatic therapy in cancer patients. CTC/DTC can show properties distinct from the primary tumor and the characterization of these cells could therefore help to select cancer patients for targeted therapies.

In particular, the HER2 oncogene has become the most prominent target for biological therapies in breast cancer and a humanized anti-HER2 monoclonal antibody (trastuzumab) was recently approved by the FDA.[42,82] Currently, all patients are stratified to this targeted therapy by primary tumor analysis only. However, recent reports have shown that HER2-positive DTC and CTC can also be detected in patients with HER2-negative primary tumors.[44,83,84] These findings are consistent with our previous data on the high frequency and prognostic relevance of HER2 expression on DTC in BM[43] and they suggest that additional patients who could benefit from HER2-directed therapies.[83] Ongoing clinical studies will reveal whether the HER2 status of DTC or CTC may predict response to trastuzumab or other HER2-directed therapies.

CONCLUSIONS

Recently reported studies suggest that CTC levels may serve both as a prognostic marker and for early assessment of therapeutic response in patients with metastatic breast cancer. However, in early stage breast cancer, the impact of CTC is less well established than the presence of DTC in BM where several clinical studies demonstrated that such cells are an independent prognostic factor at primary diagnosis.

The characterization of DTC/CTC has shed new light on the complex process underlying early tumor cell dissemination and metastatic progression in cancer patients. Characterization of DTC should help to identify novel targets for biological therapies aimed to prevent metastatic relapse and to monitor the efficacy of these therapies. In addition, understanding tumor "dormancy" and identifying metastatic stem cells might result in the development of new therapeutic concepts.

ACKNOWLEDGMENT

This work was supported by grants from the Ministère de l'Economie des Finances et de l'Industrie (MINEFI); the University Medical Center of Montpellier, France; The Deutsche Forschungsgemeinschaft (PA 341/15-2), Bonn, Germany; and the European Commission (DISMAL-project, contract no. LSHC-CT-2005-018911).

REFERENCES

1. Herbert GS, Sohn VY, Brown TA. The impact of nodal isolated tumor cells on survival of breast cancer patients. Am J Surg 2007; 193(5): 571–3; discussion 3–4.
2. Imoto S, Ochiai A, Okumura C et al. Impact of isolated tumor cells in sentinel lymph nodes detected by immunohistochemical staining. Eur J Surg Oncol 2006; 32(10): 1175–9.
3. Kahn HJ, Hanna WM, Chapman JA et al. Biological significance of occult micrometastases in histologically negative axillary lymph nodes in breast cancer patients using the recent American Joint Committee on Cancer breast cancer staging system. Breast J 2006; 12(4): 294–301.
4. Gebauer G, Fehm T, Merkle E et al. Epithelial cells in bone marrow of breast cancer patients at time of primary surgery: clinical outcome during long-term follow-up. J Clin Oncol 2001; 19(16): 3669–74.
5. Landys K, Persson S, Kovarik J et al. Prognostic value of bone marrow biopsy in operable breast cancer patients at the time of initial diagnosis: results of a 20-year median follow-up. Breast Cancer Res Treat 1998; 49(1): 27–33.
6. Gerber B, Krause A, Muller H et al. Simultaneous immunohistochemical detection of tumor cells in lymph nodes and bone marrow aspirates in breast cancer and its correlation with other prognostic factors. J Clin Oncol 2001; 19(4): 960–71.
7. Pierga JY, Bonneton C, Magdelenat H et al. Real-time quantitative PCR determination of urokinase-type plasminogen activator receptor (uPAR) expression of isolated micrometastatic cells from bone marrow of breast cancer patients. Int J Cancer 2005; 114(2): 291–8.
8. Braun S, Vogl FD, Naume B et al. A pooled analysis of bone marrow micrometastasis in breast cancer. N Engl J Med 2005; 353(8): 793–802.
9. Pantel K, Felber E, Schlimok G. Detection and characterization of residual disease in breast cancer. J Hematother 1994; 3(4): 315–22.
10. Braun S, Pantel K, Muller P et al. Cytokeratin-positive cells in the bone marrow and survival of patients with stage I, II, or III breast cancer. N Engl J Med 2000; 342(8): 525–33.

11. Borgen E, Beiske K, Trachsel S et al. Immunocyto-chemical detection of isolated epithelial cells in bone marrow: non-specific staining and contribution by plasma cells directly reactive to alkaline phosphatase. J Pathol 1998; 185(4): 427–34.

12. Braun S, Pantel K. Micrometastatic bone marrow involvement: detection and prognostic significance. Med Oncol 1999; 16(3): 154–65.

13. Borgen E, Naume B, Nesland JM et al. Standardization of the immunocytochemical detection of cancer cells in BM and blood: I. Establishment of objecive criteria for the evaluation of immunostained cells. Cytometry 1999; 1(5): 377–88.

14. Fehm T, Braun S, Müller V et al. A concept for the standardized detection of disseminated tumor cells in bone marrow of patients with primary breast cancer and its clinical implementation. Cancer 2006; 107(5): 885–92.

15. Zach O, Lutz D. Tumor cell detection in peripheral blood and bone marrow. Curr Opin Oncol 2006; 18(1): 48–56.

16. Paterlini-Brechot P, Benali NL. Circulating tumor cells (CTC) detection: clinical impact and future directions. Cancer Lett 2007; 18(253): 180–204.

17. Pinzani P, Salvadori B, Simi L et al. Isolation by size of epithelial tumor cells in peripheral blood of patients with breast cancer: correlation with real-time reverse transcriptase-polymerase chain reaction results and feasibility of molecular analysis by laser microdissection. Hum Pathol 2006; 37(6): 711–18.

18. Wong NS, Kahn HJ, Zhang L et al. Prognostic significance of circulating tumour cells enumerated after filtration enrichment in early and metastatic breast cancer patients. Breast Cancer Res Treat 2006; 99(1): 63–9.

19. Rosenberg R, Gertler R, Friederichs J et al. Comparison of two density gradient centrifugation systems for the enrichment of disseminated tumor cells in blood. Cytometry 2002; 49(4): 150–8.

20. Witzig TE, Bossy B, Kimlinger T et al. Detection of circulating cytokeratin-positive cells in the blood of breast cancer patients using immunomagnetic enrichment and digital microscopy. Clin Cancer Res 2002; 8(5): 1085–91.

21. Wiedswang G, Borgen E, Karesen R et al. Detection of isolated tumor cells in bone marrow is an independent prognostic factor in breast cancer. J Clin Oncol 2003; 21(18): 3469–78.

22. Woelfle U, Breit E, Zafrakas K et al. Bi-specific immunomagnetic enrichment of micrometastatic tumour cell clusters from bone marrow of cancer patients. J Immunol Methods 2005; 300(1–2): 136–45.

23. Kraeft SK, Ladanyi A, Galiger K et al. Reliable and sensitive identification of occult tumor cells using the improved rare event imaging system. Clin Cancer Res 2004; 10(9): 3020–8.

24. Borgen E, Naume B, Nesland JM et al. Use of automated microscopy for the detection of disseminated tumor cells in bone marrow samples. Cytometry 2001; 46(4): 215–21.

25. Kraeft SK, Sutherland R, Gravelin L et al. Detection and analysis of cancer cells in blood and bone marrow using a rare event imaging system. Clin Cancer Res 2000; 6(2): 434–42.

26. Bauer KD, de la Torre-Bueno J, Diel IJ et al. Reliable and sensitive analysis of occult bone marrow metastases using automated cellular imaging. Clin Cancer Res 2000; 6(9): 3552–9.

27. Mehes G, Luegmayr A, Ambros IM et al. Combined automatic immunological and molecular cytogenetic analysis allows exact identification and quantification of tumor cells in the bone marrow. Clin Cancer Res 2001; 7(7): 1969–75.

28. Cristofanilli M, Budd GT, Ellis MJ et al. Circulating tumor cells, disease progression, and survival in metastatic breast cancer. N Engl J Med 2004; 351(8): 781–91.

29. Riethdorf S, Fritsche H, Müller V et al. Detection of circulating tumor cells in peripheral blood of patients with metastatic breast cancer: a validation study of the CellSearch system. Clin Cancer Res 2007; 13(3): 920–8.

30. Symmans WF, Liu J, Knowles DM et al. Breast cancer heterogeneity: evaluation of clonality in primary and metastatic lesions. Hum Pathol 1995; 26: 210–16.

31. Braun S, Hepp F, Sommer HL et al. Tumor-antigen heterogeneity of disseminated breast cancer cells: implications for immunotherapy of minimal residual disease. Int J Cancer 1999; 84(1): 1–5.

32. Datta YH, Adams PT, Drobyski WR et al. Sensitive detection of occult breast cancer by the reverse-transcriptase polymerase chain reaction. J Clin Oncol 1994; 12(3): 475–82.

33. Zippelius A, Kufer P, Honold G et al. Limitations of reverse-transcriptase polymerase chain reaction analyses for detection of micrometastatic epithelial cancer cells in bone marrow. J Clin Oncol 1997; 15(7): 2701–8.

34. Bostick PJ, Chatterjee S, Chi DD et al. Limitations of specific reverse-transcriptase polymerase chain reaction markers in the detection of metastases in the lymph nodes and blood of breast cancer patients. J Clin Oncol 1998; 16(8): 2632–40.

35. Jung R, Kruger W, Hosch S et al. Specificity of reverse transcriptase polymerase chain reaction assays designed for the detection of circulating cancer cells is influenced by cytokines in vivo and in vitro. Br J Cancer 1998; 78(9): 1194–8.

36. Lankiewicz S, Rivero BG, Bocher O. Quantitative real-time RT-PCR of disseminated tumor cells in combination with immunomagnetic cell enrichment. Mol Biotechnol 2006; 34(1): 15–27.

37. Pantel K, Alix-Panabieres C. The clinical significance of circulating tumor cells. Nat Clin Pract Oncol 2007; 4(2): 62–3.

38. Czerkinsky C, Moldoveanu Z, Mestecky J et al. A novel two colour ELISPOT assay. I. Simultaneous detection of distinct types of antibody-secreting cells. J Immunol Meth 1988; 115(1): 31–7.

39. Alix-Panabières C, Vendrell J-P, Pellé O et al. Detection and characterization of putative metastatic precursor cells in cancer patients. Clin Chem 2007; 53(3): 537–9.

40. Brandt B, Roetger A, Heidl S et al. Isolation of blood-borne epithelium-derived c-erbB-2 oncoprotein-positive clustered cells from the peripheral blood of breast cancer patients. Int J Cancer 1998; 76(6): 824–8.

41. Fehm T, Sagalowsky A, Clifford E et al. Cytogenetic evidence that circulating epithelial cells in patients with carcinoma are malignant. Clin Cancer Res 2002; 8(7): 2073–84.

42. Piccart-Gebhart MJ, Procter M, Leyland-Jones B et al. Trastuzumab after adjuvant chemotherapy in HER2-positive breast cancer. N Engl J Med 2005; 353(16): 1659–72.

43. Braun S, Schlimok G, Heumos I et al. ErbB2 overexpression on occult metastatic cells in bone marrow predicts poor clinical outcome of stage I–III breast cancer patients. Cancer Res 2001; 61: 1890–5.

44. Wülfing P, Borchard J, Buerger H et al. HER2-positive circulating tumor cells indicate poor clinical outcome in stage I to III breast cancer patients. Clin Cancer Res 2006; 12(6): 1715–20.

45. Pantel K, Schlimok G, Braun S et al. Differential expression of proliferation-associated molecules in individual micrometastatic carcinoma cells. J Natl Cancer Inst 1993; 85(17): 1419–24.

46. Müller V, Stahmann N, Riethdorf S et al. Circulating tumor cells in breast cancer: correlation to bone marrow micrometastases, heterogeneous response to systemic therapy and low proliferative activity. Clin Cancer Res 2005; 11(10): 3678–85.

47. Klein CA, Blankenstein TJF, Schmidt-Kittler O et al. Genetic heterogeneity of single disseminated tumour cells in minimal residual cancer. The Lancet 2002; 360: 683–9.

48. Gangnus R, Langer S, Breit E et al. Genomic profiling of viable and proliferative micrometastatic cells from early-stage breast cancer patients. Clin Cancer Res 2004; 10(10): 3457–64.

49. Woelfle U, Cloos J, Sauter G et al. Molecular signature associated with bone marrow micrometastasis in human breast cancer. Cancer Res 2003; 63(18): 5679–84.

50. Bernards R, Weinberg RA. A progression puzzle. Nature 2002; 418: 823.

51. Ramaswamy S, Ross KN, Lander ES et al. A molecular signature of metastasis in primary solid tumors. Nat Genet 2003; 33: 1–6.

52. Pantel K, Brakenhoff RH. Dissecting the metastatic cascade. Nat Rev Cancer 2004; 4: 448–56.

53. Muller A, Homey B, Soto H et al. Involvement of chemokine receptors in breast cancer metastasis. Nature 2001; 410(6824): 50–6.

54. Kaifi JT, Yekebas EF, Schurr P et al. Tumor-cell homing to lymph nodes and bone marrow and CXCR4 expression in esophageal cancer. J Natl Cancer Inst 2005; 97(24): 1840–7.

55. Generali D, Berruti A, Brizzi MP et al. Hypoxia-inducible factor-1alpha expression predicts a poor response to primary chemoendocrine therapy and disease-free survival in primary human breast cancer. Clin Cancer Res 2006; 12(15): 4562–8.

56. Braun S, Vogl FD, Naume B et al. International pooled analysis of prognostic significance of bone marrow micrometastasis in patients with stage I, II, or III breast cancer. N Engl J Med 2005; 353(8): 793–802.

57. Janni W, Rack B, Schindlbeck C et al. The persistence of isolated tumor cells in bone marrow from patients with breast carcinoma predicts an increased risk for recurrence. Cancer 2005; 103(5): 884–91.

58. Naumov GN, Bender E, Zurakowski D et al. A model of human tumor dormancy: an angiogenic switch from the nonangiogenic phenotype. J Natl Cancer Inst 2006; 98(5): 316–25.

59. Meng S, Tripathy D, Frenkel EP et al. Circulating tumor cells in patients with breast cancer dormancy. Clin Cancer Res 2004; 10(24): 8152–62.

60. Marches R, Scheuermann R, Uhr J. Cancer dormancy: from mice to man. Cell Cycle 2006; 5(16): 1772–8.

61. Apostolaki S, Perraki M, Pallis A et al. Circulating HER2 mRNA-positive cells in the peripheral blood of patients with stage I and II breast cancer after the administration of adjuvant chemotherapy: evaluation of their clinical relevance. Ann Oncol 2007; 18(10): 1623–31.

62. Shackleton M, Vaillant F, Simpson KJ et al. Generation of a functional mammary gland from a single stem cell. Nature 2006; 439(7072): 84–8.

63. Clarke MF, Fuller M. Stem cells and cancer: two 1faces of eve. Cell 2006; 124(6): 111–15.

64. Liu R, Wang X, Chen GY et al. The prognostic role of a gene signature from tumorigenic breast-cancer cells. N Engl J Med 2007; 356(3): 217–26.

65. Becker S, Becker-Pergola G, Wallwiener D et al. Detection of cytokeratin-positive cells in the bone marrow of breast cancer patients undergoing adjuvant therapy. Breast Cancer Res Treat 2006; 97(1): 91–6.

66. Becker S, Solomayer E, Becker-Pergola G et al. Primary systemic therapy does not eradicate disseminated tumor cells in breast cancer patients. Breast Cancer Res Treat 2007; 106(2): 239–43.

67. Balic M, Lin H, Young L et al. Most early disseminated cancer cells detected in bone marrow of breast cancer patients have a putative breast cancer stem cell phenotype. Clin Cancer Res 2006; 12(19): 5615–21.

68. Wicha MS. Cancer stem cells and metastasis: lethal seeds. Clin Cancer Res 2006; 12(19): 5606–7.

69. Braun S, Kentenich C, Janni W et al. Lack of effect of adjuvant chemotherapy on the elimination of single dormant tumor cells in bone marrow of high-risk breast cancer patients. J Clin Oncol 2000; 18(1): 80–6.

70. Wiedswang G, Borgen E, Karesen R et al. Isolated tumor cells in bone marrow three years after diagnosis in disease-free breast cancer patients predict unfavorable clinical outcome. Clin Cancer Res 2004; 10(16): 5342–8.

71. Müller V, Hayes D, Pantel K. Recent translational research: circulating tumor cells in breast cancer patients. Breast Can Res 2006; 8: 110.

72. Mehes G, Witt A, Kubista E et al Circulating breast cancer cells are frequently apoptotic. Am J Pathol 2001; 159(1): 17–20.

73. Hayes DF, Cristofanilli M, Budd GT et al. Circulating tumor cells at each follow-up time point during therapy of metastatic breast cancer patients predict progression-free and overall survival. Clin Cancer Res 2006; 12(14): 4218–24.

74. Budd GT, Cristofanilli M, Ellis MJ et al. Circulating tumor cells versus imaging – predicting overall survival in metastatic breast cancer. Clin Cancer Res 2006; 12(21): 6403–9.

75. Cristofanilli M, Mendelsohn J. Circulating tumor cells in breast cancer: advanced tools for "tailored" therapy? Proc Natl Acad Sci USA 2006; 103(46): 17,073–4.

76. Ntoulia M, Stathopoulou A, Ignatiadis M et al. Detection of mammaglobin A-mRNA-positive circulating tumor cells in peripheral blood of patients with operable breast cancer with nested RT-PCR. Clin Biochem 2006; 39(9): 879–87.

77. Xenidis N, Perraki M, Kafousi M et al. Predictive and prognostic value of peripheral blood cytokeratin-19 mRNA-positive cells detected by real-time polymerase chain reaction in node-negative breast cancer patients. J Clin Oncol 2006; 24(23): 3756–62.

78. Quintela-Fandino M, Lopez JM, Hitt R et al. Breast cancer-specific mRNA transcripts presence in peripheral blood after adjuvant chemotherapy predicts poor survival among high-risk breast cancer patients treated with high-dose chemotherapy with peripheral blood stem cell support. J Clin Oncol 2006; 24(22): 3611–18.

79. Pierga JY, Bonneton C, Vincent-Salomon A et al. Clinical significance of immunocytochemical detection of tumor cells using digital microscopy in peripheral blood and bone marrow of breast cancer patients. Clin Cancer Res 2004; 10(4): 1392–400.

80. Benoy IH, Elst H, Philips M et al. Real-time RT-PCR detection of disseminated tumour cells in bone marrow has superior prognostic significance in comparison with circulating tumour cells in patients with breast cancer. Br J Cancer 2006; 94(5): 672–80.

81. Wiedswang G, Borgen E, Schirmer C et al. Comparison of the clinical significance of occult tumor cells in blood and bone marrow in breast cancer. Int J Cancer 2006; 118(8): 2013–19.

82. Romond EH, Perez EA, Bryant J et al. Trastuzumab plus adjuvant chemotherapy for operable HER2-positive breast cancer. N Engl J Med 2005; 353(16): 1673–84.

83. Solomayer EF, Becker S, Pergola-Becker G et al. Comparison of HER2 status between primary tumor and disseminated tumor cells in primary breast cancer patients. Breast Cancer Res Treat 2006; 98(2): 179–84.

84. Meng S, Tripathy D, Shete S et al. uPAR and HER-2 gene status in individual breast cancer cells from blood and tissues. Proc Natl Acad Sci USA 2006; 103(46): 17,361–5.

85. Schlimok G, Funke I, Holzmann B et al. Micrometastatic cancer cells in bone marrow: in vitro detection with anti-cytokeratin and in vivo labeling with anti-17-1A monoclonal antibodies. Proc Natl Acad Sci USA 1987; 84(23): 8672–6.

86. Cote RJ, Rosen PP, Lesser ML et al. Prediction of early relapse in patients with operable breast cancer by detection of occult bone marrow micrometastases. J Clin Oncol 1991; 9(10): 1749–56.

87. Harbeck N, Untch M, Pache L et al. Tumour cell detection in the bone marrow of breast cancer patients at primary therapy: results of a 3-year median follow-up. Br J Cancer 1994; 69(3): 566–71.

88. Diel IJ, Kaufmann M, Costa SD et al. Micrometastatic breast cancer cells in bone marrow at primary surgery: prognostic value in comparison with nodal status. J Natl Cancer Inst 1996; 88(22): 1652–8.

89. Molino A, Pelosi G, Turazza M et al. Bone marrow micrometastases in 109 breast cancer patients: correlations with clinical and pathological features and prognosis. Breast Cancer Res Treat 1997; 42(1): 23–30.

90. Mansi JL, Gogas H, Bliss JM et al. Outcome of primary-breast-cancer patients with micrometastases: a long-term follow-up study. Lancet 1999; 354(9174): 197–202.

Plasma tumor DNA in determining breast cancer behavior

8

Jacqueline A Shaw, Karen Page, Natasha Hava and
R Charles Coombes

INTRODUCTION

Breast cancer is the most common malignancy in women and accounts for 30% of all female cancer.[1] The prevalence of the disease has increased in recent decades in part due to in an increasingly aging population and to increased detection following the introduction of mammographic screening. In addition, Western lifestyle changes have had an impact on established risk factors such as age at menarche, first pregnancy and menopause.[2,3] The introduction of new treatments has led to improved patient survival and so the rate of mortality has not risen as sharply as the prevalence. However, the development of novel and improved strategies for reducing mortality remain a priority. Alternative approaches to breast cancer detection are needed both for developing countries, where the high cost of mammography precludes the use of this approach, and for the detection of premenopausal breast cancer. Accumulating data from studies of tumor-specific alterations in circulating cell-free DNA suggest that analysis of nucleic acids in blood could provide noninvasive tests for diagnosis and monitoring of breast cancers. The aim of this chapter is to review progress in the investigation of the clinical utility of plasma DNA and RNA analysis for determining breast cancer behavior and for early detection of breast cancer.

DETECTION OF DISSEMINATED TUMOR CELLS AND CIRCULATING TUMOR CELLS

Both early diagnosis of breast cancer and identification of metastases can improve the success of breast cancer treatment.[4] Two approaches currently under close scrutiny for diagnostic and prognostic use are detection of disseminated tumor cells (DTCs) and detection of circulating tumor cells (CTCs), as discussed in Chapter 7. Although the risk of invasive bone marrow aspiration has made its routine use for breast cancer screening and follow-up problematic for patients, a number of groups have successfully detected DTCs in the bone marrow in primary breast cancer patients (reviewed by Slade and Coombes[5]). Detection of CTCs in the blood is obviously a much less invasive procedure. Their presence probably reflects a relapse or metastasis; hence, detection of CTCs may be most useful in metastatic disease and for monitoring of the adjuvant situation.[6] However, CTCs have been detected at a low frequency in early stage disease[7] and recently CTCs were detected in 10 of 35 (29%) stage I patients using a sensitive quantitative (q) reverse transcription polymerase chain reaction (RT-PCR) assay.[8] These data highlight the need for larger scale studies comparing detection of DTCs and CTCs in early stage disease, and comparing sensitivity and specificity with assessment of cell-free nucleic acids in the circulation.

DETECTION OF CIRCULATING NUCLEIC ACIDS IN PLASMA OR SERUM

The first description of DNA in plasma or serum was by Mandel and Métais in 1948.[9] Using a perchloric acid precipitation method, they detected both DNA and RNA at a concentration of between 0.3 to 1.0 mg/l of plasma in healthy and sick individuals. This concentration is higher than that reported in more recent studies, probably reflecting both methodological and sample differences. It was not until the 1960s that the field was revisited when high levels of DNA were reported in the serum of patients with systemic lupus erythematosis.[10] Subsequent studies showed increased concentrations of free DNA in plasma or serum from patients with rheumatoid arthritis, pancreatitis, pulmonary embolism, ulcerative colitis, inflammatory bowel disease, peptic ulcer, and other inflammatory conditions.[11–14] Increasingly sensitive assays were also able to detect small amounts of free DNA, up to 30 ng of soluble DNA/ml, in the serum and plasma of healthy individuals.[15]

Subsequently, patients with cancer were shown to have higher levels of free circulating plasma DNA than those with nonmalignant disease, often >100 ng/ml of plasma.[11,16–18] Leon et al[16] used a radioimmunoassay to study the level of free DNA in the serum of 173 patients with cancer and 55 healthy individuals. The mean DNA concentration was 13 ng/ml in the healthy controls and 180 ng/ml in the cancer patients.[16] Similar levels were reported for 26 patients with breast cancer, where the mean concentration of DNA in plasma was 211 ng/ml but was only 21 ng/ml for 92 healthy female controls (p <0.01) matched closely for age and menopausal status.[19]

For the 173 cancer patients studied by Leon et al,[16] subsequent studies found no correlation between the level of free DNA in serum and either the size or location of the primary tumor. However, significantly higher levels of free DNA were found in the serum of patients with metastases compared to those with localized disease. Lymphomas, lung, ovarian, endometrial, and cervical carcinomas that responded to radiotherapy were shown to have up to a 90% decrease in DNA levels in serum, whereas persistently high or increasing DNA levels were associated with a lack of response to treatment.[20] Hence, quantitative analysis of circulating nucleic acids might be useful for disease monitoring.

RECENT QUANTITATIVE AND QUALITATIVE ANALYSES OF BREAST CANCER PLASMA DNA

With the now widespread availability of real-time qPCR a number of research groups have developed quantitative assays to determine the level of cell-free DNA in plasma and serum. These assays measure the concentration of a known gene (typically glyceraldehyde 3-phosphate dehydrogenase (GAPDH); Genbank Accession No. J04038) in either plasma or serum samples relative to a serial dilution curve starting with a known concentration of human genomic DNA. Gal et al[21] analyzed serum samples from 96 patients with primary breast cancer and compared these to 24 healthy controls. The DNA concentration in the serum of the patients differed significantly from the controls. The medians were 221 ng/ml and 63 ng/ml of serum, respectively (p <0.001), and serum DNA levels were elevated in cancer independently of the size of the primary tumor or lymph node metastases. However, others have cautioned against the use of serum to monitor the concentration of cell-free DNA in a patient's circulation since most cell-free DNA in serum samples may be generated during the process of clotting in the original collection tube.[22] This is supported by the consistent finding of lower amounts of cell free-DNA in plasma than in serum.

Huang et al[23] reported the median plasma DNA concentration of 61 breast cancer patients as 65 ng/ml. This was shown to be significantly higher than that in either 31 patients with benign breast disease (median 22 ng/ml, p <0.05) or 27 healthy controls (median 13 ng/ml). There was no association with plasma DNA concentration or clinicopathological parameters.[23] A similar study compared

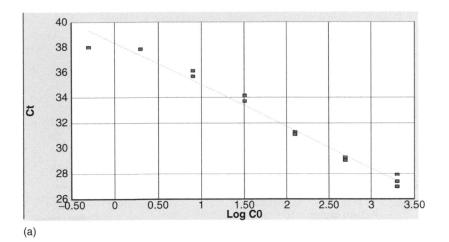

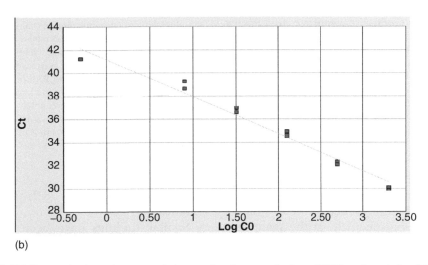

Figure 8.1 GAPDH quantitative polymerase chain reaction for quantitation of DNA and analysis of DNA integrity. Measurement of reaction efficiency: (a) 96bp amplicon R2 = 0.98, slope = −3.31, efficiency = 100%; (b) 291bp amplicon R2 = 0.98, slope = −3.2, efficiency = 105%.

plasma DNA from 33 patients with breast cancer, 32 females with benign breast lesions and 50 healthy female controls. The results showed that the level of cell-free DNA in the breast cancer group was significantly higher than in either the benign breast lesion or the control groups (p = 0.007 and 0.013, respectively), and higher DNA levels were associated with malignant tumor size.[24]

We, and others, have shown that there is also a qualitative difference, with increased DNA integrity in plasma being associated with cancer.[25,26] Using PCR analysis of increasing sized amplicons, we were able to amplify >500bp amplicons in plasma DNA from breast cancer patients compared to <300bp in healthy female controls.[26] In a cohort of both high risk (HR; >3 nodes positive at the time of diagnosis) and low risk (LR; T1/node-negative) cases, DNA fragments >512bp were detected in 16 of 22 HR samples and 13 of 16 LR samples (K Page, personal communication). However, none of 28 healthy female control samples had amplifiable DNA fragments >272bp in size.

Recently, we have developed a real-time qPCR assay using a common probe to detect two GAPDH amplicons of 96bp and 291bp in

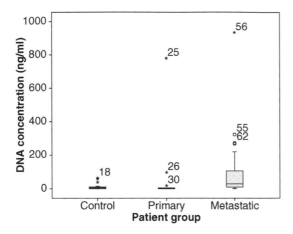

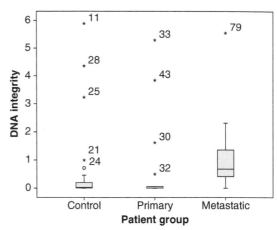

Figure 8.2   Measurement of DNA concentration (ng/ml) in control, primary, and metastatic breast cancer plasma DNA samples by quantitative polymerase chain reaction analysis of 96bp amplicon. The upper and lower limits of the boxes and the line inside the box represents the 75th and 25th percentiles and the median, respectively. The upper and lower horizontal bars denote the 90th and 10th percentiles, respectively. The metastatic plasma DNA group was significantly different to the control group (p = <0.001 Mann-Whitney nonparametric test).

Figure 8.3   Measurement of the DNA integrity index in control, metastatic, and primary breast cancer plasma DNA samples by quantitative polymerase chain reaction analysis. The DNA integrity index was calculated as the ratio of the concentration of the 291bp and 96bp amplicons. The upper and lower limits of the boxes and the line inside the box represents the 75th and 25th percentiles and the median, respectively. The upper and lower horizontal bars denote the 90th and 10th percentiles, respectively. The metastatic plasma DNA group was significantly different to the control group (p = 0.003 Mann-Whitney).

size. The assay uses a sensitive Minor Groove Binder TaqMan probe, which enables increased probe specificity at the same time as using a shorter DNA probe. Figure 8.1 shows standard curves produced from serial dilutions of cell line genomic DNA for the 96bp and 291bp amplicons. Since the efficiency of the two assays is approximately equal, it is possible calculate the ratio of the concentration of the two amplicons as a measure of DNA integrity. Using these assays we have compared DNA concentration and integrity for 33 early stage primary breast cancers, 30 metastatic breast cancers, and 25 healthy female controls. The mean plasma DNA concentration (Table 8.1) and DNA integrity was shown to be significantly higher in metastatic breast cancers than in controls (p <0.001 and 0.003, respectively). However, there was clear overlap between the early stage primary patient group and the controls when comparing both DNA concentration

(Table 8.1 and Figure 8.2) and integrity (Figure 8.3).

Similar findings have been reported for cell-free DNA in serum. Using real-time qPCR analysis of ALU DNA repeats, the mean serum DNA integrity was shown to be significantly higher in late-stage breast cancers (assessed as American Joint Committee on Cancer stage II–IV disease) than healthy females, but not in early stage (stage 0 or stage I) cancers.[27] The study also assessed 15 females with postoperative recurrence of breast cancer and found a high mean serum DNA integrity, similar to that of patients with stage III or IV primary breast cancer. Large-scale studies are now needed to more fully evaluate the utility of plasma and/or serum quantitative and integrity analyses for breast cancer screening and monitoring. However, whilst these real-time qPCR assays are simple and rapid, we suggest caution with their use as a predictive test in individual cases, since

Table 8.1 Mean concentration of plasma DNA measured by quantitative polymerase chain reaction using 96bp GAPDH amplicon relative to serial dilutions of cell line DNA: 33 primary breast cancers; 30 metastatic breast cancers; 25 healthy female controls

Sample	Mean plasma DNA (ng/ml); (range)	±SEM
Control group	9.86 (0.0031–63.44)	7.74
Metastatic breast cancer	101.34 (1.23–932.21)	34.4
Primary (early) breast cancer	51.41 (0.01–777.08)	42.92

single measurements may overlap between the different groups.

DETECTION OF TUMOR-SPECIFIC ALTERATIONS IN CELL-FREE DNA IN PLASMA/SERUM

Stroun et al[28] were the first to characterize circulating DNA from the plasma of cancer patients. They used a 32P-labeled human DNA probe to show that it was human in origin and comprised of double-stranded fragments of up to 21kb in length.[28] Detectable amounts of circulating DNA were found predominantly in patients with advanced malignancies bearing a large tumor cell burden. They then went on to demonstrate that plasma DNA from cancer patients had decreased strand stability, in common with DNA of cancer cells, and was of tumor origin,[29] hence paving the way for analysis of tumor-specific alterations in plasma DNA.

Two key studies published back-to-back in 1996 first demonstrated that tumor-specific loss of heterozygosity (LOH) could be detected by PCR in the plasma and serum of patients with advanced small cell lung cancer, and head and neck cancer, respectively.[30,31] Tumor specific LOH were subsequently detected in the plasma of breast cancer[32,33] and colon cancer patients;[34] and K-ras and p53 gene mutations,[35–37] and aberrant promoter hypermethylation of tumor-suppressor genes including p16^{INK4a} were demonstrated in non-small cell lung cancer and liver cancer patients, respectively.[38,39]

Many studies have attempted to correlate tumor-specific alterations in plasma DNA with prognosis. Some studies report high detection rates of tumor-specific alterations, whilst others report very low detection rates. For example, LOH was detected in the plasma DNA of 32 of 57 melanoma cases (56%). For stage III disease, the presence of LOH in preoperative plasma DNA was shown to be an independent variable associated with an increased risk of death ($p = 0.05$). Furthermore, LOH at the D1S228 marker in the plasma of patients with advanced disease correlated significantly ($p = 0.0009$) with a poorer survival after surgical resection.[40] However, in 91 head and neck squamous cell carcinomas, tumor-derived DNA was unambiguously detected in the plasma of only 17 patients. Moreover, the presence of circulating tumor-derived DNA could not be correlated with disease outcome or other clinical parameters, suggesting that the particular alterations studied had no prognostic significance.[41] The most useful tumor-specific DNA markers remain to be defined and validated for each cancer type.

For colorectal cancer, Diehl et al[42] showed that mutant adenomatous polyposis coli (APC) molecules were detected in the plasma of >60% of patients with early colorectal cancers.[42,43] However, they were not able to detect mutant DNA in the plasma of patients with premalignant adenomas. The levels of mutant APC molecules in the plasma were low, averaging only 11% of the total DNA molecules, even in very large adenomas. Therefore, they suggested caution against reliable detection of LOH in plasma, at least in colorectal cancers. However, the sensitivity of mutation detection remains to be more fully assessed in a wider range of cancer types and a larger series of cases.

TUMOR-SPECIFIC GENETIC ALTERATIONS IN SERUM/PLASMA DNA OF BREAST CANCER PATIENTS

Most studies of breast cancer plasma DNA have focused on detection of LOH and/or p53 mutation. Silva et al[33] first analyzed 62 breast cancer cases for LOH and/or microsatellite instability (MSI) at 6 polymorphic markers, p53 mutations, and promoter methylation of p16[INK4a]. They identified 56 cases (90%) with at least one molecular event in tumor DNA, 41 (66%) of which showed a similar alteration in plasma DNA. The presence of plasma DNA with tumor-specific alterations showed a statistically significant correlation with parameters associated with poor prognosis: high proliferative index, 3 or more positive lymph nodes, infiltrating ductal carcinoma (IDC) type, and grade III tumors with peritumoral vessel involvement and lymph node metastasis. The concordance between plasma and tumor DNA alterations varied from 42% for point mutations in p53 to 100% for LOH at the TH2 marker. In subsequent studies of 147 patients on follow-up, 61 cases showed concurrent alterations in tumor and plasma DNA, and 74% of the recurrences were in patients with circulating tumor DNA.[44] Univariate statistical analysis showed that tumor plasma DNA was a predictor of both disease-free survival[44] and overall survival.[45]

Chen et al[32] studied 61 breast cancer patients in three subgroups using different markers: 23 of the cases were analyzed with 11 markers; 81% of the tumor samples showed LOH; and 48% had LOH in the corresponding serum sample. Three patients who had metastatic disease at the time of diagnosis displayed LOH in plasma or serum at more than 1 locus; otherwise no obvious correlation was found between detection of plasma/serum with tumor-specific alterations and any clinicopathological parameters. However, two patients with small grade 1 tumors and one case of ductal carcinoma in situ (DCIS) also displayed specific DNA alterations in serum/plasma DNA, suggesting that circulating tumor-specific DNA may appear at an early pathological stage. Thus far, there have been no other large-scale studies reported to substantiate these findings.

p53 mutations have been reported in 50–75% of breast carcinomas,[46] suggesting that p53 mutation may constitute a useful tumor marker.[42] Shao et al[48] identified 30 of 46 patients (65.1%) with p53 mutations in the primary tumor which had the same mutation in plasma DNA.[49] These plasma DNA mutations were correlated with clinical stage, tumor size, lymph node metastasis and estrogen receptor (ER) status ($p < 0.05$). Moreover, patients with both primary tumor and plasma p53 mutations had the poorest survival: 13 of 22 patients with recurrence and/or metastasis later had detectable p53 mutations in their plasma DNA.

In our studies we identified 10 of 32 patients (31%) with primary breast cancer showing the same LOH (6 of 32) or MSI (4 of 32) between plasma and tumor DNA. There were no significant differences observed in terms of node involvement or tumor size between the 10 patients that displayed LOH or MSI in plasma DNA and the 22 patients who had no tumor-specific alterations detected. Where follow-up blood samples were available ($n = 21$), the second plasma and lymphocyte DNA samples showed the same genotypes as the preoperative sample.[50] In a separate study of 16 patients, using 24 microsatellite markers, no association was found between plasma LOH and tumor stage or the clinical status at time of blood collection. Although plasma LOH was concordant with the primary tumor for 12 cases, detection of LOH was not consistent between serial samples from 5 cases, despite stable clinical conditions.[51] More suitable markers and larger cohorts of patients need to be studied to resolve these differences.

Of the 10 patients in our study with primary breast cancer with LOH or MSI in plasma DNA, 5 patients had no involved lymph nodes and 8 showed no evidence of lymphovascular invasion. This contrasts with the data of Silva et al[33] who found a significant correlation between microsatellite alterations and involvement of ≥3 lymph nodes. Importantly, our findings suggest that tumor cell access to the vasculature exist, even in breast cancers where none can be seen by conventional histology. The origin of this circulating DNA remains unknown; lysis of primary tumor and/or circulating tumor cells, apoptosis of some tumor cells, and necroses of tumor cells have all been proposed previously.[52] It is likely that active cell destruction is required to generate cell-free plasma DNA.[49] The follow up of a larger cohort of cases is currently ongoing in our group in order to establish whether variations in plasma tumor DNA might anticipate clinical diagnosis and predict clinical behavior.

DETECTION OF EPIGENETIC CHANGE

DNA methylation at CpG dinucleotides in the promoter region of many genes is commonly associated with transcriptional gene silencing. Gene hypermethylation is therefore another mechanism for inactivation of tumor-suppressor genes,[53] and has been shown to be a frequent and early alteration in many tumor types, including breast cancers.[54–56] Hence, early methylation changes might prove to be useful markers for cancer screening if they are also tumor specific. A number of tumor-suppressor genes, including RAS-associated domain family protein 1A (RASSF1a)[57] and adenomatous polyposis coli (APC),[58] have been shown to be hypermethylated in breast cancers but unmethylated in normal cells, and these and other targets are currently being studied as potential cancer-specific biomarkers in both serum and plasma.

Thus far, there have been five studies published, which have examined promoter hypermethylation in paired tumor and serum, or plasma DNA from breast cancer patients using PCR-based approaches (summarized in Table 8.2). In total, 12 different loci have been investigated, with p16, APC, and RASSF1a common to more than one study.[59–63] Using just two markers, p16 and CDH1, Hu et al[59] were first to demonstrate common methylation in

plasma and tumor DNA for 9 of 36 (25%) breast cancers.[59] Moreover, the other 25 cases without methylation in tumor DNA did not show any epigenetic change in plasma. Tumor suppressor promoter hypermethylation was then detected in preinvasive DCIS.[60] However, the study also detected methylation in a small proportion (13%) of the 76 female controls studied, suggesting that the particular methylation events were not tumor specific. Recently, Sharma et al[63] reported high sensitivity and demonstrated concordant hypermethylation between tumor and serum DNA for 30 of 36 (83%) breast cancers. These studies hold some promise for methylation-based cancer screening and monitoring. However, issues remain to be resolved in terms of assay sensitivity and specificity, and additional studies are needed to fully validate hypermethylation-based screening in a larger number of cases and to examine HR populations.

CELL-FREE RNA

Circulating cell-free RNA has also been found in the plasma and serum of healthy individuals,[64] with increased levels detected in cancer patients,[65–67] including breast cancers.[68] Fewer studies have been published than for circulating DNA, in part due to RNA stability problems in stored and freeze-thawed samples,[69] and reproducibility problems with RNA analyses.[70] Silva et al[71] used nested RT-PCR to detect the presence of cytokeratin 19 (CK19) and mammoglobin RNA in plasma as markers of tumor epithelial cell RNA: 27 (60%) and 22 (49%) of 45 breast cancer patients were positive for CK19 and mammoglobin RNA, respectively. The presence of either mRNA alone or combined with plasma correlated with poor pathological parameters (tumor size and proliferative index) and with the presence of circulating tumor cells. Since telomerase activity has been detected in almost all types of cancer tissue, it has been proposed as a new reliable tumor marker. Among 25 breast cancer patients, telomerase RNA for human Telomerase RNA (hTR) and human Telomerase Reverse Transcriptase

Table 8.2   Promoter hypermethylation in serum/plasma of breast cancer patients

Number of cases studied	Markers analyzed	Method	Hypermethylation in tumor	Hypermethylation in serum/plasma
36	p16, CDH1	MSP	11 (31%)	9 (25%) plasma[59]
34	RASSF1A, APC, DAP-kinase	MSP	32 (94%)	26/34 (76%) serum[60]
84	APC, GSTP1, RASSF1A, RARβ2	qMSP	48 (87%)	32 (67%) plasma[61]
50	TMS1, BRCA1, ERα PRB	MSP	36 (72%)	32 (64%) serum[62]
36	p16, p14(ARF), cyclin D2, Slit2	MSP	31 (86%)	30 (83%) serum[63]

MSP, Methylation-specific polymerase chain reaction (PCR); qMSP, quantitative methylation-specific PCR.

(hTERT) subunits was detected in the plasma of 23 and 12 patients, respectively.[72] In a recent study, erbB2 mRNA was detectable in the plasma of 46 of 106 (43.3%) breast cancer patients, whereas only 5 of 50 healthy subjects in the control group (10%) were positive ($p = 0.001$).[73] However, the presence of erbB2 mRNA in the plasma was not associated with erbB2 expression in the primary tumor, but was significantly associated with negative ER and progesterone receptor (PR) status of the primary tumor ($p = 0.031$ and 0.026, respectively). Further studies are needed to determine whether circulating cell-free mRNA may serve as a complementary tumor marker for breast cancer monitoring.

CONCLUSIONS AND POSSIBLE FUTURE PERSPECTIVES

Early detection of cancer must ultimately move towards population screening for asymptomatic cases. A blood-based assay is clearly an attractive idea for the future, which should be acceptable to the general population. Such an assay might focus on the detection of a combination of factors, identifiable in both circulating tumor cells and circulating nucleic acids. However, before a multibiomarker test can be developed and validated, a number of key issues remain to be resolved. Although the majority of plasma/serum DNA alterations concur with those seen in tumor DNA, several studies have shown alterations in plasma or tumor only (e.g. Silva et al[37] and Shaw et al[50]). Garcia et al[74] showed that heterogeneous tumor clones, and not PCR artefacts, could explain some nonmatched alterations between plasma and tumor DNA. Clearly, molecular markers which show homogeneous alterations in tumor are desired for analysis in plasma DNA. DNA methylation-based biomarkers, and detection of common mutations, are probably the most attractive for development, although each will require close scrutiny of assay sensitivity and specificity. DNA changes have the advantage of being qualitative (present or absent) rather than quantitative, such as for mRNA and protein.[50] However, given the differences in amounts of free DNA detected between cancers and controls, it might be useful to combine both qualitative and quantitative criteria for detection of tumor-specific DNA in blood. A number of research groups, including our own, are currently following up different cohorts of patients with a range of molecular markers and assays. However, additional studies will be needed in order to validate the most useful markers for plasma/serum DNA and/or RNA analysis in large cohorts of breast cancer patients and other tumor types. Ultimately, the development of a high-throughput sensitive blood-based test may well be achievable for early detection of breast cancer.

REFERENCES

1. Breast Cancer Campaign, 2007. http://www.breast-cancercampaign.org/breastcancer/breast_cancer_facts//

2. Miller BA, Feur EJ, Hankey BF Breast cancer. N Engl J Med 1992; 327: 1756–7.

3. Veronesi U, Goldhirsch A, Yarnold J. Breast Cancer. In: Peckham M, Pinedo HM, Veronesi U eds. Oxford Textbook of Oncolgy. New York: Oxford University Press, 1995; 2: 1243–89.

4. Pantel K, Muller V, Auer M et al. Detection and clinical implications of early systemic tumour cell dissemination in breast cancer. Clin Cancer Res 2003; 9: 6326–34.

5. Slade MJ, Coombes RC. The clinical significance of disseminated tumor cells in breast cancer. Nat Clin Pract Oncol 2007; 4: 30–41.

6. Hauch S, Zimmermann S, Lankiewicz S et al. The clinical significance of circulating tumour cells in breast cancer and colorectal cancer patients. Anticancer Res 2007; 27: 1337–41.

7. Muller V, Stahmann S, Riethdorf S et al. Circulating tumour cells in breast cancer: correlation to bone marrow metastases, heterogeneous response to systemic therapy and low proliferative activity. Clin Cancer Res 2005; 11: 3678–85.

8. Nakagawa T, Martinez SR, Goto Y et al. Detection of circulating tumor cells in early-stage breast cancer metastasis to axillary lymph nodes. Clin Cancer Res 2007; 13: 4105–10.

9. Mandel P, Métias P. Les acides nucléiques du plasma sanguin chez l'homme. CR Acad Sci Paris 1948; 142: 241–3.

10. Tan EM, Schur PH, Carr RI et al. Deoxyribonucleic acid (DNA) and antibodies to DNA in the serum of patients with systemic lupus erythematosus. J Clin Invest 1966; 45: 1732–40.

11. Shapiro B, Chakrabarty M, Cohn EM, Leon SA. Determination of circulating DNA levels in patients with benign or malignant gastrointestinal disease. Cancer 1983; 51: 2116–20.

12. Koffler D, Agnello V, Winchester R, Kunkel H. The occurrence of single stranded DNA in the serum of patients with SLE and other diseases. J Clin Invest 1973; 52: 198–204.

13. Davis GL, Davis JS. Detection of circulating DNA by counter immunoelectrophoresis (CIE). Arthritis Rheum 1973; 16: 52–5.

14. Leon SA, Revach M, Ehrlich GE et al. DNA in synovial fluid and the circulation of patients with arthritis. Arthritis Rheum 1981; 24: 1142–50.

15. Steinman CR. Free DNA in serum and plasma from normal adults. J Clin Invest 1975; 56: 512–15.

16. Leon SA, Green A, Yaros MJ et al. Radioimmunoassey for nanogram quantities of DNA. J Immunol Meth 1975; 9: 157–64.

17. Stroun M, Anker P, Lyautey J. Isolation and characterization of DNA from the plasma of cancer patients. Eur J Cancer Clin Oncol 1987; 23: 707–12.

18. Maebo A. Plasma DNA level as a tumour marker in primary lung cancer. Jpn J Thorac Dis 1990; 28: 1085–91.

19. Shao ZM, Wu J, Shen ZZ et al. p53 mutation in plasma DNA and its prognostic value in breast cancer patients. Clin Cancer Res 2001; 8: 2222–7.

20. Leon SA, Shapiro B, Sklaroff D et al. Free DNA in the serum of cancer patients and the effect of therapy. Cancer Res 1977; 37: 646–50.

21. Gal S, Fidler C, Lo YM et al. Quantitation of circulating DNA in the serum of breast cancer patients by real-time PCR. Br J Cancer 2004; 90: 1211–15.

22. Lee TH, Montalvo L, Chrebtow V et al. Quantitation of genomic DNA in plasma and serum samples: higher concentrations of genomic DNA found in serum than in plasma. Transfusion 2001; 41: 276–82.

23. Huang ZH, Li LH, Hua D. Quantitative analysis of plasma circulating DNA at diagnosis and during follow-up of breast cancer patients. Cancer Lett 2006; 243: 64–70.

24. Zhong XY, Ladewig A, Schmid S et al. Elevated level of cell-free plasma DNA is associated with breast cancer. Arch Gynecol Obstet 2007 (e-pub ahead of print).

25. Wang BG, Huang HY, Chen YC et al. Increased plasma DNA integrity in cancer patients. Cancer Res 2003; 63: 3966–8.

26. Page K, Powles T, Slade MJ et al. The importance of careful blood processing in isolation of cell-free DNA. Ann NY Acad Sci 2006; 1075: 313–17.

27. Umetani N, Giuliano AE, Hiramatsu SH et al. Prediction of breast tumor progression by integrity of free circulating DNA in serum. J Clin Oncol 2006; 24: 4270–6.

28. Stroun M, Anker P, Lyautey J. Isolation and characterization of DNA from the plasma of cancer patients. Eur J Cancer Clin Oncol 1987; 23: 707–12.

29. Stroun M, Anker P, Maurice P et al. Neoplastic characteristics of the DNA found in the plasma of cancer patients. Oncology 1989; 46: 318–22.

30. Chen XQ, Stroun M, Magnenat JL et al. Microsatellite alterations in plasma DNA of small cell lung cancer patients. Nat Med 1996; 2: 1033–5.

31. Nawroz H, Koch W, Anker P et al. Microsatellite alterations in serum DNA of head and neck patients. Nat Med 1996; 2: 1035–7.

32. Chen X, Bonnefoi H, Diebold-Berger S et al. Detecting tumour-related alterations in plasma or serum DNA of patients diagnosed with breast cancer. Clin Cancer Res 1999; 5: 2297–303.

33. Silva JM, Dominguez G, Garcia JM et al. Presence of tumour DNA in plasma of breast cancer patients: clinicopathological correlations. Cancer Res 1999; 59: 3251–6.

34. Anker P, Lefort F, Vasioukhin V et al. K-ras gene mutations in the plasma of colorectal cancer patients. Gastroenterology 1997; 112: 1114–20.

35. Kopreski MS, Benko FA, Kwee C et al. Detection of mutant K-ras DNA in plasma or serum of patients with colorectal cancer. Br J Cancer 1997; 76: 1293–9.

36. Mulcahy H, Anker P, Lyautey J et al. K-ras gene mutations in the plasma of pancreatic patients. Clin
Cancer Res 1998; 4: 271–5.

37. Silva JM, Gonzalez R, Dominguez G et al. TP53 gene
mutations in plasma DNA of cancer patients. Genes
Chromosomes Cancer 1999; 24: 160–1.

38. Sanchex-Cespedes EM, Rossell M, Sidransky D et al.
Detection of aberrant promoter hypermethylation
of tumour suppressor genes in serum DNA from
non-small cell lung cancer patients. Cancer Res
1999; 59: 67–70.

39. Wong IH, Lo YM, Zhang J et al. Detection of aberrant p16 methylation in the plasma and serum of
liver cancer patients. Cancer Res 1999; 59: 71–3.

40. Taback B, Fujiwara Y, Wang HJ et al. Prognostic significance of circulating microsatellite markers in the
plasma of melanoma patients. Cancer Res 2001; 61:
5723–6.

41. Nunes DN, Kowalski LP, Simpson AJ. Circulating
tumour-derived DNA may permit the early diagnosis
of head and neck squamous cell carcinomas. Int J
Cancer 2001; 2: 214–19.

42. Diehl F, Li M, Dressman D et al. Detection and quantification of mutations in the plasma of patients with
colorectal tumors. Proc Natl Acad Sci USA 2005;
102: 16,368–73.

43. Schmidt K, Diehl F. A blood-based DNA test for colorectal cancer screening. Discov Med 2007; 7: 7–12.

44. Silva JM, Silva J, Sanchez A et al. Tumor DNA in
plasma at diagnosis of breast cancer patients is
a valuable predictor of disease-free survival. Clin
Cancer Res 2002; 8: 3761–6.

45. Garcia JM, Garcia V, Silva J et al. Extracellular tumor
DNA in plasma and overall survival in breast cancer
patients. Genes Chromosomes Cancer 2006; 45:
692–701.

46. Hollstein M, Sidransky D, Vogelstein B et al. p53 mutations in human cancer. Science 1991; 253: 49–53.

47. Linderholm BK, Lindahl T, Holmberg L et al. The
expression of vascular endothelial growth factor correlates with mutant p53 and poor prognosis in
human breast cancer. Cancer Res 2001; 61: 256–60.

48. Shao ZM, Wu J, Shen ZZ et al. p53 mutation in
plasma DNA and its prognostic value in breast cancer patients. Clin Cancer Res 2001; 8: 2222–7.

49. Levenson VV. Biomarkers for early detection of
breast cancer: what, when, and where? Biochim
Biophys Acta 2007; 1770: 847–56.

50. Shaw JA, Smith BM, Walsh T et al. Microsatellite
alterations plasma DNA of primary breast cancer
patients. Clin Cancer Res 2000; 6: 1119–24.

51. Wang Q, Larson PS, Schlechter BL et al. Loss of
heterozygosity in serial plasma DNA samples during
follow-up of women with breast cancer. Int J Cancer
2003; 106: 923–9.

52. Anker P. Quantitative aspects of plasma/serum
DNA in cancer patients. Ann NY Acad Sci 2000; 906:
5–7.

53. Baylin SB, Herman JG, Graff JR et al. Alterations in
DNA methylation: a fundamental aspect of neoplasia. Adv Cancer Res 1998; 72: 141–96.

54. Ferguson AT, Evron E, Umbricht CB et al. High frequency of hypermethylation at the 14–3–3 sigma
locus leads to gene silencing in breast cancer. Proc
Natl Acad Sci USA 2000; 97: 6049–54.

55. Umbricht CB, Evron E, Gabrielson E et al. Hypermethylation of 14–3–3 sigma (stratifin) is an early event
in breast cancer. Oncogene 2001; 20: 3348–53.

56. Lehmann U, Länger F, Feist H et al. Quantitative assessment of promoter hypermethylation during breast cancer development. Am J Pathol 2002; 160: 605–12.

57. Dammann R, Yang G, Pfeifer GP. Hypermethylation
of the cpG island of Ras association domain family
1A (RASSF1A), a putative tumor suppressor gene
from the 3p21.3 locus, occurs in a large percentage
of human breast cancers. Cancer Res 2001; 61:
3105–9.

58. Esteller M, Sparks A, Toyota M et al. Analysis of adenomatous polyposis coli promoter hypermethylation
in human cancer. Cancer Res 2000; 60: 4366–71.

59. Hu XC, Wong IH, Chow LW. Tumor-derived aberrant methylation in plasma of invasive ductal breast
cancer patients: clinical implications. Oncol Rep
2003; 10: 1811–15.

60. Dulaimi E, Hillinck J, Ibanez de Caceres I et al.
Tumor suppressor gene promoter hypermethylation
in serum of breast cancer patients. Clin Cancer Res
2004; 10: 6189–93.

61. Hoque MO, Feng Q, Toure P et al. Detection of
aberrant methylation of four genes in plasma DNA
for the detection of breast cancer. J Clin Oncol 2006;
24: 4262–9.

62. Mirza S, Sharma G, Prasad CP et al. Promoter hypermethylation of TMS1, BRCA1, ERalpha and PRB in
serum and tumor DNA of invasive ductal breast carcinoma patients. Life Sci 2007; 81: 280–7.

63. Sharma G, Mirza S, Prasad CP et al. Promoter hypermethylation of p16INK4A, p14ARF, CyclinD2 and
Slit2 in serum and tumor DNA from breast cancer
patients. Life Sci 2007; 80: 1873–81.

64. Guin LW, Griswold KE, Patton S. Electrophoretic
characterization of plasma RNA. Biochem Med
1975; 13: 224–30.

65. Wieczorek AJ, Sitaramam V, Machleidt W.
Diagnostic and prognostic value of RNA-proteolipid
in sera of patients with malignant disorders following therapy: first clinical evaluation of a novel tumor
marker. Cancer Res 1987; 47: 6407–12.

66. Kopreski MS, Benko FA, Kwak LW et al. Detection
of tumor messenger RNA in the serum of patients
with malignant melanoma. Clin Cancer Res 1999; 5:
1961–5.

67. Lo KW, Lo YM, Leung SF. Analysis of cell-free
Epstein-Barr virus associated RNA in the plasma of
patients with nasopharyngeal carcinoma. Clin Chem
1999; 45: 1292–4.

68. Chen XQ, Bonnefoi H, Pelte MF et al. Telomerase RNA as a detection marker in the serum of breast cancer patients. Clin Cancer Res 2000; 6: 3823–6.

69. Tsui NB, Ng EK, Lo YM. Stability of endogenous and added RNA in blood specimens, serum, and plasma. Clin Chem 2002; 48: 1647–53.

70. El-Hefnawy T, Raja S, Kelly L et al. Characterization of amplifiable, circulating RNA in plasma and its potential as a tool for cancer diagnostics. Clin Chem 2004; 50: 564–73.

71. Silva JM, Dominguez G, Silva J et al. Detection of epithelial messenger RNA in the plasma of breast cancer patients is associated with poor prognosis tumour characteristics. Clin Cancer Res 2001; 7: 2821–5.

72. Novakovic S, Hocevar M, Zgajnar J et al. Detection of telomerase RNA in the plasma of patients with breast cancer, malignant melanoma or thyroid cancer. Oncol Rep 2004; 11: 245–52.

73. Xu Y, Yao L, Li H et al. Presence of erbB2 mRNA in the plasma of breast cancer patients is associated with circulating tumor cells and negative estrogen and progesterone receptor status. Breast Cancer Res Treat 2006; 97: 49–55.

74. Garcia JM, Silva JM, Dominguez G et al. Heterogeneous tumour clones as an explanation of discordance between plasma DNA and tumour DNA alterations. Genes Chromosomes Cancer 2000; 31: 300–1.

9

Steroid receptors and associated transcriptional cofactors in predicting the response to endocrine therapy

Sandra Ghayad and Pascale A Cohen

ENDOCRINE THERAPIES FOR BREAST CANCER

Breast cancer is the most common female cancer in the Western world (accounting for 28% of all cancers) and the leading cause of death by cancer in women (approximately 20%). Although the mortality rate has stabilized or decreased, the incidence of breast cancer is still rising in all European countries.[1] Around two-thirds of breast cancers are hormone (estrogen)-dependent as they are positive for estrogen receptor alpha (ERα) and/or progesterone receptor (PR). As estrogen is the principal molecule stimulating the proliferation of these ER-positive tumors, blocking estrogen signaling has been the main endocrine therapy for patients with ER-positive breast cancer.

Over the past three decades, the antiestrogen tamoxifen, which belongs to the first generation of selective ER modulators (SERMs) and which acts as an estrogen antagonist on the breast, has been the gold standard for the endocrine treatment of all stages of these cancers. Tamoxifen acts as a SERM by blocking the AF-2 domain of ER but does not inhibit AF-1 activity (Figure 9.1). The benefits of tamoxifen and chemotherapy in women who have node-negative ERα-positive breast cancer have been demonstrated in large clinical trials such as the National Surgical Adjuvant Breast and Bowel Project (NSABP) trials B-14 and B-20.[2,3] Five years of tamoxifen started immediately after surgery for early stage ER-positive breast cancer was shown to reduce recurrence by 51% and mortality by 28%.[4] Tamoxifen can also be used as a chemopreventive agent to reduce the incidence of breast cancer in high-risk women and to treat patients with ductal carcinoma in situ (DCIS), reducing the incidence of invasive cancer and second primaries.[5]

However, tamoxifen is only partially effective because of intrinsic or acquired tumor resistance. Approximately 40% of patients with ER-positive breast cancer will not respond to tamoxifen (de novo resistance). Moreover, long-term follow-up and clinical trials have demonstrated that up to 62% of cancers initially responsive to endocrine therapy subsequently escaped control with the patient requiring salvage surgery.[6,7] To circumvent such tamoxifen resistance, drugs such as aromatase inhibitors (AIs) have been developed. AIs reduce peripheral estrogen synthesis, and include the irreversible steroidal AI exemestane (Aromasin) and the reversible non-steroidal inhibitors anastrozole (Arimidex) and letrozole (Femara). Recently, third-generation AIs have proved to be more effective than tamoxifen for treating both advanced and early hormone-sensitive breast cancers in postmenopausal women, as either first- or second-line therapy.[8,9] The greater efficacy of AIs compared with tamoxifen in small-scale studies of postmenopausal women with early breast

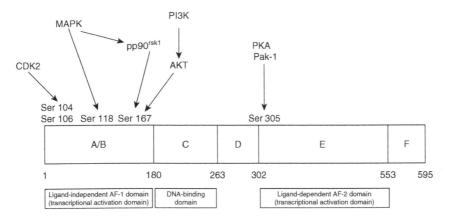

Figure 9.1   Structural and functional domains of estrogen receptor α; CDK, cyclin-dependent kinase; MAPK, mitogen-activated protein kinase; PI3K, phosphoinositide kinase-3; PKA, protein kinase A; Ser, serine.

cancer led to large-scale trials demonstrating that third-generation AIs are effective in the neoadjuvant, adjuvant and extended adjuvant settings. While AIs may replace tamoxifen as first-line endocrine therapy for most post-menopausal women, tamoxifen will continue to play a role in premenopausal women, as second-line therapy in postmenopausal women, and as chemoprevention in all age groups.[10] Another newer endocrine therapy has recently emerged with the selective estrogen receptor downregulator (SERD) fulvestrant (Faslodex, formerly known as ICI 182,780). This steroidal ER antagonist lacks any agonist effect but binds, blocks and accelerates the degradation of ER protein. Fulvestrant has been shown to be as effective as anastrozole and tamoxifen in the treatment of advanced ER-positive breast carcinoma (in second-line and first-line treatment, respectively).[11,12] Other clinical trials have also shown that, when used in patients with advanced breast cancer progressing on prior endocrine therapy with tamoxifen or an AI, fulvestrant yielded a clinical benefit in 43% and 30% of patients, respectively.[11,13,14] These clinical data underline both the importance of fulvestrant in the therapeutic arsenal against ER-positive breast cancers and the fact that fulvestrant is also prone to resistance.

ENDOCRINE RESISTANCE AND BIOLOGY OF THE ESTROGEN RECEPTOR FUNCTION

As resistance to endocrine therapy is one of the main challenges in the treatment of ER-positive breast cancer, understanding such processes is of major importance. In particular, deciphering the biology of the ER function, and the proteins which participate in estrogen signaling, it is hoped to improve our knowledge of the events which cause a response to endocrine therapy and thus identify accurate predictive markers for responsiveness to treatment.

In early studies, ER was identified as a transcription factor regulating the expression of specific genes in the nucleus. Some of these genes are important in breast physiology, and others for the proliferation and survival of breast cancer cells. This estrogen-mediated action in the nucleus is termed nuclear-initiated steroid signaling (NISS), or genomic activity of the ER. Recent evidence also suggests that estrogen can bind ERs located in or near the plasma membrane and rapidly activate other signaling pathways. This is called membrane-initiated steroid signaling (MISS), or nongenomic activity of the ER.

Nuclear-initiated steroid signaling

ER is a hormone-regulated nuclear transcription factor which can induce the expression of a number of genes (e.g. progesterone receptor (PR)). After the binding of estrogen, ERs bind to estrogen response elements (EREs) in target genes, recruits a transcriptional coregulator complex, then regulates the transcription of specific genes.[15] ER can also function as a transcriptional regulator in an unconventional manner without DNA binding by tethering to other transcription factor complexes including AP1, SP1 and USF.[16–18] ER action is controlled by coregulatory proteins termed coactivators and corepressors, which recruit enzymes which modulate chromatin structure to facilitate or repress gene transcription.[19] The varied cellular response to SERMs such as tamoxifen may be related to tissue-specific levels of different coregulatory proteins.[20] Other stimuli in addition to estrogen can enhance NISS in a ligand-independent manner. One of the mechanisms for such activation may be phosphorylation of ER, or its coregulators, at specific sites induced by growth factors and stress-related kinases (see also Chapter 10): (ERK) 1/2 and p38 mitogen-activated protein kinases (MAPKs); cyclin-dependent kinase (CDK) 2, CDK7; c-SRC; protein kinase A (PKA); pp90[rsk1]; and AKT (for a review, see Normanno et al[21]). Phosphorylation of ERα at serine (Ser) residues clustered at its amino terminus (Ser104/106, −118, and −167) enhances transcriptional transactivating activity arising from the ligand-independent AF-1 domain[21] (Figure 9.1).

Membrane-initiated steroid signaling

Growing evidence showing that estrogen can exert rapid cellular effects within minutes, long before its effects on gene transcription, suggests that other mechanisms of action are also involved. ER can be detected in or near the plasma membrane where it can interact directly with, and modulate, several signaling molecules, including the insulin-like growth factor-1 receptor (IGF1-R), phosphatidylinositol-3-kinase (PI3K), insulin receptor substrate-1 (IRS1), and

Shc and Src.[22–25] The exact consequences of such events are currently under investigation and the functional significance has yet to be deciphered.

The molecular mechanism that leads to tamoxifen resistance is still not fully understood, and multifactorial changes leading to a survival system for the cancer cells seem to be involved, rather than a gain-of-function and/ or a loss-of-function mechanism.[26] Cellular disturbances have been reported as possibly involved in the emergence of tamoxifen resistance, including modifications in tamoxifen metabolism;[27] ER mutation;[28] altered ERα or ER beta (ERβ) expression;[29,30] qualitative and/ or quantitative changes in transcriptional corepressors or coactivators;[31,32] and phosphorylation of ERα by MAPK,[33] PI3K/AKT[34] or PKA.[35] Compelling evidence has also been found that close crosstalk between growth factor signaling and the ER pathway is associated with the emergence of endocrine resistance (see also Chapter 10). Hence, inappropriate activation of growth factor signaling cascades (e.g. by overexpression of heregulins, transforming growth factor beta (TGFβ), epidermal growth factor receptor (EGFR), human epidermal growth factor receptor 2 (HER2/ erbb2) could promote endocrine resistance. Supporting data show that MAPK activity correlates with a shorter response to endocrine therapy in clinical breast cancer.[36] Compelling data also suggest that activation of the PI3K/AKT pathway is associated with: resistance to endocrine therapy; worse outcome in breast cancer patients;[37] and relapse and death in ER-positive breast patients treated with tamoxifen.[38]

By a NISS mechanism of action, ERα can also induce the expression of transcripts for amphiregulin,[39] which is able to bind and activate EGFR, leading to activation of MAPK and AKT pathways.[40] Conversely, the cytoplasmic kinases may phosphorylate coactivators which can modify ERα activity.[41] Finally, ERα can be phosphorylated and its transactivation function activated by a ligand-independent mechanism. In particular, ERα is phosphorylated at key positions (Ser118 and -167) in the AF-1 domain after activation of the MAPK or PI3K/AKT pathways[34,42] (Figure 9.1). An important step in the progression of tamoxifen resistance is the loss of tamoxifen's anti-estrogenic activity to the benefit of an agonist activity.[43] Phosphorylation of the AF-1 domain or qualitative/quantitative changes in transcriptional coregulators are possible mechanisms involved in this genomic agonist activity of tamoxifen.

Less information is currently available for the other drugs used in endocrine therapy. Clinical studies have shown that tamoxifen-resistant breast tumors are often sensitive to the SERM fulvestrant.[11,13] A possible mechanism in such phenotypes is that the tamoxifen resistance developed by these tumors could be due to phosphorylation of the ER by PKA (Figure 9.1), which would convert the antagonist action of tamoxifen into an agonist, while the cells remain sensitive to fulvestrant.[35] Other studies have suggested that nuclear factor kappa B (NFKB),[44] MAPK,[45] and neural precursor cell expressed developmentally downregulated 8 (NEDD8) PI3K/AKT[46] pathways may also be involved in the development of fulvestrant resistance.[47] Little is known concerning resistance to AIs, but the activation of HER2- and MAPK-mediated signaling pathways, and phosphorylation of ERα at Ser118, have been observed in xenograft models of letrozole resistance.[48]

STEROID RECEPTORS AND ASSOCIATED TRANSCRIPTIONAL COFACTORS IN PREDICTING RESPONSE TO ENDOCRINE THERAPY

Estrogen receptor alpha

There are two isoforms of ER, ERα and ERβ, encoded by two different genes. Studies in rodents have shown that both ERα and ERβ are expressed in the normal mammary gland[49] and that expression of ERα, but not ERβ, is critical for normal mammary gland ductal development.[50] ER is also expressed in the normal human breast and a dramatic increase in ERα expression is seen in early hyperproliferative premalignant lesions.[51]

The presence or absence of ERα is a well-established prognostic marker of breast cancer (at least in the early years following diagnosis) and a predictive marker for endocrine therapy.[52–54] This has led clinicians to distinguish between ER-positive and ER-negative breast tumors when coming to clinical decisions. In the adjuvant setting, a meta-analysis showed that tamoxifen significantly reduces recurrence and death only in patients with ER-positive tumors.[55] Similar results have been observed in trials prospectively designed to test the value of tamoxifen in ER-negative tumors,[3,4] and also in retrospective studies.[56] Prevention trials have shown that tamoxifen reduces the risk of contralateral endocrine-responsive breast cancer by almost 50%, but has no effect on ER-negative tumors.[2,57] The conclusion was that tamoxifen does not provide a clear benefit in ER-negative tumors. The response to tamoxifen in ER-positive tumors is directly related to ER levels,[58] but responses have been obtained in tumors that have as little as 4–10 fmol/mg of ER protein, or as few as 1–10% of cells positive for ER as shown by immunohistochemistry.[59] One of the adjuvant AI studies that provides additional data about ER as a predictive factor is the ATAC trial, since 16% of randomized patients were ER-negative or ER unknown.[60,61] Hence, a subgroup analysis showed that these patients had no benefit in receiving an AI, as previously shown for tamoxifen.

Phosphorylation of estrogen receptor alpha

ERα possesses several different phosphorylation sites which may modulate ERα action and activate transactivation functions through a ligand-independent mechanism. In particular, ERα is phosphorylated in the AF-1 domain at Ser118 following activation of the MAPK pathway and at Ser167 by AKT or p90RSK.[34,42,62] In ER-positive breast cancers, high levels of phosphoMAPK have been correlated with a poor response to endocrine therapy and decreased patient survival.[36] Immunohistochemical studies of phosphoSer118-ERα have found expression to be associated with better disease outcome in women treated with tamoxifen[63] and higher levels to be present in cancers that responded then progressed on tamoxifen.[64] These data suggest that phosphoSer118-ERα may be a useful marker of an intact ligand-dependent ER signaling pathway. Conversely, high levels of phosphoSer118-ERα have also been detected in ER-positive breast cancers which do not respond to endocrine therapy,[65] and increased levels have been found in biopsies taken from patients who relapsed whilst on tamoxifen.[64] Another recent study found that ER phosphorylated at Ser118 had no predictive value for the response to endocrine therapy.[66]

AKT activation (high levels of phospho-Ser473-AKT) has been shown to be associated with decreased overall survival rates in patients receiving endocrine therapy.[38,67] However, phosphoSer167-ERα has been shown to be a good prognostic factor in primary breast cancer.[68] PhosphoSer167-ERα has also been found to be predictive of response to endocrine therapy, as patients with primary breast tumors with high phosphorylation levels of ERα at Ser167 responded significantly to endocrine therapy and had a better survival rate after relapse.[66] These data suggested that phosphorylation of ERα at Ser167 could be helpful in selecting patients who may benefit from endocrine therapy.

Taken together, these data clearly illustrate the complexity of assessing ER phosphorylation, with different findings for pharmacological response and the emergence of endocrine resistance. This question should be addressed in future prospective studies. Also, given the complexity of the crosstalk between ER and growth factor signaling, assessing the phosphorylation status of ER at different key residues might be more informative in the delineation of subgroups of patients with different responses to endocrine therapy.

Estrogen receptor beta

The recent discovery of a second ER, called ERβ,[69] and of several of its variants, raised the question of the relative value of ERα and ERβ in predicting tamoxifen resistance or sensitivity in breast cancer patients. ERα and ERβ both mediate gene transcription via ERE. However, while ERα can also activate gene transcription from the AP-1 site, ERβ cannot.[70] ERβ binds estrogens with similar affinity as ERα, but binds antiestrogens and their hydroxylated metabolites with a higher affinity than does ERα.[71] Unlike ERα, antiestrogen-occupied ERβ can activate transcription via nonclassical ER signaling pathways, leading some investigators to speculate that ERβ could play a role in tamoxifen resistance through the agonist activity of tamoxifen.

Contradictory results have been obtained concerning the predictive value of ERβ in breast cancer. Initially, it was proposed that ERβ mRNA could predict endocrine resistance, and some studies seemed to prove this as elevated ERβ transcripts correlated with tamoxifen resistance.[29,72] However, antibody-based studies have shown that low ERβ protein expression is associated with tamoxifen resistance.[73–75] Only one prospective clinical study has investigated the relationship between ERβ mRNA expression and the response to endocrine therapy.[76] In this study, ERβ mRNA expression failed to predict the response to toremifene. Finally, a recent study provided new information by showing that ERβ protein expression may be an independent marker of a favorable prognosis after adjuvant tamoxifen treatment in ERα-negative breast cancer patients,[77] suggesting that patients diagnosed with ERα-negative/ERβ-positive breast carcinoma may benefit from adjuvant tamoxifen.

More recently, studies have been conducted to consider the role of specific ERβ isoforms. ERβ2, also known as ERβcx, is the best characterized of the five known ERβ variants and is identical to ERβ through exons 1–7 but contains an alternative exon 8.[78] This predicts replacement of the C-terminal 61 amino acids of ERβ encoding the terminal part of the ligand-binding domain, and the entire AF-2 domain with a unique 26 amino acid sequence, enabling this receptor to bind to tamoxifen. Given that ERβ2 can, through heterodimerization, inhibit the transcriptional activity of both ERα and ERβ,[79] with a preference for ERα, this variant may well be significant in regulating ER signaling in the mammary gland. Significantly higher ERβ2 expression in DCIS and in invasive breast cancer than in normal breast has been reported.[80] In areas of breast tumors with strong ERα positivity, a significant correlation has also been observed with ERβ2 expression and PR negativity.[81]

Rather than full-length ERβ alone, splice variants of ERβ may be more valuable assessors of the biological status of individual breast cancers. This was illustrated in a subset of patients receiving adjuvant tamoxifen where ERβ2 mRNA (more than full-length ERβ) predicted their response to endocrine therapy and was associated with relapse-free survival.[82] Supporting data showed that ERβ2 protein expression correlated with a favorable response to endocrine therapy, with patients having ERβ2-positive tumors showing increased survival.[83] Finally, in breast cancers with low PR expression, ERβ2 protein expression was found to correlate with a poor response to tamoxifen, suggesting that evaluating ERβ2 and PR may contribute to a better characterization of ERα-positive breast cancers.[81] However, a contradictory study concluded that ERβ2 protein expression was not predictive of tamoxifen resistance.[75] More recently, a further level of complexity was added as ERβ2 mRNA levels, but not protein levels, were found independently to be predictive of outcome in tamoxifen-treated ERα-positive breast tumors.[84]

Finally, two recent studies failed to prove that an association exists between either ERβ or ERβ2 protein expression and tamoxifen resistance.[66,85] Taken together, these studies, with apparently contradictory results, clearly illustrate the difficulties encountered when attempting to validate the predictive value of ERβ and/or ERβ variants in endocrine therapy responsiveness. One of the reasons for these discrepancies is certainly the lack of universally and well-validated antibodies against ERβ proteins, and this question must be addressed in the future.

Transcriptional estrogen receptor coregulators

At the nuclear level, ERs directly control the expression of a number of specific genes through binding to ERE located in the regulatory region of target gene promoters. Depending on the ligand, ER interacts with either corepressors or coactivators which inhibit or enhance ER transcriptional activity. The current view suggests that the ligand-bound receptor exists in a dynamic equilibrium with coactivator and corepressor proteins, affording a regular and tightly controlled regulation of ER-mediated gene expression. These coregulators are also able to regulate the relative agonist/antagonist activity of the SERM tamoxifen, and it has been suggested that the coactivator:corepressor ratio may be important both in endocrine therapy responsiveness and the development of resistance. Indeed, high levels of coactivator expression may enhance the agonist activity of tamoxifen.[20,86,87] Assessing coregulator expression and activity may thus be essential in the prognosis and for predicting response to endocrine therapy.[31] The most striking findings have been obtained with the two coactivators AIB1 and SRC-1, and the corepressor NCOR1.

AIB1 – also called SRC-3, RAC3, ACTR, or p/CIP – is an ER coactivator which is thought to be important in breast cancer. It is overexpressed in breast cancer cells compared with normal duct epithelial cells and is amplified in a small proportion of breast tumors.[88,89] AIB1, like the ER itself, is phosphorylated and thereby is functionally activated by MAPKs; therefore, high levels of activated AIB1 may reduce the antagonist effects of tamoxifen, especially in tumors which also overexpress the HER2 receptor which activates MAPKs.[87] To explore these hypotheses, AIB1 protein levels and HER2 levels were measured in extracts of frozen breast tumors from 316 patients with long-term clinical follow-up.[32] Nearly all of these tumors were ER-positive. AIB1 protein expression did not correlate with the quantity of ER but it was inversely correlated with PR expression. AIB1 also positively correlated with a higher S-phase fraction and higher HER2 expression. Despite the correlation between AIB1 with both S-phase and HER2 (markers of a more aggressive phenotype), high AIB1 expression was a good prognostic factor for patients treated with surgery alone without adjuvant therapy. Although high AIB1 expression was associated with improved disease-free survival in untreated patients, those patients receiving tamoxifen adjuvant therapy and having cancers with high AIB1 expression suffered worse disease-free survival. In a multivariate analysis that included the same biomarkers as described above, only the number of positive lymph nodes and AIB1 status were statistically significant predictors of outcome, consistent with the hypothesis that high AIB1 expression reduces tamoxifen's antagonist activity. When AIB1 expression was considered together with HER2 expression, even more impressive results were obtained, as only those patients with tumors which expressed high AIB1 and high HER2 had adverse disease-free survival with tamoxifen. Finally, patients with low expression of one or both of these proteins showed significantly better disease-free survival with tamoxifen adjuvant therapy.

SRC-1 (or NCOA1) is also an ER coactivator and its expression has been investigated by immunohistochemical analysis in breast tumors (ER- and/or PR-positive) in relation to HER2 status in patients treated with chemotherapy and tamoxifen. A multivariate analysis showed that SRC-1 expression was associated with disease recurrence only in HER2-positive breast tumors.[90] This study supports the hypothesis that SRC-1 is involved in tamoxifen resistance only in a specific subset of breast tumors, and underlines the necessity to take into account the expression status of previously identified tamoxifen resistance markers such as HER2. Interestingly, an inverse relationship between SRC-1 and ERβ was also found to predict outcome in endocrine-resistant breast cancer.[91]

ER-associated corepressors include the NCOR proteins which recruit histone deacetylases such as HDAC2 and HDAC4, and inhibit gene transcription.[92] In vitro studies have shown that NCOR1 protein binds ER and inhibits the partial agonist activity of tamoxifen,[93] and that HDAC activity is required for the transrepressive effect of SERMs.[94] Additionally, expression of dominant-negative NCOR in MCF-7 cells was found to both enhance the transcriptional activity of tamoxifen bound to ER and induce cell growth.[95] In further studies, MCF-7 cells were implanted into nude mice which were then treated with tamoxifen. A decrease in tumor NCOR levels was associated with acquired resistance in these tumors, with loss of the antiproliferative effects of tamoxifen.[96] An investigation of NCOR1 mRNA expression in tamoxifen-treated ER-positive patients showed that low NCOR1 mRNA expression status was associated with shorter relapse-free survival.[31] In the same study, by combining NCOR1 and HER2 mRNA expression, it was found that patients with the best prognosis were those with high NCOR1 expression and normal HER2 expression, suggesting that NCOR1 expression may provide an accurate predictive marker of endocrine therapy responsiveness.

In conclusion, the balance between coactivators and corepressors seems to play a key role in the prevention of breast tumor proliferation by tamoxifen, and supports this as a mechanism associated with endocrine resistance. Recent in vitro data showed that endocrine resistance is also associated with the progressive loss of ER coregulator recruitment.[97] In another recent study, it was observed that ER phosphorylation status may be involved in the recruitment of coregulators.[98] As phosphorylation by PKA at Ser305 of ERα altered the orientation between ERα and its coactivator SRC-1, the transcription complex was rendered active in the presence of tamoxifen.[98] Taken together, these results support the idea that transcriptional ER coregulators may be valuable markers of endocrine therapy response.

Progesterone receptor

About 65–75% of primary breast cancers express ER; over half of these also express PR, and <10% of tumors express PR in the absence of ER.[99] When PR was first identified as an ER-regulated gene product, it was proposed that the presence of PR might indicate a functioning ER pathway and a tumor which is highly dependent on estrogen for growth, and, consequently, one that would respond to endocrine therapy.[100] Thus, ER-positive tumors lacking PR would be less dependent on estrogen and would therefore be less responsive to endocrine therapy.

Retrospective studies of patients with metastatic disease, most receiving tamoxifen, supported this idea.[58] PR-negative tumors consistently respond less well to endocrine therapy than PR-positive tumors, although some do benefit. Elevated PR levels significantly and independently correlate with a higher probability of response, longer time to treatment failure, and longer overall survival in patients with metastatic disease treated with tamoxifen.[56,101] Data confirming the predictive value of PR also come from adjuvant and neoadjuvant trials showing that, in agreement with the studies in metastatic disease, patients with ER-positive/PR-positive tumors benefited far more from tamoxifen than those with PR-negative tumors.[54,102–105] Recent supporting data also showed that PR status provides predictive value for adjuvant endocrine therapy in older ER-positive breast cancer patients.[106] In all these studies, both ER and PR were independent predictors of outcome in multivariate analyses. PR was still predictive even when ER was considered as a continuous variable, indicating that the predictive information is independent of quantitative ER levels, an important result considering that the presence of PR is directly related to quantitative levels of ER.[102] When resistance to endocrine therapy evolves, PR levels decrease dramatically, with up to half of tumors completely losing PR expression.[107,108] These ER-positive/PR-negative metastatic tumors then follow a far more aggressive course, with poor patient survival after PR loss compared with those retaining PR expression.[108,109]

However, the observation that some PR-negative tumors still respond to endocrine therapy raised questions, with the most striking data derived from a retrospective analysis of the results of the ATAC trial.[60,110] This trial randomized postmenopausal women with early breast cancer to 5 years of treatment with the AI anastrozole or tamoxifen, or a combination of the two. Time to recurrence was longer for anastrozole-treated than tamoxifen-treated patients in both ER-positive/PR-positive and ER-positive/PR-negative subgroups, but the benefit was substantially greater in the PR-negative subgroup.[111] Two neoadjuvant AI trials validated these observations.[104,112] This suggests that the overall benefit of anastrozole may be due to reduced tamoxifen efficacy in patients with PR-negative tumors. These data also indicate that ER-positive/PR-negative breast tumors are less responsive to SERM therapy than ER-positive/PR-positive tumors. Clearly, the simple theory that PR serves as an indicator of a functionally intact ER pathway fails to explain why some patients with ER-positive/PR-negative tumors still respond to tamoxifen, or differences such as those between anastrozole and tamoxifen in the ATAC trial, treatments which both target ER, albeit in different ways.

These observations are nevertheless compatible with new information on the biology of ER and PR in breast cancer. For instance, recent laboratory and clinical studies strongly support the idea that one of the mechanisms leading to PR gene downregulation is excessive growth factor receptor signaling, in particular the PI3K/AKT pathway.[113] Thus, PR levels may reflect growth factor activity within a tumor. In addition, high growth factor signaling may reduce the ability of tamoxifen to act as an antagonist, resulting in SERM resistance. It therefore follows that tumors which have activated growth factor receptor signaling would benefit less from tamoxifen and would be more likely to have little or no PR content. Recent supporting data demonstrated that HER1–3-positive and/or PR-negative patients combined as a "high-risk" group were significantly more likely to relapse on tamoxifen.[114]

Consequently, tumors with little or negative PR content would likely be more responsive to AIs than tamoxifen, as observed in the ATAC trial.[111] Taken together, these observations indicate that PR may be a better indicator than ER for predicting response to SERM therapy since levels of PR reflect the combined and integrated effects of ER and growth factor activity. This also leads to the prediction that PR may be a valuable future marker of responsiveness to growth factor receptor inhibitor therapies. Finally, PR was not found to have any predictive value in a recent study of fulvestrant responsiveness.[115]

Progesterone receptor isoforms

Another field of future investigation is to decipher the functional importance of the altered expression of PR isoforms and how this may affect the response of breast tumors to endocrine therapy. PR is expressed as two isoforms – PR-A and PR-B, which are products of a single gene but which are under the control of two distinct promoters.[116] The two isoforms possess different, promoter- and cell line-specific transactivation properties. Studies have shown that in poor prognostic tumors, the ratio between PR-A and PR-B is altered, with PR-A predominating and loss of PR-B.[117] An overabundance of PR-A may be associated with resistance to tamoxifen,[117] while functional polymorphism resulting in increased production of PR-B may be associated with an increased risk of breast cancer.[118] Other findings showed that PR-B expression was correlated with good prognostic markers and better overall survival in breast cancer.[119] In a study of T47D human breast tumor xenografts, tamoxifen preferentially inhibited the growth of PR-A tumors, whereas PR-B tumors were unaffected.[120] Recently, PR-A and PR-B were both found to be predictive of response to endocrine therapy.[66] Taken together, these findings highlight the need for future studies to decipher the functional importance of the altered expression of PR isoforms and how disrupted progesterone signaling may affect the response of breast tumors to endocrine therapy.

CONCLUSIONS

Identifying and using biomarkers to predict the response to anticancer therapies has the capacity to revolutionize the treatment of patients with cancer. While the predictive value of ERα is now universally recognized in the endocrine therapy of breast cancer, deciphering the newly discovered biological roles for ER and the complex crosstalk with growth factor signaling provides additional complexity. The discovery of new variants of ER and PR also opens up new fields of investigation. For instance, preliminary data on ERα variants (such as the ERα ERδE7 or the ERα A908G mutant) indicate that they are able either to regulate the activity of full-length ERα, or to modify the pharmacological response to estrogen or to antiestrogens (for a review, see Townson and O'Cornell[121]). For PR, several variants and polymorphisms have also been identified but, in the same manner as for ER variants, little data has been published regarding their effect on clinical outcome. An important question to be addressed in future studies is therefore the impact of ER and/or PR variants expression on the response to endocrine therapy. One future challenge is also to improve the detection of ER and PR isoforms and variants to provide important predictive and/or prognostic clinical information. Taken together, these data highlight the complex impact of ER-mediated signaling on clinical outcome and emphasize that multifactorial approaches may be required to identify factors associated with improved endocrine therapy responsiveness. One of the most promising strategies is certainly the recent development of high throughput screening methods in genomics and proteomics, which should help to identify new predictive markers of endocrine therapy.[122–124]

ACKNOWLEDGMENTS

This work was supported by the Entente Cordiale Program (France/UK), the Ligue Nationale Contre le Cancer (France) and the ARC (Association pour la Recherche sur le

Cancer, France). Thanks to M Jones for presubmission editorial assistance.

REFERENCES

1. Botha JL, Bray F, Sankila R et al. Breast cancer incidence and mortality trends in 16 European countries. Eur J Cancer 2003; 39: 1718–29.

2. Fisher B, Costantino JP, Wickerham DL et al. Tamoxifen for prevention of breast cancer: report of the National Surgical Adjuvant Breast and Bowel Project P-1 Study. J Natl Cancer Inst 1998; 90: 1371–88.

3. Fisher B, Anderson S, Tan-Chiu E et al. Tamoxifen and chemotherapy for axillary node-negative, estrogen receptor-negative breast cancer: findings from National Surgical Adjuvant Breast and Bowel Project B-23. J Clin Oncol 2001; 19: 931–42.

4. EBCTC Group. Tamoxifen for early breast cancer: an overview of the randomised trials. Early Breast Cancer Trialists' Collaborative Group. Lancet 1998; 351: 1451–67.

5. Fisher B, Dignam J, Wolmark N et al. Tamoxifen in treatment of intraductal breast cancer: National Surgical Adjuvant Breast and Bowel Project B-24 randomised controlled trial. Lancet 1999; 353: 1993–2000.

6. Horobin JM, Preece PE, Dewar JA et al. Long-term follow-up of elderly patients with locoregional breast cancer treated with tamoxifen only. Br J Surg 1991; 78: 213–17.

7. Fennessy M, Bates T, MacRae K et al. Late follow-up of a randomized trial of surgery plus tamoxifen versus tamoxifen alone in women aged over 70 years with operable breast cancer. Br J Surg 2004; 91: 699–704.

8. Johnston SR, Dowsett M. Aromatase inhibitors for breast cancer: lessons from the laboratory. Nat Rev Cancer 2003; 3: 821–31.

9. Wong ZW, Ellis MJ. First-line endocrine treatment of breast cancer: aromatase inhibitor or antioestrogen? Br J Cancer 2004; 90: 20–5.

10. Wolmark N, Dunn BK. The role of tamoxifen in breast cancer prevention: issues sparked by the NSABP Breast Cancer Prevention Trial (P-1). Ann NY Acad Sci 2001; 949: 99–108.

11. Howell A, Robertson JF, Quaresma Albano J et al. Fulvestrant, formerly ICI 182,780, is as effective as anastrozole in postmenopausal women with advanced breast cancer progressing after prior endocrine treatment. J Clin Oncol 2002; 20: 3396–403.

12. Dodwell D, Vergote I. A comparison of fulvestrant and the third-generation aromatase inhibitors in the second-line treatment of postmenopausal women with advanced breast cancer. Cancer Treat Rev 2005; 31: 274–82.

13. Osborne CK, Pippen J, Jones SE et al. Double-blind, randomized trial comparing the efficacy and tolerability of fulvestrant versus anastrozole in postmenopausal women with advanced breast cancer progressing on prior endocrine therapy: results of a North American trial. J Clin Oncol 2002; 20: 3386–95.

14. Perey L, Paridaens R, Hawle H et al. Clinical benefit of fulvestrant in postmenopausal women with advanced breast cancer and primary or acquired resistance to aromatase inhibitors: final results of phase II Swiss Group for Clinical Cancer Research Trial (SAKK 21/00). Ann Oncol 2007; 18: 64–9.

15. Klein-Hitpass L, Ryffel GU, Heitlinger E et al. A 13 bp palindrome is a functional estrogen responsive element and interacts specifically with estrogen receptor. Nucleic Acids Res 1988; 16: 647–63.

16. Kushner PJ, Agard DA, Greene GL et al. Estrogen receptor pathways to AP-1. J Steroid Biochem Mol Biol 2000; 74: 311–17.

17. Safe S. Transcriptional activation of genes by 17 beta-estradiol through estrogen receptor-Sp1 interactions. Vitamoxifen Horm 2001; 62: 231–52.

18. Xing W, Archer TK. Upstream stimulatory factors mediate estrogen receptor activation of the cathepsin D promoter. Mol Endocrinol 1998; 12: 1310–21.

19. Smith CL, O'Malley BW. Coregulator function: a key to understanding tissue specificity of selective receptor modulators. Endocr Rev 2004; 25: 45–71.

20. Smith CL, Nawaz Z, O'Malley BW. Coactivator and corepressor regulation of the agonist/antagonist activity of the mixed antiestrogen, 4-hydroxytamoxifen. Mol Endocrinol 1997; 11: 657–66.

21. Normanno N, Di Maio M, De Maio E et al. Mechanisms of endocrine resistance and novel therapeutic strategies in breast cancer. Endocr Relat Cancer 2005; 12: 721–47.

22. Kahlert S, Nuedling S, van Eickels M et al. Estrogen receptor alpha rapidly activates the IGF-1 receptor pathway. J Biol Chem 2000; 275: 18,447–53.

23. Simoncini T, Hafezi-Moghadam A, Brazil DP et al. Interaction of oestrogen receptor with the regulatory subunit of phosphatidylinositol-3-OH kinase. Nature 2000; 407: 538–41.

24. Morelli C, Garofalo C, Bartucci M et al. Estrogen receptor-alpha regulates the degradation of insulin receptor substrates 1 and 2 in breast cancer cells. Oncogene 2003; 22: 4007–16.

25. Song RX, McPherson RA, Adam L et al. Linkage of rapid estrogen action to MAPK activation by ERalpha-Shc association and Shc pathway activation. Mol Endocrinol 2002; 16: 116–27.

26. Brockdorff BL, Heiberg I, Lykkesfeldt AE. Resistance to different antiestrogens is caused by different multi-factorial changes and is associated with reduced expression of IGF receptor Ialpha. Endocr Relat Cancer 2003; 10: 579–90.

27. Osborne CK. Mechanisms for tamoxifen resistance in breast cancer: possible role of tamoxifenoxifen metabolism. J Steroid Biochem Mol Biol 1993; 47: 83–9.

28. Mahfoudi A, Roulet E, Dauvois S et al. Specific mutations in the estrogen receptor change the properties of antiestrogens to full agonists. Proc Natl Acad Sci USA 1995; 92: 4206–10.

29. Speirs V, Malone C, Walton DS et al. Increased expression of estrogen receptor beta mRNA in tamoxifen-resistant breast cancer patients. Cancer Res 1999; 59: 5421–4.

30. Johnston SR, Saccani-Jotti G, Smith IE et al. Changes in estrogen receptor, progesterone receptor, and pS2 expression in tamoxifen-resistant human breast cancer. Cancer Res 1995; 55: 3331–8.

31. Girault I, Lerebours F, Amarir S et al. Expression analysis of estrogen receptor alpha coregulators in breast carcinoma: evidence that NCOR1 expression is predictive of the response to tamoxifen. Clin Cancer Res 2003; 9: 1259–66.

32. Osborne CK, Bardou V, Hopp TA et al. Role of the estrogen receptor coactivator AIB1 (SRC-3) and HER2/neu in tamoxifen resistance in breast cancer. J Natl Cancer Inst 2003; 95: 353–61.

33. Kato S, Endoh H, Masuhiro Y et al. Activation of the estrogen receptor through phosphorylation by mitogen-activated protein kinase. Science 1995; 270: 1491–4.

34. Campbell RA, Bhat-Nakshatri P, Patel NM et al. Phosphatidylinositol 3-kinase/AKT-mediated activation of estrogen receptor alpha: a new model for anti-estrogen resistance. J Biol Chem 2001; 276: 9817–24.

35. Michalides R, Griekspoor A, Balkenende A et al. Tamoxifen resistance by a conformational arrest of the estrogen receptor alpha after PKA activation in breast cancer. Cancer Cell 2004; 5: 597–605.

36. Gee JM, Robertson JF, Ellis IO et al. Phosphorylation of ERK1/2 mitogen-activated protein kinase is associated with poor response to anti-hormonal therapy and decreased patient survival in clinical breast cancer. Int J Cancer 2001; 95: 247–54.

37. Perez-Tenorio G, Stal O. Activation of AKT/PKB in breast cancer predicts a worse outcome among endocrine treated patients. Br J Cancer 2002; 86: 540–5.

38. Kirkegaard T, Witton CJ, McGlynn LM et al. AKT activation predicts outcome in breast cancer patients treated with tamoxifen. J Pathol 2005; 207: 139–46.

39. Martinez-Lacaci I, Saceda M, Plowman GD et al. Estrogen and phorbol esters regulate amphiregulin expression by two separate mechanisms in human breast cancer cell lines. Endocrinology 1995; 136: 3983–92.

40. Salomon DS, Normanno N, Ciardiello F et al. The role of amphiregulin in breast cancer. Breast Cancer Res Treat 1995; 33: 103–14.

41. Wu RC, Qin J, Yi P et al. Selective phosphorylations of the SRC-3/AIB1 coactivator integrate genomic responses to multiple cellular signalling pathways. Mol Cell 2004; 15: 937–49.

42. Bunone G, Briand PA, Miksicek RJ et al. Activation of the unliganded estrogen receptor by EGF involves the MAP kinase pathway and direct phosphorylation. Embo J 1996; 15: 2174–83.

43. Ring A, Dowsett M. Mechanisms of tamoxifen resistance. Endocr Relat Cancer 2004; 11: 643–58.

44. Riggins RB, Zwart A, Nehra R et al. The nuclear factor kappa B inhibitor parthenolide restores ICI 182,780 (Faslodex; fulvestrant)-induced apoptosis in antiestrogen-resistant breast cancer cells. Mol Cancer Ther 2005; 4: 33–41.

45. McClelland RA, Barrow D, Madden TA et al. Enhanced epidermal growth factor receptor signalling in MCF7 breast cancer cells after long-term culture in the presence of the pure antiestrogen ICI 182,780 (Faslodex). Endocrinology 2001; 142: 2776–88.

46. Frogne T, Jepsen JS, Larsen SS et al. Antiestrogen-resistant human breast cancer cells require activated protein kinase B/Akt for growth. Endocr Relat Cancer 2005; 12: 599–614.

47. Fan M, Bigsby RM, Nephew KP. The NEDD8 pathway is required for proteasome-mediated degradation of human estrogen receptor (ER)-alpha and essential for the antiproliferative activity of ICI 182,780 in ERalpha-positive breast cancer cells. Mol Endocrinol 2003; 17: 356–65.

48. Macedo LF, Sabnis G, Brodie A. Preclinical modeling of endocrine response and resistance: focus on aromatase inhibitors. Cancer 2007; 112: 679–88.

49. Saji S, Jensen EV, Nilsson S et al. Estrogen receptors alpha and beta in the rodent mammary gland. Proc Natl Acad Sci USA 2000; 97: 337–42.

50. Bocchinfuso WP, Korach KS. Mammary gland development and tumorigenesis in estrogen receptor knockout mice. J Mammary Gland Biol Neoplasia 1997; 2: 323–34.

51. Allred DC, Mohsin SK, Fuqua SA. Histological and biological evolution of human premalignant breast disease. Endocr Relat Cancer 2001; 8: 47–61.

52. Pichon MF, Broet P, Magdelenat H et al. Prognostic value of steroid receptors after long-term follow-up of 2257 operable breast cancers. Br J Cancer 1996; 73: 1545–51.

53. Henry JA, Nicholson S, Farndon JR et al. Measurement of oestrogen receptor mRNA levels in human breast tumours. Br J Cancer 1988; 58: 600–5.

54. Ferno M, Stal O, Baldetorp B et al. Results of two or five years of adjuvant tamoxifen correlated to steroid receptor and S-phase levels. South Sweden Breast Cancer Group, and South-East Sweden Breast Cancer Group. Breast Cancer Res Treat 2000; 59: 69–76.

55. EBCTC Group. Systemic treatment of early breast cancer by hormonal, cytotoxic, or immune therapy. 133 randomised trials involving 31,000 recurrences and 24,000 deaths among 75,000 women. Early Breast Cancer Trialists' Collaborative Group. Lancet 1992; 339: 71–85.

56. Elledge RM, Green S, Pugh R et al. Estrogen receptor (ER) and progesterone receptor (PgR), by ligand-binding assay compared with ER, PgR and pS2, by immuno-histochemistry in predicting response to tamoxifen in metastatic breast cancer: a Southwest Oncology Group Study. Int J Cancer 2000; 89: 111–17.

57. Cuzick J, Forbes J, Edwards R et al. First results from the International Breast Cancer Intervention Study (IBIS-I): a randomised prevention trial. Lancet 2002; 360: 817–24.

58. Osborne CK, Yochmowitz MG, Knight WA, 3rd et al. The value of estrogen and progesterone receptors in the treatment of breast cancer. Cancer 1980; 46: 2884–8.

59. Harvey JM, Clark GM, Osborne CK et al. Estrogen receptor status by immunohistochemistry is superior to the ligand-binding assay for predicting response to adjuvant endocrine therapy in breast cancer. J Clin Oncol 1999; 17: 1474–81.

60. Baum M, Budzar AU, Cuzick J et al. Anastrozole alone or in combination with tamoxifen versus tamoxifen alone for adjuvant treatment of postmenopausal women with early breast cancer: first results of the ATAC randomised trial. Lancet 2002; 359: 2131–9.

61. Howell A, Cuzick J, Baum M et al. Results of the ATAC (Arimidex, Tamoxifen, Alone or in Combination) trial after completion of 5 years' adjuvant treatment for breast cancer. Lancet 2005; 365: 60–2.

62. Joel PB, Smith J, Sturgill TW et al. pp90rsk1 regulates estrogen receptor-mediated transcription through phosphorylation of Ser-167. Mol Cell Biol 1998; 18: 1978–84.

63. Murphy L, Cherlet T, Adeyinka A et al. Phospho-serine-118 estrogen receptor-alpha detection in human breast tumors in vivo. Clin Cancer Res 2004; 10: 1354–9.

64. Sarwar N, Kim JS, Jiang J et al. Phosphorylation of ERalpha at serine 118 in primary breast cancer and in tamoxifen-resistant tumours is indicative of a complex role for ERalpha phosphorylation in breast cancer progression. Endocr Relat Cancer 2006; 13: 851–61.

65. Gee JM, Robertson JF, Gutteridge E et al. Epidermal growth factor receptor/HER2/insulin-like growth factor receptor signalling and oestrogen receptor activity in clinical breast cancer. Endocr Relat Cancer 2005; 12 (Suppl 1): S99–S111.

66. Yamashita H, Nishio M, Kobayashi S et al. Phosphorylation of estrogen receptor alpha serine 167 is predictive of response to endocrine therapy and increases postrelapse survival in metastatic breast cancer. Breast Cancer Res 2005; 7: R753–R764.

67. Tokunaga E, Kimura Y, Oki E et al. Akt is frequently activated in HER2/neu-positive breast cancers and associated with poor prognosis among hormone-treated patients. Int J Cancer 2006; 118: 284–9.

68. Jiang J, Sarwar N, Peston D et al. Phosphorylation of estrogen receptor-alpha at Ser167 is indicative of longer disease-free and overall survival in breast cancer patients. Clin Cancer Res 2007; 13: 5769–76.

69. Gustafsson JA. Estrogen receptor beta – a new dimension in estrogen mechanism of action. J Endocrinol 1999; 163: 379–83.

70. Paech K, Webb P, Kuiper GG et al. Differential ligand activation of estrogen receptors ERalpha and ERbeta at AP1 sites. Science 1997; 277: 1508–10.

71. Kuiper GG, Carlsson B, Grandien K et al. Comparison of the ligand binding specificity and transcript tissue distribution of estrogen receptors alpha and beta. Endocrinology 1997; 138: 863–70.

72. Speirs V, Parkes AT, Kerin MJ et al. Coexpression of estrogen receptor alpha and beta: poor prognostic factors in human breast cancer? Cancer Res 1999; 59: 525–8.

73. Iwase H, Zhang Z, Omoto Y et al. Clinical significance of the expression of estrogen receptors alpha and beta for endocrine therapy of breast cancer. Cancer Chemother Pharmacol 2003; 52 (Suppl 1): S34–S38.

74. Hopp TA, Weiss HL, Parra IS et al. Low levels of estrogen receptor beta protein predict resistance to tamoxifen therapy in breast cancer. Clin Cancer Res 2004; 10: 7490–9.

75. Esslimani-Sahla M, Simony-Lafontaine J, Kramar A et al. Estrogen receptor beta (ER beta) level but not its ER beta cx variant helps to predict tamoxifen resistance in breast cancer. Clin Cancer Res 2004; 10: 5769–76.

76. Cappelletti V, Celio L, Bajetta E et al. Prospective evaluation of estrogen receptor-beta in predicting response to neoadjuvant antiestrogen therapy in elderly breast cancer patients. Endocr Relat Cancer 2004; 11: 761–70.

77. Gruvberger-Saal SK, Bendahl PO, Saal LH et al. Estrogen receptor beta expression is associated with tamoxifen response in ERalpha-negative breast carcinoma. Clin Cancer Res 2007; 13: 1987–94.

78. Moore JT, McKee DD, Slentz-Kesler K et al. Cloning and characterization of human estrogen receptor beta isoforms. Biochem Biophys Res Commun 1998; 247: 75–8.

79. Ogawa S, Inoue S, Watanabe T et al. Molecular cloning and characterization of human estrogen receptor betacx: a potential inhibitor of estrogen action in human. Nucleic Acids Res 1998; 26: 3505–12.

80. Esslimani-Sahla M, Kramar A, Simony-Lafontaine J et al. Increased estrogen receptor betacx expression during mammary carcinogenesis. Clin Cancer Res 2005; 11: 3170–4.

81. Saji S, Omoto Y, Shimizu C et al. Expression of estrogen receptor (ER) (beta)cx protein in ER(alpha)-positive breast cancer: specific correlation with progesterone receptor. Cancer Res 2002; 62: 4849–53.

82. Davies MP, O'Neill PA, Innes H et al. Correlation of mRNA for oestrogen receptor beta splice variants ERbeta1, ERbeta2/ERbetacx and ERbeta5 with outcome in endocrine-treated breast cancer. J Mol Endocrinol 2004; 33: 773–82.

83. Palmieri C, Lam EW, Mansi J et al. The expression of ER beta cx in human breast cancer and the relationship to endocrine therapy and survival. Clin Cancer Res 2004; 10: 2421–8.

84. Vinayagam R, Sibson DR, Holcombe C et al. Association of oestrogen receptor beta 2 (ER beta 2/ER beta cx) with outcome of adjuvant endocrine treatment for primary breast cancer – a retrospective study. BMC Cancer 2007; 7: 131.

85. Miller WR, Anderson TJ, Dixon JM et al. Oestrogen receptor beta and neoadjuvant therapy with tamoxifen: prediction of response and effects of treatment. Br J Cancer 2006; 94: 1333–8.

86. Smith CL, Onate SA, Tsai MJ et al. CREB binding protein acts synergistically with steroid receptor coactivator-1 to enhance steroid receptor-dependent transcription. Proc Natl Acad Sci USA 1996; 93: 8884–8.

87. Font de Mora J, Brown M. AIB1 is a conduit for kinase-mediated growth factor signaling to the estrogen receptor. Mol Cell Biol 2000; 20: 5041–7.

88. Anzick SL, Kononen J, Walker RL et al. AIB1, a steroid receptor coactivator amplified in breast and ovarian cancer. Science 1997; 277: 965–8.

89. Murphy LC, Simon SL, Parkes A et al. Altered expression of estrogen receptor coregulators during human breast tumorigenesis. Cancer Res 2000; 60: 6266–71.

90. Fleming FJ, Myers E, Kelly G et al. Expression of SRC-1, AIB1, and PEA3 in HER2 mediated endocrine resistant breast cancer; a predictive role for SRC-1. J Clin Pathol 2004; 57: 1069–74.

91. Myers E, Fleming FJ, Crotty TB et al. Inverse relationship between ER-beta and SRC-1 predicts outcome in endocrine-resistant breast cancer. Br J Cancer 2004; 91: 1687–93.

92. Shang Y, Brown M. Molecular determinants for the tissue specificity of SERMs. Science 2002; 295: 2465–8.

93. Cottone E, Orso F, Biglia N et al. Role of coactivators and corepressors in steroid and nuclear receptor signaling: potential markers of tumor growth and drug sensitivity. Int J Biol Markers 2001; 16: 151–66.

94. Margueron R, Duong V, Bonnet S et al. Histone deacetylase inhibition and estrogen receptor alpha levels modulate the transcriptional activity of partial antiestrogens. J Mol Endocrinol 2004; 32: 583–94.

95. Fujita T, Kobayashi Y, Wada O et al. Full activation of estrogen receptor alpha activation function-1 induces proliferation of breast cancer cells. J Biol Chem 2003; 278: 26,704–14.

96. Lavinsky RM, Jepsen K, Heinzel T et al. Diverse signaling pathways modulate nuclear receptor recruitment of N-CoR and SMRT complexes. Proc Natl Acad Sci USA 1998; 95: 2920–5.

97. Naughton C, MacLeod K, Kuske B et al. Progressive loss of estrogen receptor alpha cofactor recruitment in endocrine resistance. Mol Endocrinol 2007; 21: 2615–26.

98. Zwart W, Griekspoor A, Berno V et al. PKA-induced resistance to tamoxifen is associated with an altered orientation of ERalpha towards co-activator SRC-1. Embo J 2007; 26: 3534–44.

99. McGuire WL. Hormone receptors: their role in predicting prognosis and response to endocrine therapy. Semin Oncol 1978; 5: 428–33.

100. Horwitz KB, Koseki Y, McGuire WL. Estrogen control of progesterone receptor in human breast cancer: role of estradiol and antiestrogen. Endocrinology 1978; 103: 1742–51.

101. Ravdin PM, Green S, Dorr TM et al. Prognostic significance of progesterone receptor levels in estrogen receptor-positive patients with metastatic breast cancer treated with tamoxifen: results of a prospective Southwest Oncology Group study. J Clin Oncol 1992; 10: 1284–91.

102. Bardou VJ, Arpino G, Elledge RM et al. Progesterone receptor status significantly improves outcome prediction over estrogen receptor status alone for adjuvant endocrine therapy in two large breast cancer databases. J Clin Oncol 2003; 21: 1973–9.

103. Lamy PJ, Pujol P, Thezenas S et al. Progesterone receptor quantification as a strong prognostic determinant in postmenopausal breast cancer women under tamoxifen therapy. Breast Cancer Res Treat 2002; 76: 65–71.

104. Ellis MJ, Coop A, Singh B et al. Letrozole is more effective neoadjuvant endocrine therapy than tamoxifenoxifen for ErbB-1- and/or ErbB-2-positive, estrogen receptor-positive primary breast cancer: evidence from a phase III randomized trial. J Clin Oncol 2001; 19: 3808–16.

105. Dowsett M, Harper-Wynne C, Boeddinghaus I et al. HER2 amplification impedes the antiproliferative effects of hormone therapy in estrogen receptor-positive primary breast cancer. Cancer Res 2001; 61: 8452–8.

106. Yu KD, Liu GY, Di GH et al. Progesterone receptor status provides predictive value for adjuvant endocrine therapy in older estrogen receptor-positive breast cancer patients. Breast 2007; 16: 307–15.

107. Hull DF, 3rd, Clark GM, Osborne CK et al. Multiple estrogen receptor assays in human breast cancer. Cancer Res 1983; 43: 413–16.

108. Gross GE, Clark GM, Chamness GC et al. Multiple progesterone receptor assays in human breast cancer. Cancer Res 1984; 44: 836–40.

109. Balleine RL, Earl MJ, Greenberg ML et al. Absence of progesterone receptor associated with secondary breast cancer in postmenopausal women. Br J Cancer 1999; 79: 1564–71.

110. Baum M, Howell A, Cuzick J et al. Adjuvant endocrine therapy in postmenopausal women with early breast cancer: Where are we now? Results of the ATAC

(Arimidex, Tamoxifenoxifen, Alone or in Combination) trial after completion of 5 years' adjuvant treatment for breast cancer. Anastrozole alone or in combination with tamoxifen versus tamoxifen alone for adjuvant treatment of postmenopausal women with early breast cancer: first results of the ATAC randomised trial. Eur J Cancer 2005; 365: 60–2.

111. Dowsett M, Cuzick J, Wale C et al. Retrospective analysis of time to recurrence in the ATAC trial according to hormone receptor status: an hypothesis-generating study. J Clin Oncol 2005; 23: 7512–17.

112. Smith IE, Dowsett M, Ebbs SR et al. Neoadjuvant treatment of postmenopausal breast cancer with anastrozole, tamoxifen, or both in combination: the Immediate Preoperative Anastrozole, Tamoxifen, or Combined with Tamoxifen (IMPACT) multicenter double-blind randomized trial. J Clin Oncol 2005; 23: 5108–16.

113. Cui X, Zhang P, Deng W et al. Insulin-like growth factor-I inhibits progesterone receptor expression in breast cancer cells via the phosphatidylinositol 3-kinase/Akt/mammalian target of rapamycin pathway: progesterone receptor as a potential indicator of growth factor activity in breast cancer. Mol Endocrinol 2003; 17: 575–88.

114. Tovey S, Dunne B, Witton CJ et al. Can molecular markers predict when to implement treatment with aromatase inhibitors in invasive breast cancer? Clin Cancer Res 2005; 11: 4835–42.

115. Bartsch R, Wenzel C, Altorjai G et al. Her2 and progesterone receptor status are not predictive of response to fulvestrant treatment. Clin Cancer Res 2007; 13: 4435–9.

116. Kraus WL, Montano MM, Katzenellenbogen BS. Cloning of the rat progesterone receptor gene 5'-region and identification of two functionally distinct promoters. Mol Endocrinol 1993; 7: 1603–16.

117. Hopp TA, Weiss HL, Hilsenbeck SG et al. Breast cancer patients with progesterone receptor PR-A-rich tumors have poorer disease-free survival rates. Clin Cancer Res 2004; 10: 2751–60.

118. De Vivo I, Hankinson SE, Colditz GA et al. A functional polymorphism in the progesterone receptor gene is associated with an increase in breast cancer risk. Cancer Res 2003; 63: 5236–8.

119. McCormack O, Chung WY, Fitzpatrick P et al. Progesterone receptor B (PRB) promoter hypermethylation in sporadic breast cancer: progesterone receptor B hypermethylation in breast cancer. Breast Cancer Res Treat 2007 (in press).

120. Sartorius CA, Shen T, Horwitz KB. Progesterone receptors A and B differentially affect the growth of estrogen-dependent human breast tumor xenografts. Breast Cancer Res Treat 2003; 79: 287–99.

121. Townson SM, O'Connell P. Identification of estrogen receptor alpha variants in breast tumors: implications for predicting response to hormonal therapies. J Surg Oncol 2006; 94: 271–3.

122. Jansen MP, Foekens JA, van Staveren IL et al. Molecular classification of tamoxifen-resistant breast carcinomas by gene expression profiling. J Clin Oncol 2005; 23: 732–40.

123. Ma XJ, Wang Z, Ryan PD et al. A two-gene expression ratio predicts clinical outcome in breast cancer patients treated with tamoxifen. Cancer Cell 2004; 5: 607–16.

124. van 't Veer LJ, Dai H, van de Vijver MJ et al. Gene expression profiling predicts clinical outcome of breast cancer. Nature 2002; 415: 530–6.

Mitogen-activated protein kinase family members and endocrine response and survival in breast cancer

10

Iain R Hutcheson, Robert I Nicholson and Julia MW Gee

INTRODUCTION

Until relatively recently endocrine response pathways in breast cancer were described solely in terms of the intracellular pathways used by estrogens and the subsequent disruptive effects exerted by antihormonal treatments on estrogen receptor (ER) signaling.[1] Thus, it was frequently proposed that estrogens promoted tumor growth by binding to ERs, which then acted as nuclear transcription factors regulating the expression of genes involved in proliferation and survival mechanisms. In contrast, antihormones, acting either to reduce the amount of estrogens available to the tumor cells or binding the ER to antagonize the cellular actions of estrogens, prevented this flow of information to promote tumor remissions.[1,2]

However, a more modern view of endocrine response pathways retains the concept that estrogens acting through ERs are central to the development of breast cancer, but also recognizes that it is naïve to consider ER signaling in isolation of the remainder of the cancer cell biology.[3,4] Indeed, an increasing number of elements within the breast cancer phenotype, notably including peptide growth factors, have now been identified which modify, and can be modified by, ER signaling.[4] As such, their signal transduction has the capacity to significantly influence the sensitivity of breast cancer cells to estrogens. Importantly, however, these factors are also likely to be critical in the mechanism of response to antihormonal drugs and, moreover, may be integral in the escape from antihormone control of growth that occurs on disease relapse.

In this light, the present chapter seeks to outline the elaborate molecular biology of estrogen and growth factor-directed mitogen-activated protein (MAP) kinase interactions which are likely to play a central role in hormone-sensitive breast tumor growth. It subsequently examines how changes often present in the breast cancer phenotype would severely perturb the balance of such signaling, thus providing a possible explanatory hypothesis for the tumor growth associated with the phenomena of de novo and acquired endocrine resistance. Routine monitoring of MAP kinase signaling in breast cancer specimens would thus be predicted to prove not only prognostically valuable but also relevant in defining a new and important therapeutic target to improve the actions of antihormonal drugs in breast cancer.

GROWTH FACTOR-INDUCED MITOGEN-ACTIVATED PROTEIN KINASE SIGNALING

The MAP kinase signal transduction pathways are highly conserved signaling cascades which exert a profound effect on cell physiology.[5–7] MAP kinase pathways can be activated by a variety of different stimuli, including growth

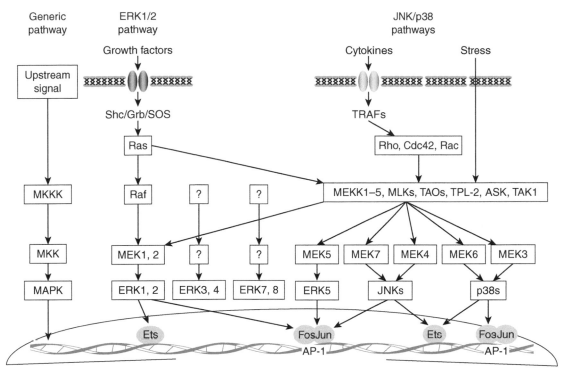

Figure 10.1   The mitogen-activated protein (MAP) kinase pathways. AP-1, Activator protein 1; ASK, apotosis signal regulating kinases; ERK, extracellular signal-regulated kinases; JNK, c-jun N-terminal kinases; MAPK, mitogen-activated protein kinase; MKK, MAP kinase kinase (MAP2K); MKKK, MAP kinase kinase kinase (MAP3K); MEK, MEK (MAP kinase or ERK kinase); MLK, mixed lineage kinases; TAK, transforming growth factor-activated kinase; TAO, thousand and one; TPL, tumor necrosis factor receptor associated factor; TRAF, tumor necrosis factor receptor associated factor.

factors, cytokines and enviromental stresses, and play a role in the regulation of cell proliferation, cell differentiation and cell death. Three families of mammalian MAP kinase have been identified; the extracellular signal-regulated kinases (ERKs); p38 MAP kinases; and c-jun N-terminal kinases (JNKs). Each family consists of a three-tiered signaling module that establishes a sequential activation pathway (Figure 10.1). The first kinase of the module is a MAP kinase kinase kinase (MAP3K), which can be activated by either a MAP3K kinase (MAP4K) or a small guanosine triphosphate (GTP)-binding protein of the Rho or Ras family. Activated MAP3K phosphorylates and activates a MAP kinase kinase (MAP2K), which in turn phosphorylates and activates a MAP kinase. The MAP kinases then phosphorylate and regulate nuclear proteins,

which coordinate gene transcription, cell cycle machinery, and cell survival/apoptotic pathways.

To date, the ERK pathway includes seven MAP kinases, ERK1–5, 7 and 8,[5,7] of which ERK1/2 are the most extensively studied. ERK1/2 are believed to play a central role in cell proliferation and their activation in response to growth factor stimulation is reasonably well understood. For example, binding of epidermal growth factor (EGF) to its receptor stimulates the receptors intrinsic tyrosine kinase activity, resulting in autophosphorylation of tyrosine residues in its cytoplasmic domain. Phosphotyrosine residues act as docking sites for adaptor proteins which coordinate the activation of the downstream signal transduction pathways. These adaptor proteins, which include Shc and Grb2, bind to the activated EGF receptor (EGFR), and further recruit the guanine nucleotide exchange factor Son of sevenless (Sos).[8] Sos promotes the activation of Ras by stimulating the exchange of bound guanosine diphosphate (GDP) to GTP, which in turn initiates the sequential activation of the ERK1/2 pathway module, consisting of Raf-1 (the MAP3K), MEK1/2 (the MAP2Ks) and ERK1/2 (the MAP kinases).[5,8] The physiological outcome of MAP kinase signaling depends on both the magnitude and duration of kinase activation. The principal mechanism of action of ERK1/2 is increased cell proliferation as a consequence of sustained kinase activity, promotion of nuclear transcription factor expression and activation (e.g. Ets and activator protein-1 (AP-1) components), and subsequent regulation of proteins involved in the cell cycle, e.g. cyclin D1.[9,10] However, high levels of ERK1/2 activity can also lead to cell cycle arrest through induction of p21 and p27.[10] Other downstream cytoplasmic effectors of ERK1/2 include protein kinases and phosphatases, cytoskeletal elements, regulators of apoptosis, and a variety of other signaling-related molecules.[11] Components of its own signaling cascade (EGFR, Sos, Raf-1 and MAP kinase/ERK kinase MEK) are also key targets, suggesting a possible feedback inhibition mechanism.[7] The MAP kinase pathways utilizing the remaining ERK3–5, 7 and 8 remain to be fully characterized, and their roles in cell physiology have yet to be clearly established. However, recent evidence has indicated a potential role for ERK5 in mitogenic signaling as it can be activated by EGF and neuregulin stimulation, and can regulate expression of cyclin D1.[9,12]

The p38 and JNK pathways are activated by phosphorylation in response to stress ("stress-activated" MAP kinase family members; SAPKs), and may play a central role in the regulation of cell survival/apoptosis and inflammation.[6] The upstream activators of the p38 and JNK pathway modules remain unclear, although recent evidence implicates a role for the Rho family of GTPases (cdc42, rac) and the tumor necrosis factor receptor associated factor (TRAF) adaptor proteins, associated with the tumor necrosis factor (TNF) family of receptors.[6,13–15] The p38 and JNK pathway modules are better characterized, and structurally resemble the ERK pathway. The MEKK1–5 (MAP K and ERK kinase kinases), mixed lineage kinases (MLKs), apoptosis signal-regulating kinases (ASKs), Tak1, Cot and TAO kinases, all act as MAP3Ks in either the p38 or the JNK pathway modules, and activate the downstream MAP2Ks 3 ,4, 6 and 7, which in turn phosphorylate the MAP kinases.[6,7] The JNK pathway module has a potential 12 MAP kinases, 3 genes encode for JNK1–3 and each gene has four possible splice variants ($\alpha1$, $\alpha2$, $\beta1$ and $\beta2$), whereas the p38 pathway module has just 4 MAP kinase isoforms (p38α, β, γ and δ).[6,7] A prominent action of both p38 and JNK pathways is the ability to initiate apoptosis in certain cell types, possibly through recruitment of the AP-1 transcription factor or suppression of the antiapoptotic proteins Bcl2 and Bcl-XL.[6,7,9,16,17] However, these pathways alone are not sufficient to induce cell death in all systems. Other substrates for these pathways include protein kinases involved in cytoskeletal regulation (MAP kinase-activated protein kinases, p38-regulated/activated kinase), protein translation (MAP kinase-interacting kinases), gene transcription (mitogen- and stress-activated protein kinases), and insulin receptor signaling, indicating further roles for these kinases in cell invasion, proliferation, metabolism and differentiation.[16,17]

"CROSSTALK" BETWEEN ESTROGEN RECEPTOR AND MITOGEN-ACTIVATED PROTEIN KINASE-ASSOCIATED SIGNALING

Many studies have now identified that breast tumors which exhibit an effective endocrine response (i.e. complete and partial response) are often histologically low grade, well-differentiated and notably ER-positive, with a minimal level of proliferation at presentation.[18–20] The 40–50% of breast cancer patients

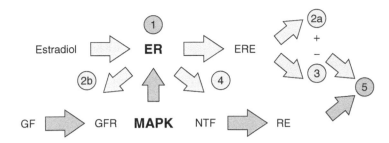

Figure 10.2 Crosstalk between estrogen receptor (ER) and mitogen-activated protein kinase (MAPK)-associated signaling. ERE, Estrogen response element; GF, growth factor; GFR, growth factor receptor; NTF, nuclear transcription factor; RE, response element.

bearing such tumors frequently enjoy a long duration of response and survival time.[21] In such tumors, it is likely that ER signaling is central to mitogenesis, with steroid hormone occupancy of the receptor efficiently driving cell growth and survival, together with expression of target genes bearing either estrogen response elements (ERE)[1,3] or response elements for other transcription factors which interact with the ER protein.[22] However, it is increasingly proposed that such events proceed most efficiently in an appropriate growth factor environment, with steroid hormone and growth factor signaling pathways "crosstalking" to reinforce each other's signaling. Notably, ERK1/2 MAP kinase is thought to be a key regulatory element in the interactions between estrogen and growth factor crosstalk. A number of these interactions are detailed below and are illustrated in Figure 10.2.

The estrogen receptor is a target for growth factor-induced kinase activity

Phosphorylation of estrogen receptors by mitogen-activated protein kinases

Numerous studies have now shown that the ER protein is subject to phosphorylation and activation by several peptide growth factors (e.g. IGF1,[23] EGF, transforming growth factorα [TGFα [24]] and heregulin[25]), events which can subsequently initiate ERE-mediated gene expression.[26,27] These events are believed to be mediated by downstream signal transduction molecules such as ERK1/2 MAP kinase.[24,28–30]

This has been consistently shown to activate ER possibly by mediating phosphorylation of serine residues 118 and 167, located in the N-terminal of the ER that contains the ligand-independent activator function-1 (AF-1) domain, thereby enhancing recruitment of coactivators and potentiating AF-1 activity.[24,28,29,31,32] Increased ER transcriptional activity may also arise as a result of p38-mediated phosphorylation at threonine residue 311, which has been shown to promote nuclear localization of the receptor.[33] Similarly, growth factor-driven ERK1/2 activity has also been shown to promote nuclear localization of ER through an AF-1-dependent mechanism;[34] however, increased ERK1/2 activity resulting from HER2 overexpression has also been reported to reduce nuclear transcriptional activity by promoting relocalization of ER to the cytoplasm.[35] Further transduction molecules demonstrated to target the ER include casein kinase II, Akt, pp90rsk1, protein kinase C δ, protein kinase A, cyclin A/cdk2, and Rho pathway elements.[30,36] In addition, the nonreceptor tyrosine kinase Src is believed to enhance AF-1 activity not only through ER phosphorylation via ERK1/2 MAP kinase, but also via JNK signaling which acts to phosphorylate coactivators for ER, thereby activating ER in an indirect manner.[37] Significantly, growth factors and downstream signal transduction pathways appear to differentially regulate the two transcriptional activator functions of the ER (i.e. AF-1 and AF-2), with the former being highly responsive to EGF, TGFα and MAP kinase signaling.[24] While activation by these factors occurs most efficiently in the presence of estrogens, their promotion of AF-1 responses certainly appears adequate for initiating transcription in the absence of the steroid hormone. An emerging concept for steroid hormone receptors is therefore that they function not only as direct transducers of steroid hormone effects but, as members of the cellular nuclear transcription factor pool, also serve as key points of convergence for multiple signal transduction pathways.[38]

Downregulation of estrogen receptors by mitogen-activated protein kinases

Although, as established above, growth factor pathways can enhance ER phosphorylation, transcriptional activity and cell growth in a ligand-independent manner, paradoxically a decline in ER expression is also a possible outcome when growth factor signaling is extreme or sustained. Evidence for this arises from several stable transfection studies in ER-positive breast cancer cells. Such studies demonstrate that growth factor signaling elements comprising the EGFR/HER2 pathway, which share an ability to hyperactivate ERK1/2 MAP kinase, all act to impair ER function and promote ER loss when overexpressed in ER-positive breast cancer cells. In our own laboratory, we have shown that constitutive upregulation of MEK1 in MCF-7 cells leads to a substantial increase in ERK1/2 MAP kinase activation, decreased ER level, and marked loss of expression of the ER-regulated gene progesterone receptor (PR) (RA McClelland, unpublished observations). Similarly, El-Ashry and colleagues[39,40] have noted precipitous falls in ER mRNA and protein following transfection of constitutively active HER2, MEK1, Raf1 or ligand-stimulated EGFR into MCF-7 cells, all of which hyperactivate ERK1/2 MAPK. There is a parallel loss of estrogen-mediated gene expression and a marked suppression of activity of ERE-reporter gene constructs in these transient transfection experiments which is not overcome by estradiol treatment. Increased ERK1/2 activity has also been reported to mediate hypoxia-induced ER downregulation, and ERK7 has been shown to regulate hormone responsiveness

in breast cells by controlling the rate of ERα degradation.[41,42] Holloway et al[43] later demonstrated that hyperactivated ERK1/2 MAPK is able to downregulate ER via substrates including the transcription factor nuclear factor kappa B (NFκB), which is markedly increased in activity in the various transfection models and is inhibited by abrogating ERK1/2 MAPK signaling.

Estrogens stimulate positive elements of growth factor signaling pathways, which may facilitate extracellular signal-regulated kinases 1 and 2 mitogen-activated protein kinase-directed cell proliferation

Genomic mechanisms

Classically, the ER functions as a transcription factor within the nucleus, and the ability of estrogen/antiestrogens to regulate gene expression has been extensively investigated in experimental models of human breast cancer both in vitro and in vivo. Based on these studies, it is becoming increasingly evident that estrogens can promote the autocrine expression of growth factor signaling pathway elements (Figure 10.2, 2a)[44,45] – notably components of the EGFR and insulin-like growth factor receptor (IGF-1R) pathways – in estrogen-responsive and -dependent human breast cancer cell lines.[46–48] In the latter instance, the IGF-1R has also been shown to be activated by estrogen, subsequently recruiting downstream signaling components, notably including insulin receptor substrate-1 (IRS-1), which in turn may be estrogenregulated.[46,49] Such actions, which are often antagonized by antiestrogens, could significantly supplement the cellular growth responses directly primed by estrogens.[44,45,48]

Nongenomic mechanisms

In addition to its classic genomic actions, recent evidence suggests that estrogen can also mediate rapid, nongenomic signaling events through binding to ER localized at the cell membrane.[50] A small pool of ER has been shown to be tethered to the plasma membrane through either binding to the lipid raft proteins caveolin-1 and flotillin or complexing with a range of membrane-associated signal transduction proteins such as growth factor receptors and G proteins.[51] In breast cancer cells, signaling via membrane ER, or membrane-initiated steroid signaling (MISS), has been shown to involve the coupling of ER with EGFR, HER2, IGF-1R and SRC, providing important mitogenic signals to epithelial cells through the subsequent recruitment and activation of downstream p38 and ERK1/2 MAP kinase pathways (Figure 10.2, 2b).[50,51] Interestingly, MISS has also been shown to subsequently impact on ER transcriptional activity through MAP kinase-mediated phosphorylation of nuclear ER and its associated coactivator AIB-1 in human epidermal growth factor receptor 2 (HER2)-overexpressing cells, providing an integrated genomic/nongenomic signaling network which can mediate both acute and long-term actions of estrogen.[51,52]

Estrogens inhibit negative elements of growth factor signaling pathways

As well as the positive influences exerted by estrogens on growth factor signaling pathways detailed above, it is notable that in parallel they diminish (while antiestrogens induce) the expression of the growth inhibitory factor TGFβ in several estrogen-responsive human breast cancer cell lines, possibly via activation of the p38 pathway (Figure 10.2, 3).[53] Estrogens thus serve to inhibit the expression of a factor, which can act through the p38/JNK pathways, to induce programed cell death.[54,55]

Additionally, however, it is of particular significance that estrogens have been reported to inhibit expression of tyrosine phosphatases in ER-positive breast cancer cells to increase growth factor mitogenic activity, while both steroidal and nonsteroidal antiestrogens increase phosphatase activity.[56,57] Tamoxifen, for example, inhibits the mitogenic activity of EGF by promoting significant dephosphorylation of EGFR, an effect that reduces MAP

kinase signaling and is believed to be ER mediated.[56]

The estrogen receptor interacts with growth factor-induced nuclear transcription factors, coactivators/corepressors, and additional proteins to target a diversity of response elements

An important feature of growth factor signaling is its potential to activate several profiles of nuclear transcription factors, which subsequently serve to promote the expression of genes participating in a diversity of endpoints, including cell cycle progression (Figure 10.2, 4). For example, as stated previously, in addition to its phosphorylation of the ER protein, growth factor-induced MAP kinase (ERK1/2) directly activates Elk-1/p62TCF.[58] This latter transcription factor subsequently forms a ternary complex with p67SRF (serum response factor) and primes Fos expression via the c-fos serum response element.[58] Similarly, JNK phosphorylates the c-Jun protein which subsequently heterodimerises with Fos.[9,17] The resultant complex, AP-1, is of central importance since it directly targets the 12-O-tetradecanoyl-phorbol-13 acetate-responsive element (TPA-RE), a sequence found in the promoters of many genes involved in a plethora of cellular endpoints, including proliferation and survival.[59]

In light of this, it has been reported that estrogens can significantly enhance growth factor induced AP-1 activity in hormone-sensitive breast cancer cells.[60] This feature is believed to be a consequence of productive protein/protein interactions between the estrogen receptor and the AP-1 complex,[22] a phenomenon also demonstrated to occur between ER and other transcription factors such as SP-1.[61] Thus, ER appears able to activate genes containing AP-1 sites in their promoters,[62] providing a mechanism whereby ER signaling may be markedly diversified. Initial studies suggested that antiestrogens antagonized growth factor-induced AP-1 activity, with maximal inhibition by pure antiestrogens.[60] In contrast to the above, ER may repress the activity of the transcription factor NFκB,[63] which regulates expression of many cytokines and growth factors.[64]

Finally, it should be remembered that ER/ERE-mediated gene transcription is also significantly enhanced by the recruitment of several coactivators and/or by overcoming the effects of corepressor proteins. Indeed, ERK1/2 and p38 MAP kinase-mediated serine phosphorylation of coactivators such as SRC-1, GRIP1 and AIB1, and the corepressor SMRT, has been shown to regulate their ability to associate with ERα and influence its transcriptional activity.[65–69] Additional proteins also under growth factor/MAP kinase regulation have been show to interact with the ER, including the cell cycle protein cyclin D1 and the orphan member of the nuclear receptor superfamily, the estrogen-related receptor alpha (ERRalpha).[70,71] Cyclin D1 can activate ER by direct binding, as well as by recruiting coactivators of the SRC-1 family to the ER,[70] whilst ERRalpha has been shown to compete directly with ER, and consequently repress transcriptional activity via this receptor.[71]

Steroid hormone and growth factor signaling pathways influence common growth regulatory genes

In order for cells to proliferate, they initially need to be recruited into the cell cycle and then be induced to progress through it. These outcomes are orchestrated by at least two series of events, which can be jointly influenced by steroid hormone and growth factor-directed MAP kinase signaling pathways:[72] firstly, the induction of intermediate early response genes, such as c-fos,[73] c-jun,[73,74] and c-myc;[72,75] and secondly, the regulation of G1 cyclins (e.g. cyclin D1), and their partner kinases and inhibitors which are involved in restriction point control.[72,76] Joint activation of these pathways by estrogens and growth factor-induced MAP kinase would, at a minimum, reinforce mitogenic signals to responsive cells, and might even result in synergistic interactions between overlapping elements (Figure 10.2, 5).

MITOGEN-ACTIVATED PROTEIN KINASE AND BREAST CANCER MODELS OF ENDOCRINE RESPONSIVE AND UNRESPONSIVE DISEASE

Importantly, in the archetypal endocrine responsive breast cancer cell line MCF-7, growth factor signaling leads to increased MAP kinase activity, which appears critical for their growth, since substantial growth inhibition is achieved with the MEK1 inhibitor PD098059. Significantly, however, the increases in growth factor-induced MAP kinase activity, which facilitate the productive crosstalk with ER signaling described above, are only short-lived due to a highly efficient negative feedback of phosphorylation of these enzymes.[7] Such a negative-feedback system stems not only from phosphatases effectively targeting MAP kinases, but additionally from distinct nonaberrant expression patterns of growth factor receptors and intracellular signaling elements comprising the network upstream of MAP kinase activation.[77] This serves to tailor input signals to the precise growth requirements of the cells and maintain the modest levels of proliferation which are characteristic of endocrine responsive disease.

In contrast to the above, in several instances elevated activation of ERK1/2 MAP kinase and upstream regulators of this pathway have been associated with the more aggressive growth of de novo and acquired endocrine resistant cells.[40,44,45,52,78–83] Significantly, within our in-house breast cancer cell models of acquired resistance to tamoxifen and faslodex,[78,79] not only was PD098059 shown to be a highly effective inhibitor of the growth of the anti-hormone-resistant cells, but arrest of cell proliferation was also achieved with ZD1839, an EGFR selective tyrosine kinase inhibitor, and herceptin, an inhibitor of c-erbB2.[78,79] Such data indicate that these erbB receptors are direct upstream regulators of MAP kinase-induced growth regulation in these resistant cell lines. erbB receptors do not appear to be the only regulators of MAP kinase activity in tamoxifen resistance, as Cui et al[84] have reported that reduced activity of MAP kinase phosphatase 3 (MKP3), a negative regulator of ERK1/2 MAP kinase, may also play a role in the generation of the acquired tamoxifen-resistant phenotype. More recently, activation of the p38 signaling pathway has also been implicated in endocrine resistance, with enhanced levels of phosphorylated p38 being observed in a xenograft model of acquired tamoxifen-resistant MCF-7 cells.[85]

In addition to directly driving cell growth, we have also demonstrated that the increased EGFR/HER2/ERK1/2 MAP kinase signaling observed in our tamoxifen-resistant variant can efficiently phosphorylate serine 118 within the AF-1 domain of ER.[86] It is possible that such ligand-independent activation of ER may play a role in tamoxifen resistance, as cell lines resistant to this antiestrogen, in common with their clinical counterparts, continue to express ER at an equivalent level to that observed in the parental cell line.[87–91] Indeed, increased ER phosphorylation has been reported in breast cancer cell lines resistant to tamoxifen and long-term estrogen deprivation,[92–96] and more recently in ovariectomized mice bearing tumor xenografts from aromatase-transfected MCF-7 cells.[97] This MAP kinase-dependent phosphorylation of ER allows recruitment of several AF-1 coactivators, such as p68 RNA helicase, and subsequent reactivation of ER as a nuclear transcription factor, resulting in expression of detectable levels of the estrogen regulated genes, in particular amphiregulin, in our tamoxifen-resistant cell line.[86] Although the temporal sequence of these events remains to be established during the development of tamoxifen resistance, we have postulated that EGFR/MAP kinase/ER-driven increases in expression of amphiregulin may serve to establish a self-propagating autocrine signaling loop, allowing the emergence and maintenance of efficient EGFR/MAP kinase-promoted resistant growth.[86] It should also be noted that, as mentioned previously, MAP kinase signaling can directly promote phosphorylation of ER coactivators, which can result in their increased nuclear localization and enhance their impact on ER function.[65–69]

Indeed, overexpression of the coactivator AIB1 has been shown to correlate with resistance to tamoxifen in breast cancer patients, and EGFR/HER2/ERK1/2 MAP kinase-dependent phosphorylation of this coactivator has also been proposed to mediate tamoxifen resistance in HER2 overexpressing MCF-7 cells.[52,94]

Targeting the ER with the pure antiestrogen faslodex, which acts by promoting ERα degradation to deplete ERα protein expression,[1,98,99] can effectively interrupt the autocrine signaling loop established in our tamoxifen-resistant cell line, reducing activation of EGFR, c-erbB2 and MAP kinase, and potently inhibiting cell growth.[87] However, exposure of these cells to exogenous EGF ligands not only activates EGFR, c-erbB2 and ERK1/2 MAP kinase, but also supports substantial tumor cell growth in the presence of faslodex. Thus, strengthening the EGFR pathway it appears able to entirely circumvent the catastrophic effects of this antiestrogen on the ER protein in such cells.[87] EGFR ligand-treated cells are thus refractory to the growth inhibitory effects of both tamoxifen and faslodex (i.e. complete endocrine insensitivity), data which certainly implies that the primary growth regulatory role for ER in the tamoxifen-resistant cells is to maintain the efficiency of EGFR signaling. In agreement with these findings, it has recently been reported that exogenous treatment of breast cancer cells with either fibroblast growth factor-1, heregulin beta-1 or vascular endothelial growth factor, and subsequent activation of ERK1/2 MAP kinase signaling, can similarly overcome the growth inhibitory actions of faslodex.[100,101] In this context, it is also of considerable interest that Oh et al[39] have demonstrated that high levels of constitutive Raf kinase activity, leading to hyperactivation of MAP kinase, imparts MCF-7 cells with an ability to grow in the absence of estrogen. Such cells have lost their ERs and showed no activation of transfected EREs reporter gene constructs. Importantly, this effect was abrogated by inhibiting MAP kinase, thus restoring ER expression.

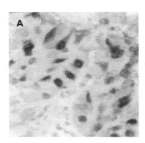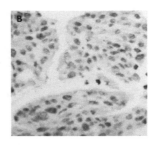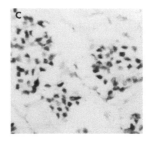

Figure 10.3   Activation of mitogen-activated protein kinase family members in clinical breast cancer: (a) phosphorylated extracellular signal regulated kinases 1 and 2; (b) phosphorylated c-jun N-terminal kinases; (c) phosphorylated p38.

Recently, Yue et al[102] have reported that ERs can also lie upstream of MAP kinase signaling in cell models of acquired endocrine resistance. They have shown that acquisition of resistance to tamoxifen and long-term estrogen deprivation in MCF-7 cells is associated with an enhanced nongenomic effect of estrogen on MAP kinase activity, which results from an increased association of ERs with EGFR/IGF-1R at the plasma membrane. In the tamoxifen-resistant variant, both tamoxifen and estrogen were found to act as an agonist on membrane ER to elicit MAP kinase activity, paralleling similar findings in HER2-overexpressing MCF-7 cells.[52,94,102]

CLINICAL ASSOCIATIONS

Extracellular signal-regulated kinases 1 and 2 mitogen-activated protein

Our previous studies, using antibodies raised to the dually phosphorylated pTEpY region within the catalytic core of the active form of ERK1 and ERK2 MAP kinase, are supportive of a pivotal role for exaggerated ERK1/2 MAP kinase activation (pMAP kinase) in ER-positive and -negative endocrine-resistant tumor growth.[103] Immunocytochemistry using such antibodies generated heterogeneous nuclear immunostaining for pMAP kinase within formalin-fixed, paraffin-embedded human breast tumor specimens (Figure 10.3), and two distinct subgroups of patients were readily identifiable based on the resultant staining.

The first group of patients demonstrated very low pMAP kinase. Many such patients exhibited objective responses (i.e. complete (CR) or partial (PR) responses) to tamoxifen as measured at 6 months after initiation of antihormonal therapy. Responses were of extended duration with a longer patient survival, as measured from the initiation of endocrine therapy. These low levels of pMAP kinase may be critical to the growth of such tumors since, using sequential tamoxifen-treated samples obtained from primary elderly breast cancer patients, we have been able to detect further decreases in pMAP kinase in parallel with the clinical tamoxifen response profile. Moreover, as stated above, we have demonstrated some cell growth inhibition of the endocrine responsive breast cancer line MCF-7 with the MEK1 inhibitor PD098059, despite only minimal activation of ERK1/2 MAP kinase. Such data again suggest that the diminished pMAP kinase levels detectable in endocrine responsive disease may be reflective of highly efficient regulation of enzyme phosphorylation. Some link has been made between pMAP kinase regulation and the IGF-1R pathway in ER-positive well-differentiated tumors, although it should be noted that there was some conflict with our own observations since higher pMAP kinase levels were reported for this patient group.[104]

The second patient subgroup in our study (72% of patients) exhibited quite substantial pMAP kinase. Such patients invariably exhibited de novo endocrine resistant (i.e. progressive) disease, or at best disease stabilization. There was a poorer survival from initiation of endocrine therapy (by univariate analysis) and a shortened time to disease relapse on such treatment (by univariate and multivariate analysis[103]). Biochemical studies using tissue homogenates confirm that hyperexpression and anomalous MAP kinase activation is a feature of a proportion of breast neoplasms.[105–108] Furthermore, a biochemical study by Mueller et al[109] reported a relationship between elevated MAP kinase activity and shortened disease-free survival in primary breast cancer, which is complementary to our own data. However, such observations remain controversial since links between increased pMAP kinase and good outcome have also been reported.[110] The reasons underlying such variations in results remain unknown; however, localization appears critical to the observations since, while nuclear ERK correlates with shortened patient survival, cytoplasmic staining is favorable.[111]

What mechanisms might underlie any exaggeration of pMAP kinase in poorer prognosis de novo endocrine resistant clinical breast cancer? Mutation, overexpression or constitutive activity of ERK1/2 MAP kinase,[105,106,108,112] or indeed of any of the key regulators identified in cell models of endocrine resisitance such as growth factor receptors (EGFR, HER2) and phosphatases (MKP3), might feasibly explain this phenomenon. Indeed, an increasing number of anomalies in erbB/ERK1/2 MAP kinase signaling have been identified within such tumors.[113] Associations have been made between endocrine independence and exaggeration of EGFR and HER2,[113] and very recent studies have shown that activation of HER2 correlates with pMAP kinase (and also with the alternative kinase p38[114]), while inhibition of EGFR and/or HER2 with agents such as lapatinib and gefitinib can deplete pMAP kinase, and thereby proliferation in breast cancer, suggesting interlinked pathways.[115] It is also interesting that elevated levels and/or activity of many additional intracellular molecules impinging on the ERK 1/2 MAP kinase signaling pathway (including pp60c-src, Grb2, RHAMM, Ras, Raf, protein kinase C) have been observed in malignant breast cells, commonly associating with a poorer patient prognosis.[106,116–119]

Interestingly, we noted that increased pMAP kinase was particularly common in the poorer prognosis, endocrine-unresponsive ER-negative patient subgroup.[103] Such tumors are reported to employ elevated EGFR signaling for their expansion.[44,45,113,120,121] Interestingly, these findings parallel the evidence derived from cell models implicating MAP kinase signaling in driving ER negativity. In these tumors, we observed associations between pMAP kinase, EGFR positivity, and the activated AP-1 component c-Jun,[122] data implicating pMAP kinase as a key intermediary of elevated EGFR signaling which impinges on AP-1-mediated events, and thereby growth of ER-negative disease. Our in vivo observations are complemented by in vitro studies, which have similarly demonstrated enhanced tyrosine phosphorylation,[74] and marked ERK1/2 MAP kinase activation in ER-negative MDA-MB-231 breast cancer cells.[123]

Importantly, however, we noted that associations between increased pMAP kinase and hormone refractory disease in the clinic were also retained within ER-positive patients.[103] Multivariate analysis confirmed significant associations with earlier relapse on endocrine therapy and poorer survival time in these patients. Further studies have also linked increased MAPK activity and impaired tamoxifen response in ER-positive patients,[124] although, as stated above, observations linking MAPK activation to adverse outcome remain controversial. Our clinical data are complimented by many in vitro observations equating enhanced MAP kinase activity with the acquisition of steroid hormone independence or antihormone resistance by ER-positive breast cancer cells, including our own panel of endocrine resistant MCF-7 sublines.[78,79] Indeed, we have recently observed increased pMAP kinase at the time of acquisition of tamoxifen resistance and disease relapse in ER-positive, initially responsive, clinical disease. In total, these data offer considerable support of a central role for exaggerated pMAP kinase in sustaining antihormonal-resistant ER-positive tumor growth. As observed in the model systems, there is also emerging clinical evidence that pMAP kinase may be able to promote ER activity in

ER-positive breast cancer. Prominent activation of ER serine 118 has been reported to correlate with more differentiated disease and better clinical outcome on tamoxifen.[113,125,126] However, such ER activity is also readily detectable in ER-positive de novo and acquired tamoxifen-resistant breast cancer (moreover at elevated levels in relapse samples). Interestingly, both increased EGFR and pMAP kinase correlate with phosphorylation of serine 118 ER in clinical disease,[113,126] while Polychronis et al[127] observed that neoadjuvant gefitinib treatment of ER-positive/EGFR-positive disease depletes both pMAP kinase and serine 118 ER phosphorylation. In total, these data suggest EGFR/MAP kinase regulation of ER activation may be important to tamoxifen-resistant phenotypes in vivo as in breast cancer cell models.[113,125] Surprisingly, our study showed that there was a lack of direct correlation between pMAP kinase and expression of a panel of "classically" estrogen regulated genes (i.e. PgR, pS2 and bcl-2), although some association was noted between TGFα, a known estrogen responsive gene, and pMAP kinase.[103] These data indicate that the mechanisms involving pMAP kinase priming of ER activity are far from simple, and may selectively influence specific subsets of estrogen-regulated genes more integral in tumor growth processes. Moreover, while initially entering into positive crosstalk with ER, at its most extreme, hyperactivation of MAP kinase may ultimately act to inhibit ER expression, thereby producing completely endocrine refractory growth.

The "stress-activated" mitogen-activated protein kinases JNK and p38

As stated above, significant influences on ER and AP-1 signaling may also occur following phosphorylation of the SAPK members Jun kinase (JNK) and p38. While the endpoints of such signaling are likely to be as diverse as for ERK1/2 MAP kinase, as stated above, significant in vitro associations with negative growth regulation in breast cancer cells have been reported for JNK and p38.[16,17,53] If represented

in clinical breast cancer, therefore, JNK and p38 signaling would perhaps be predicted to substantially impact on patient prognosis and endocrine response in a manner diametrically opposed to pMAP kinase. Again, our studies immunocytochemically employing phospho-specific antibodies for JNK and p38 in clinical breast cancer have proved interesting in this regard.[128] We noted that nuclear activation of JNK or p38 was not uncommon within clinical breast cancer (Figure 10.3). Significant expression of activated p38 and JNK appeared to confer an advantage on duration of survival and endocrine response, an observation in marked contrast to our observations with pMAP kinase. This was particularly apparent within tumors where the relationship between response to endocrine therapy and elevated pMAP kinase activation proved imperfect. Thus, approximately 15% of objective responders with elevated pMAP kinase activation in their tumors coexpressed activated JNK or p38.[128] These data suggest that activation of p38 and JNK may serve as a "counterbalance" in some breast cancers for the undesirable positive influences of pMAP kinase, thereby facilitating the growth inhibitory activity of endocrine agents.[129]

However, our observations with SAPKs in clinical breast cancer remain controversial. Paradoxically, increases in both p38 and JNK activity have also been associated with disease progression with activity elevated in effusions compared with primary tumors and lymph node metastases, and p38 relating to reduced overall survival[130] and to shortened progression-free survival in lymph node-positive breast cancer.[131] Moreover, our preliminary studies also noted some increases in activity of both JNK and p38 at the time of disease relapse of ER-positive endocrine responsive clinical breast cancer when treated with tamoxifen. Increased JNK activity has similarly been measured by others in acquired tamoxifen-resistant clinical breast cancer,[132,133] while Gutierrez et al[85] reported that some ER-positive, acquired tamoxifen-resistant patients (and xenografts) show increased p38 activation alongside modest gains in HER2 amplification. The latter study also revealed strong correlations between ER, p38 and ERK, data cumulatively implying crosstalk between ER, HER2, p38 (and ERK) which contributes to tamoxifen-resistant growth. Indeed, evidence of such crosstalk has been demonstrated in a xenograft model of acquired tamoxifen-resistant MCF-7 cells.[85] It is feasible that a positive role for stress-activated kinases such as p38 in driving clinical-resistant disease may occur via their regulation of AP-1 activity, which can also be increased in such material[122,132,133] or perhaps via activation of ER or its coactivators to enhance agonism of the tamoxifen–ER complex.[85]

THE FUTURE OF MITOGEN-ACTIVATED PROTEIN KINASE AS A THERAPEUTIC TARGET AND PROGNOSTIC MARKER

The clinical data described above regarding activation of ERK1/2 MAP kinase and the SAPKs JNK and p38 suggest that these signaling elements have prognostic potential. However, more definitive studies with greater access to appropriate clinical sample sets, including samples taken during response and at relapse, are required to confirm these initial findings. It should also be noted that this data may also have important therapeutic implications. For example, breast tumors derived from patients exhibiting de novo endocrine resistance and an unfavorable prognosis may be candidates for challenge with pharmacological agents disruptive of ERK1/2 MAP kinase signaling. The recent development of inhibitors of MEK1 activation,[134,135] as well as further agents disruptive of the upstream erbB signaling network, notably including tyrosine kinase inhibitors such as "ZD1839/Iressa" and targeted antibody therapies such as Herceptin,[136] could be valuable additions to the pharmacological armory appropriate in future management of the disease. Moreover, our observation that coexpression of activated JNK or p38 in clinical breast cancer is associated with a perturbation of the relationship between phosphorylated ERK 1/2 MAP kinase and poor

outlook may ultimately provide some rationale for therapeutic manipulation of SAPKs to dampen any undesirable impact of elevated ERK 1/2 MAP kinase signaling. However, it should also be noted that the identification of a role for p38 and JNK in acquired tamoxifen resistance[85,132,133] also identifies them, alongside ERK1/2 MAP kinase, as potential therapeutic targets for the treatment of this condition.

REFERENCES

1. Seery LT, Gee JMW, Dewhurst OL et al. Molecular mechanisms of antiestrogen action. In: Oettel M, Schillinger E, eds. Pharmacological Handbook. Berlin: Springer-Verlag, 1999: 201–20.
2. Nicholson RI, Manning DL, Gee JMW. New anti-hormonal approaches to breast cancer therapy. Drugs of Today 1993; 29: 363–72.
3. Nicholson RI, McClelland RA, Robertson JFR et al. Involvement of steroid hormone and growth factor cross-talk in endocrine response in breast cancer. Endocr Rel Cancer 1999; 6: 373–87.
4. Nicholson RI, Gee JWM. Oestrogen and growth factor cross-talk and endocrine insensitivity and acquired resistance in breast cancer. Br J Cancer 2000; 82: 501–13.
5. Widmann C, Gibson S, Jarpe MB et al. Mitogen-activated protein kinase: conservation of a three-kinase module from yeast to human. Physiol Rev 1999; 79(1): 143–80.
6. Kyriakis JM, Avruch J. Mammalian mitogen-activated protein kinase signal transduction pathways activated by stress and inflammation. Physiol Rev 2001; 81(2): 807–69.
7. Dhillon AS, Hagan S, Rath O et al. MAP kinase signalling pathways in cancer. Oncogene 2007; 26: 3279–90.
8. Schlessinger J. Cell signalling by receptor tyrosine kinases. Cell 2000; 103: 211–25.
9. Turjanski AG, Vaqué JP, Gutkind JS. MAP kinases and the control of nuclear events. Oncogene 2007; 26: 3240–53.
10. Meloche S, Pouysségur J. The ERK1/2 mitogen-activated protein kinase pathway as a master regulator of the G1- to S-phase transition. Oncogene 2007; 26: 3227–39.
11. Yoon S, Seger R. The extracellular signal-regulated kinase: multiple substrates regulate diverse cellular functions. Growth Factors 2006; 24: 21–44.
12. Wang X, Tournier C. Regulation of cellular functions by the ERK5 signalling pathway. Cell Signal 2006; 18: 753–60.
13. Bagrodia S, Derijard B, Davis RJ et al. Cdc42 and PAK-mediated signalling leads to Jun kinase and p38 mitogen-activated protein kinase activation. J Biol Chem 1995; 270(47): 27,995–8.

134 PROGNOSTIC AND PREDICTIVE FACTORS IN BREAST CANCER

14. Yuasa T, Ohno S, Kehrl JH et al. Tumour necrosis factor signalling to stress-activated protein kinase (SAPK)/Jun NH2-terminal kinase (JNK) and p38. Germinal center kinase couples TRAF2 to mitogen-activated protein kinase/ERK kinase kinase 1 and SAPK while receptor interacting protein associates with a mitogen-activated protein kinase kinase kinase upstream of MKK6 and p38. J Biol Chem 1998; 273(35): 22,681–92.

15. Fanger GR, Johnson NL, Johnson GL. MEK kinases are regulated by EGF and selectively interact with Rac/Cdc42. EMBO J 1997; 16(16): 4961–72.

16. Zarubin T, Han J. Activation and signalling of the p38 MAP kinase pathway. Cell Res 2005; 15: 11–18.

17. Weston CR, Davis RJ. The JNK signal transduction pathway. Curr Opin Cell Biol 2007; 19: 142–9.

18. Robertson JF, Williams MR, Todd J et al. Factors predicting the response of patients with advanced breast cancer to endocrine (Megace) therapy. Eur J Cancer Clin Oncol 1989; 25: 469–75.

19. Nicholson RI, Bouzubar N, Walker KJ et al. Hormone sensitivity in breast cancer: influence of heterogeneity of oestrogen receptor expression and cell proliferation. Eur J Cancer 1991; 27: 908–13.

20. Locker AP, Birrell K, Bell JA et al. Ki67 immunoreactivity in breast carcinoma: relationships to prognostic variables and short term survival. Eur J Surg Oncol 1992; 18: 224–9.

21. Nicholson RI, Wilson DW, Richards G et al. Biological and clinical aspects of oestrogen receptor measurements in rapidly progressing breast cancer. In: Paton W, Mitchell J, Turner P, eds. Proceedings of the IUPHAR 9th International Congress of Pharmacology. Volume 3. London: McMillan Press, 1984: 75–9.

22. Kushner PJ, Agard DA, Greene GL et al. Estrogen receptor pathways to AP-1. J Steroid Biochem Mol Biol 2000; 74: 311–17.

23. Aronica SM, Katzenellenbogen BS. Stimulation of estrogen receptor-mediated transcription and alteration in the phosphorylation state of the rat uterine estrogen receptor by estrogen, cyclic adenosinemonophosphate, and insulin-like growth factor-I. Mol Endocrinol 1993; 7(6): 743–52.

24. Bunone G, Briand PA, Miksicek RJ et al. Activation of the unliganded estrogen receptor by EGF involves the MAP k pathway and direct phosphorylation. EMBO J 1996; 15: 2174–83.

25. Pietras RJ, Arboleda J, Reese DM et al. HER-2 tyrosine k pathway targets estrogen receptor and promotes hormone-independent growth in human breast cancer cells. Oncogene 1995; 10: 2435–46.

26. Lee AV, Weng CN, Jackson JG et al. Activation of estrogen receptor-mediated gene transcription by IGF-I in human breast cancer cells. J Endocrinol 1997; 152(1): 39–47.

27. Ignar-Trowbridge DM, Pimentel M, Parker MG et al. Peptide growth factor cross-talk with the estrogen receptor requires the A/B domain and occurs independently of protein k C or estradiol. Endocrinology 1996; 137(5): 1735–44.

28. Joel PB, Smith J, Sturgill TW et al. pp90rsk1 regulates estrogen receptor-mediated transcription through phosphorylation of Ser-167. Mol Cell Biol 1998; 18: 1978–84.

29. Kato S, Endoh H, Masuhiro Y et al. Activation of the estrogen receptor through phosphorylation by mitogen-activated protein kinase. Science 1995; 270: 1491–94.

30. Lannigan DA. Estrogen receptor phosphorylation. Steroids 2003; 68: 1–9.

31. Likhite VS, Stossi F, Kim K et al. Kinase-specific phosphorylation of the estrogen receptor changes receptor interactions with ligand, deoxyribonucleic acid, and coregulators associated with alterations in estrogen and tamoxifen activity. Mol Endocrinol 2006; 20: 3120–32.

32. Weigel NL, Moore NL. Kinases and protein phosphorylation as regulators of steroid hormone action. Nucl Recept Signal 2007; 5: e005.

33. Lee H, Bai W. Regulation of estrogen receptor nuclear export by ligand-induced and p38-mediated receptor phosphorylation. Mol Cell Biol 2002; 22: 5835–45.

34. Takahashi T, Ohmichi M, Kawagoe J et al. Growth factors change nuclear distribution of estrogen receptor-alpha via mitogen-activated protein kinase or phosphatidylinositol 3-kinase cascade in a human breast cancer cell line. Endocrinology 2005; 146: 4082–9.

35. Yang Z, Barnes CJ, Kumar R. Human epidermal growth factor receptor 2 status modulates subcellular localization of and interaction with estrogen receptor alpha in breast cancer cells. Clin Cancer Res 2004; 10: 3621–8.

36. Le Goff P, Montano MM, Schodin DJ et al. Phosphorylation of the human estrogen receptor. Identification of hormone-regulated sites and examination of their influence on transcriptional activity. J Biol Chem 1994; 269: 4458–66.

37. Feng W, Webb P, Nguyen P et al. Potentiation of estrogen receptor activation function 1 (AF-1) by Src/JNK through a serine 118-independent pathway. Mol Endocrinol 2001; 15: 32–45.

38. McDonnell DP, Dana SL, Hoener PA et al. Cellular mechanisms which distinguish between hormone- and antihormone-activated estrogen receptor. Ann N Y Acad Sci 1995; 761: 121–37.

39. Oh AS, Lorant LA, Holloway JN et al. Hyper-activation of MAPK induces loss of ERalpha expression in breast cancer cells. Mol Endocrinol 2001; 15: 1344–59.

40. Creighton CJ, Hilger AM, Murthy S et al. Activation of mitogen-activated protein kinase in estrogen receptor alpha-positive breast cancer cells in vitro induces an in vivo molecular phenotype of estrogen receptor alpha-negative human breast tumors. Cancer Res 2006; 66: 3903–11.

41. Henrich LM, Smith JA, Kitt D et al. Extracellular signal-regulated kinase 7, a regulator of hormone-dependent estrogen receptor destruction. Mol Cell Biol 2003; 23: 5979–88.

42. Kronblad A, Hedenfalk I, Nilsson E et al. ERK1/2 inhibition increases antiestrogen treatment efficacy by interfering with hypoxia-induced downregulation of ERalpha: a combination therapy potentially targeting hypoxic and dormant tumour cells. Oncogene 2005; 24: 6835–41.

43. Holloway JN, Murthy S, El-Ashry D. A cytoplasmic substrate of mitogen-activated protein kinase is responsible for estrogen receptor-alpha down-regulation in breast cancer cells: the role of nuclear factor-kappaB. Mol Endocrinol 2004; 18: 1396–410.

44. Nicholson RI, Gee JWM. Growth factors and modulation of endocrine response in breast cancer. In: Vedeckis WV, ed. Hormones and Cancer. Boston: Birkhauser, 1996: 227–61.

45. Gee JWM, McClelland RA, Nicholson RI. Growth factors and endocrine sensitivity in breast cancer. In: Pasqualini JR, Katzenellenbogen BS, eds. Molecular and Clinical Endocrinology. Marcel Dekker Publishing, 1996: 169–97.

46. Bates SE, Davidson NE, Valverius EM et al. Expression of transforming growth factor-alpha and its mRNA in human breast cancer: its regulation by oestrogen and its possible functional significance. Mol Endocrinol 1988; 2: 543–55.

47. Berthois Y, Dong XF, Martin PM. Regulation of epidermal growth factor receptor by oestrogen and antioestrogen in the human breast cancer cell line MCF-7. Biochem Biophys Res Commun 1989; 159: 126–31.

48. Hamelers IH, Steenbergh PH. Interactions between estrogen and insulin-like growth factor signaling pathways in human breast tumor cells. Endocr Relat Cancer 2003; 10: 331–45.

49. Richards RG, DiAugustine RP, Petrusz P et al. Estradiol stimulates tyrosine phosphorylation of the insulin-like growth factor-1 receptor and insulin receptor substrate-1 in the uterus. Proc Natl Acad Sci USA 1996; 93: 12,002–7.

50. Nemere I, Pietras RJ, Blackmore PF. Membrane receptors for steroid hormones: signal transduction and physiological significance. J Cell Biochem 2003; 88: 438–45.

51. Levin ER, Pietras RJ. Estrogen receptors outside the nucleus in breast cancer. Breast Cancer Res Treat 2008; 108: 351–61.

52. Schiff R, Osborne CK. Endocrinology and hormone therapy in breast cancer: new insight into estrogen receptor-alpha function and its implication for endocrine therapy resistance in breast cancer. Breast Cancer Res 2005; 7: 205–11.

53. Buck MB, Knabbe C. TGF-beta signalling in breast cancer. Ann NY Acad Sci 2006; 1089: 119–26.

54. Perry RR, Kang Y, Greaves BR. Relationship between tamoxifen-induced transforming growth factor beta 1 expression, cytostasis and apoptosis in human breast cancer cells. Br J Cancer 1995; 72: 1441–6.

55. Hill CS. Signalling to the nucleus by members of the transforming growth factor-beta (TGF-beta) superfamily. Cell Signal 1996; 8: 533–44.

56. Freiss G, Vignon F. Antiestrogens increase protein tyrosine phosphatase activity in human breast cancer cells. Mol Endocrinol 1994; 8: 1389–96.

57. Freiss G, Puech C, Vignon F. Extinction of insulin-like growth factor-I mitogenic signalling by anti-estrogen-stimulated Fas-associated protein tyrosine phosphatase-1 in human breast cancer cells. Mol Endocrinol 1998; 12: 568–79.

58. Gille H, Kortenjann M, Thomae O et al. ERK phosphorylation potentiates Elk-1-mediated ternary complex formation and transactivation. EMBO J 1995; 14: 951–62.

59. Eferl R, Wagner EF. AP-1: a double-edged sword in tumourigenesis. Nat Rev Cancer 2003; 3: 859–68.

60. Philips A, Chalbos D, Rochefort H. Estradiol increases and anti-estrogens antagonize the growth factor-induced activator protein-1 activity in MCF7 breast cancer cells without affecting c-fos and c-jun synthesis. J Biol Chem 1993; 268: 14,103–8.

61. Porter W, Saville B, Hoivik D et al. Functional synergy between the transcription factor Sp1 and the estrogen receptor. Mol Endocrinol 1997; 11: 1569–80.

62. Webb P, Lopez GN, Uht RM et al. Tamoxifen activation of the estrogen receptor/AP-1 pathway: potential origin for the cell-specific estrogen-like effects of antiestrogens. Mol Endocrinol 1995; 9: 443–56.

63. Nakshatri H, Bhat-Nakshatri P, Martin DA et al. Constitutive activation of NF-kappaB during progression of breast cancer to hormone-independent growth. Mol Cell Biol 1997; 17: 3629–39.

64. Sharma HW, Narayanan R. The NF-kappaB transcription factor in oncogenesis. Anticancer Res 1996; 16: 589–96.

65. Font de Mora J, Brown M. AIB1 is a conduit for kinase-mediated growth factor signalling to the estrogen receptor. Mol Cell Biol 2000; 20: 5041–7.

66. Rowan BG, Weigel NL, O'Malley BW. Phosphorylation of steroid receptor coactivator-1. Identification of the phosphorylation sites and phosphorylation through the mitogen-activated protein kinase pathway. J Biol Chem 2000; 275: 4475–83.

67. Lopez GN, Turck CW, Schaufele F et al. Growth factors signal to steroid receptors through mitogen-activated protein kinase regulation of p160 coactivator activity. J Biol Chem 2001; 276: 22,177–82.

68. Jonas BA, Privalsky ML. SMRT and N-CoR corepressors are regulated by distinct kinase signalling pathways. J Biol Chem 2004; 279: 54,676–86.

69. Frigo DE, Basu A, Nierth-Simpson EN et al. p38 mitogen-activated protein kinase stimulates estrogen-mediated transcription and proliferation through the phosphorylation and potentiation of

the p160 coactivator glucocorticoid receptor-interacting protein 1. Mol Endocrinol 2006; 20: 971–83.

70. Zwijsen RM, Buckle RS, Hijmans EM et al. Ligand-independent recruitment of steroid receptor coactivators to estrogen receptor by cyclin D1. Genes Dev 1998; 12: 3488–98.

71. Kraus RJ, Ariazi EA, Farrell ML et al. Estrogen-related receptor alpha 1 actively antagonizes estrogen receptor-regulated transcription in MCF-7 mammary cells. J Biol Chem 2002; 277: 24,826–34.

72. Butt AJ, McNeil CM, Musgrove EA et al. Downstream targets of growth factor and oestrogen signalling and endocrine resistance: the potential roles of c-Myc, cyclin D1 and cyclin E. Endocr Relat Cancer 2005; 12 (Suppl 1): S47–S59.

73. Morishita S, Niwa K, Ichigo S et al. Overexpressions of c-fos/jun mRNA and their oncoproteins (Fos/Jun) in the mouse uterus treated with three natural estrogens. Cancer Lett 1995; 97: 225–31.

74. Mohamood AS, Gyles P, Balan KV et al. Estrogen receptor, growth factor receptor and protooncogene protein activities and possible signal transduction crosstalk in estrogen dependent and independent breast cancer cell lines. J Submicrosc Cytol Pathol 1997; 29: 1–17.

75. Dubik D, Shiu RP. Mechanism of estrogen activation of c-myc oncogene expression. Oncogene 1992; 7: 1587–94.

76. Lukas J, Bartkova J, Bartek J. Convergence of mitogenic signalling cascades from diverse classes of receptors at the cyclin D-cyclin-dependent k-pRb-controlled G1 checkpoint. Mol Cell Biol 1996; 16: 6917–25.

77. Cohen BD, Siegall CB, Bacus S et al. Role of epidermal growth factor receptor family members in growth and differentiation of breast carcinoma. Biochem Soc Symp 1998; 63: 199–210.

78. Knowlden JM, Hutcheson IR, Jones HE et al. Elevated levels of epidermal growth factor receptor/c-erbB2 heterodimers mediate an autocrine growth regulatory pathway in tamoxifen-resistant MCF-7 cells. Endocrinology 2003; 144: 1032–44.

79. McClelland RA, Barrow D, Madden TA et al. Enhanced epidermal growth factor receptor signaling in MCF7 breast cancer cells after long-term culture in the presence of the pure antiestrogen ICI 182,780 (Faslodex). Endocrinology 2001; 142: 2776–88.

80. Coutts AS, Murphy LC. Elevated mitogen-activated protein kinase activity in estrogen-nonresponsive human breast cancer cells. Cancer Res 1998; 58: 4071–4.

81. Jeng MH, Yue W, Eischeid A et al. Role of MAP kinase in the enhanced cell proliferation of long-term estrogen deprived human breast cancer cells. Breast Cancer Res Treat 2000; 62: 167–75.

82. Donovan JCH, Milic A, Slingerland JM. Constitutive MEK/MAPK activation leads to p27Kip1 deregulation and antiestrogen resistance in human breast cancer cells. J Biol Chem 1997; 276: 40,888–95.

83. Kurokawa H, Lenferink AEG, Simpson JF et al. Inhibition of HER/neu (erbB-2) and mitogen-activated protein kinases enhances tamoxifen action against HER2-overexpressing, tamoxifen resistant breast cancer cells. Cancer Res 2000; 60: 5887–94.

84. Cui Y, Parra I, Zhang M et al. Elevated expression of mitogen-activated protein kinase phosphatase 3 in breast tumors: a mechanism of tamoxifen resistance. Cancer Res 2006; 66: 5950–59.

85. Gutierrez MC, Detre S, Johnston S et al. Molecular changes in tamoxifen-resistant breast cancer: relationship between estrogen receptor, HER-2, and p38 mitogen-activated protein kinase. J Clin Oncol 2005; 23: 2469–76.

86. Britton DJ, Hutcheson IR, Knowlden JM et al. Bidirectional cross talk between ERalpha and EGFR signalling pathways regulates tamoxifen-resistant growth. Breast Cancer Res Treat 2006; 96: 131–46.

87. Hutcheson IR, Knowlden JM, Madden TA et al. Oestrogen receptor-mediated modulation of the EGFR/MAPK pathway in tamoxifen-resistant MCF-7 cells. Breast Cancer Res Treat 2003; 81: 81–93.

88. Lykkesfeldt AE, Mogens MW, Briand P. Altered expression of estrogen-regulated genes in a tamoxifen-resistant and ICI 164,384 and ICI 182,780 sensitive human breast cancer cell line, MCF-7/TAM R-1. Cancer Res 1994; 54: 1587–95.

89. Brunner N, Frandesen TL, Holst-Hansen C et al. MCF7/LCC2: a 4-hydroxytamoxifen resistant human breast cancer variant that retains sensitivity to the steroidal antiestrogen ICI 182,780. Cancer Res 1993; 53: 3229–32.

90. Johnston SR, Lu B, Dowsett M et al. Comparison of estrogen receptor DNA binding in untreated and acquired antiestrogen-resistant human breast tumors. Cancer Res 1997; 57: 3723–7.

91. Robertson JF. Oestrogen receptor: a stable phenotype in breast cancer. Br J Cancer 1996; 73: 5–12.

92. Martin LA, Farmer I, Johnston SR et al. Enhanced estrogen receptor (ER) alpha, ERBB2 and MAPK signal transduction pathways operate during the adaptation of MCF-7 cells to long term oestrogen deprivation. J Biol Chem 2003; 278: 30,458–68.

93. Campbell RA, Bhat-Nakshatri P, Patel NM et al. Phosphatidylinositol 3-kinase/AKT-mediated activation of estrogen receptor alpha: a new model for antiestrogen resistance. J Biol Chem 2001; 276: 9817–24.

94. Shou J, Massarweh S, Osborne CK et al. Mechanisms of tamoxifen resistance: increased estrogen receptor-HER2/neu cross-talk in ER/HER2-positive breast cancer. J Natl Cancer Inst 2004; 96: 926–35.

95. Chan CM, Martin LA, Johnston SR et al. Molecular changes associated with the acquisition of oestrogen hypersensitivity in MCF-7 breast cancer cells on long-term oestrogen deprivation. J Steroid Biochem Mol Biol 2002; 81: 333–41.

96. Vendrell JA, Bieche I, Desmetz C et al. Molecular changes associated with the agonist activity of hydroxy-tamoxifen and the hyper-response to estradiol in hydroxy-tamoxifen-resistant breast cancer cell lines. Endocr Relat Cancer 2005; 12: 75–92.

97. Brodie A, Sabnis G, Jelovac D. Aromatase and breast cancer. J Steroid Biochem Mol Biol 2006; 102: 97–102.

98. Gibson MK, Nemmers LA, Beckman WC Jr et al. The mechanism of ICI 164,384 antiestrogenicity involves rapid loss of estrogen receptor in uterine tissue. Endocrinology 1991; 129: 2000–10.

99. Dauvois S, Danielian PS, White R et al. Antiestrogen ICI 164,384 reduces cellular estrogen receptor content by increasing its turnover. Proc Natl Acad Sci USA 1992; 89: 4037–41.

100. Liang Y, Brekken RA, Hyder SM. Vascular endothelial growth factor induces proliferation of breast cancer cells and inhibits the anti-proliferative activity of anti-hormones. Endocr Relat Cancer 2006; 13: 905–19.

101. Thottassery JV, Sun Y, Westbrook L et al. Prolonged extracellular signal-regulated kinase 1/2 activation during fibroblast growth factor 1- or heregulin beta1-induced antiestrogen-resistant growth of breast cancer cells is resistant to mitogen-activated protein/extracellular regulated kinase kinase inhibitors. Cancer Res 2004; 64: 4637–47.

102. Yue W, Fan P, Wang J et al. Mechanisms of acquired resistance to endocrine therapy in hormone-dependent breast cancer cells. J Steroid Biochem Mol Biol 2007; 106: 102–10.

103. Gee JM, Robertson JF, Ellis IO et al. Phosphorylation of ERK1/2 mitogen-activated protein kinase is associated with poor response to anti-hormonal therapy and decreased patient survival in clinical breast cancer. Int J Cancer 2001; 95: 247–54.

104. Ueda S, Tsuda H, Sato K et al. Alternative tyrosine phosphorylation of signaling kinases according to hormone receptor status in breast cancer overexpressing the insulin-like growth factor. Cancer Sci 2006; 97: 597–604.

105. Sivaraman VS, Wang H, Nuovo GJ et al. Hyperexpression of mitogen-activated protein kinase in human breast cancer. J Clin Invest 1997; 99: 1478–83.

106. Wang C, Thor AD, Moore DH 2nd et al. The overexpression of RHAMM, a hyaluronan-binding protein that regulates Ras signalling, correlates with overexpression of mitogen-activated protein kinase and is a significant parameter in breast cancer progression. Cancer Res 1998; 4: 567–76.

107. Maemura M, Iino Y, Koibuchi Y et al. Mitogen-activated protein kinase cascade in breast cancer. Oncology 1999; 57: 37–44.

108. Salh B, Marotta A, Matthewson C et al. Investigation of the MEK-MAP kinase-Rsk pathway in human breast cancer. Anticancer Res 1999; 19: 731–40.

109. Mueller H, Flury N, Eppenberger-Castori S et al. Potential prognostic value of mitogen-activated protein kinase activity for disease-free survival of primary breast cancer patients. Int J Cancer (Pred Oncol) 2000; 89: 384–8.

110. Milde-Langosch K, Bamberger AM, Rieck G et al. Expression and prognostic relevance of activated extracellular-regulated kinases (ERK1/2) in breast cancer. Br J Cancer 2005; 92: 2206–15.

111. Nakopoulou L, Mylona E, Rafailidis P et al. Effect of different ERK2 protein localizations on prognosis of patients with invasive breast carcinoma. APMIS 2005; 113: 693–701.

112. Hoshino R, Chatani Y, Yamori T et al. Constitutive activation of the 41/43-kDa mitogen-activated protein kinase signalling pathway in human tumours. Oncogene 1999; 18: 813–22.

113. Gee JM, Robertson JF, Gutteridge E et al. Epidermal growth factor receptor/HER2/insulin-like growth factor receptor signalling and oestrogen receptor activity in clinical breast cancer. Endocr Relat Cancer 2005; 12 (Suppl 1): S99–S111.

114. Giuliani R, Durbecq V, Di Leo A et al. Phosphorylated HER-2 tyrosine kinase and Her-2/neu gene amplification as predictive factors of response to trastuzumab in patients with HER-2 overexpressing metastatic breast cancer (MBC). Eur J Cancer 2007; 43: 725–35.

115. Baselga J, Albanell J, Ruiz A et al. Phase II and tumor pharmacodynamic study of gefitinib in patients with advanced breast cancer. J Clin Oncol 2005; 23: 5323–33.

116. Lehrer S, O'Shaughnessy J, Song HK et al. Activity of pp60c-src protein kinase in human breast cancer. Mt Sinai J Med 1989; 56: 83–5.

117. Yip SS, Crew AJ, Gee JM et al. Up-regulation of the protein tyrosine phosphatase SHP-1 in human breast cancer and correlation with GRB2 expression. Int J Cancer 2000; 88: 363–8.

118. Callans LS, Naama H, Khandelwal M et al. Raf-1 protein expression in human breast cancer cells. Ann Surg Oncol 1995; 2: 38–42.

119. Gordge PC, Hulme MJ, Clegg RA et al. Elevation of protein kinase A and protein kinase C activities in malignant as compared with normal human breast tissue. Eur J Cancer 1996; 32A: 2120–6.

120. Nicholson RI, McClelland RA, Finlay P et al. Relationship between EGF-R, c-erbB-2 protein expression and Ki67 immunostaining in breast cancer and hormone sensitivity. Eur J Cancer 1993; 29A: 1018–23.

121. Nicholson RI, McClelland RA, Gee JM et al. Transforming growth factor-alpha and endocrine sensitivity in breast cancer. Cancer Res 1994; 54: 1684–9.

122. Gee JM, Barroso AF, Ellis IO et al. Biological and clinical associations of c-jun activation in human breast cancer. Int J Cancer 2000; 89: 177–86.

123. Zhou JN, Ljungdahl S, Shoshan MC et al. Activation of tissue-factor gene expression in breast carcinoma

cells by stimulation of the RAF-ERK signalling pathway. Mol Carcinog 1998; 21: 234–43.

124. Svensson S, Jirström K, Rydén L et al. ERK phosphorylation is linked to VEGFR2 expression and Ets-2 phosphorylation in breast cancer and is associated with tamoxifen treatment resistance and small tumours with good prognosis. Oncogene 2005; 24: 4370–9.

125. Sarwar N, Kim JS, Jiang J et al. Phosphorylation of ERalpha at serine 118 in primary breast cancer and in tamoxifen-resistant tumours is indicative of a complex role for ERalpha phosphorylation in breast cancer progression. Endocr Relat Cancer 2006; 13: 851–61.

126. Murphy LC, Niu Y, Snell L et al. Phospho-serine-118 estrogen receptor-alpha expression is associated with better disease outcome in women treated with tamoxifen. Clin Cancer Res 2004; 10: 5902–6.

127. Polychronis A, Sinnett HD, Hadjiminas D et al. Preoperative gefitinib versus gefitinib and anastrozole in postmenopausal patients with oestrogen-receptor positive and epidermal-growth-factor- receptor-positive primary breast cancer: a double-blind placebo-controlled phase II randomised trial. Lancet Oncol 2005; 6: 383–91.

128. Gee JM, Robertson JF, Ellis IO et al. Impact of activation of MAP kinase family members on endocrine response and survival in clinical breast cancer. Eur J Cancer 2000; 36 (Suppl 4): 105.

129. Zhang CC, Shapiro DJ. Activation of the p38 mitogen-activated protein kinase pathway by estrogen or by 4-hydroxytamoxifen is coupled to estrogen receptor-induced apoptosis. J Biol Chem 2000; 275: 479–86.

130. Davidson B, Konstantinovsky S, Kleinberg L et al. The mitogen-activated protein kinases (MAPK) p38 and JNK are markers of tumour progression in breast carcinoma. Gynecol Oncol 2006; 102: 453–61.

131. Esteva FJ, Sahin AA, Smith TL et al. Prognostic significance of phosphorylated P38 mitogen-activated protein kinase and HER-2 expression in lymph node-positive breast carcinoma. Cancer 2004; 100: 499–506.

132. Johnston SR, Lu B, Scott GK et al. Increased activator protein-1 DNA binding and c-Jun NH2-terminal kinase activity in human breast tumours with acquired tamoxifen resistance. Clin Cancer Res 1999; 5: 251–6.

133. Schiff R, Reddy P, Ahotupa M et al. Oxidative stress and AP-1 activity in tamoxifen-resistant breast tumours in vivo. J Natl Cancer Inst 2000; 92: 1926–34.

134. Duesbery NS, Webb CP, Vande Woude GF. MEK wars, a new front in the battle against cancer. Nature Med 1999; 5: 736–7.

135. Sebolt-Leopold JS, Herrera R. Targeting the mitogen-activated protein kinase cascade to treat cancer. Nat Rev Cancer 2004; 4: 937–47.

136. Slichenmyer WJ, Fry DW. Anticancer therapy targeting the erbB family of receptor tyrosine kinases. Semin Oncol 2001; 28: 67–79.

Gene expression profiles, prognosis and prediction of responses to endocrine therapy and chemotherapy

11

Lajos Pusztai and Christos Sotiriou

INTRODUCTION

The goal of medicine has been, since its inception, to provide treatment recommendations tailored to the illness of an individual. Some of the earliest medical writings clearly document that different empirical therapies were recommended for different constellations of symptoms. For example, the Ebers' papyrus written in 1500BC recommends that "… for a person who suffers from abdominal obstruction and you find (on physical examination) that it goes-and-comes under your fingers like oil-in-tube, then prepare for him fruit-of-the-dompalm, dissolve in semen, crush and cook in oil and honey." On the other hand, if a person suffers from abdominal obstruction and you find that "… his stomach is swollen and his chest asthmatic, then make for him wormwood, elderberries, sebesten, sesa chips, crush and cook in beer…".[1] Thus, personalized medicine was born. The subsequent history of medicine is intricately intertwined with technological developments in diagnostic methods which aim to define disease ever more narrowly and predict clinical outcome with or without particular therapies with increasing precision.

Current medical decision-making takes place in a four-dimensional decision space (Figure 11.1). Physicians and patients need to consider: the clinical outcome in the absence of treatment (i.e. prognosis); the probability of benefit from therapy; and the risks of

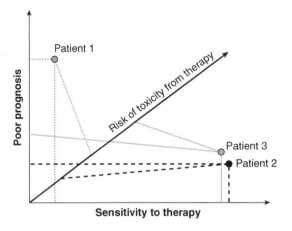

Figure 11.1 Three-dimensional decision space of predicted prognosis, predicted response to therapy and risk of toxicity/patient preference. Treatment can be equally appropriate because of high risk of relapse, even if the predicted benefit is modest, or because of modest risk of relapse but high likelihood of benefit from therapy.

adverse events from an intervention. An important fourth dimension is patient preference. A person's willingness to accept therapy is influenced by her/his risk tolerance for adverse events from the disease and from the treatment.[2] It is assumed that the more accurate the prognostic and response predictions and toxicity estimates are then the more personalized treatment recommendation can be made for an individual.

There are several diagnostic tools which are commonly used in the context of breast cancer to gauge patient preference, and to

Table 11.1 Historical tools to aid medical decision-making in breast cancer

Variable	Method to elicit outcome estimates
Patient preferences	Medical interview
Risk of adverse events	Medical history Simple organ function tests (BUN, creatinin, liver enzymes, and complete blood count) Electrocardiogram, echocardiogram
Prognosis	Tumor, node, metastasis staging system (TNM) stage Histologic grade Adjuvant Online software
Probability of benefit from therapy	Estrogen receptor, progesterone receptor immunohistochemistry[*] HER2 fluorescent in situ hybridization or immunohistochemistry[†]

*For endocrine therapy.
[†] For trastuzumab therapy.

estimate the risk of recurrence and the probability of benefit from endocrine or trastuzumab therapies (Table 11.1). Patient preferences are elicited through the medical interview. The risk of adverse events is estimated, rather subjectively, based on age, comorbid illnesses and results from simple organ function tests. The risk of recurrence is primarily determined by lymph node status, tumor size, and histological grade. Estrogen receptor (ER) and progesterone receptor (PR) immunohistochemistry results are used to define the subset of individuals who may benefit from endocrine therapy, and human epidermal growth factor receptor 2 (HER2) immunohistochemistry or fluorescent in situ hybridization (FISH) results are used to select patients for trastuzumab treatment. Several of these clinical and pathological features can be combined into a practically useful and validated multivariable outcome prediction model – see Adjuvant Online at www.adjuvantonline.com. This freely available web-based tool estimates the risk of recurrence (or death) with locoregional therapy alone and with various systemic adjuvant treatments, including endocrine therapy and/or chemotherapy.[3]

However, current prediction models are suboptimal, individual predictive variables have limited accuracy, and the actual clinical outcomes remain heterogeneous in any given prognostic group. EC and HER2 status are helpful to identify patients who are not eligible

for endocrine or trastuzumab therapies by virtue of their high negative predictive values and high sensitivities. However, only a minority of ER- or HER2-positive patients respond to receptor-targeted therapy. The positive predictive values of these tests are <50%. Currently, there are no accepted molecular predictors of response to various chemotherapy drugs. We also have limited ability to predict adverse events despite the relatively high toxicity and modest activity of cytotoxic drugs. These limitations have driven biomarker research to develop more accurate molecular predictors of clinical outcome.

NOVEL MOLECULAR TESTS IN THE CLINIC

Breast cancer is a clinically heterogeneous disease and it is generally accepted that the different clinical course of patients with histologically similar tumors is due to molecular differences among cancers. Therefore, detailed molecular analysis of the cancer could yield information that may improve clinical outcome prediction. It is also increasingly recognized that molecules which determine the behavior of neoplastic cells act in concert and form complex regulatory networks. Any individual gene may only contain limited information about the activity of the entire network. It is reasonable to hypothesize that examining many genes simultaneously will

Table 11.2 Examples of emerging molecular diagnostic tests to aid decision-making in breast cancer

Function	Test	Commercial availability for diagnostic use in the US
Prognostic tests	Mammaprint[TM 5,6]	No, FDA cleared in 2007
	76-gene signature[7,8]	No
	5-antibody, Mammostrat[TM 13]	No
Probability of benefit from endocrine therapy	Oncotype Dx[TM 9-11]	Yes
	200-gene signature[13]	No
Probability of benefit from chemotherapy	30-gene signature[17]	No

yield more accurate information about the biological behavior of the tumor. High-throughput genomic technologies, including multiplex reverse transcriptave-polymerase chain reaction (RT-PCR) and DNA microarrays, allow investigators to directly test this hypothesis.[4]

Recently, several novel multigene molecular diagnostic tests became commercially available, or are near to commercial introduction, in the USA and Europe (Table 11.2). The routine adoption of these tests would be straightforward and ubiquitous if they had perfect sensitivity, specificity and 100% positive and negative predictive values. Naturally, no test ever meets such high performance standards; therefore, the pressing question is, in what clinical situations do these tests provide added value? For many patients with newly diagnosed breast cancer, existing clinical and pathologic markers may provide sufficient information to make an appropriate treatment recommendation. For example, most patients with positive lymph nodes represent a high enough risk for recurrence that recommendations for adjuvant chemotherapy are appropriate. However, some of these individuals are frail, have multiple comorbid conditions, and may have ER-positive disease. So, a more precise prediction of sensitivity to chemotherapy and endocrine therapy could help to make the best treatment recommendation. Similarly, a substantial minority of lymph node-negative patients relapse despite adequate locoregional therapy, and better prognostic predictions could help to identify those who could benefit from systemic

chemotherapy. It would be helpful in this situation as well to understand endocrine and chemotherapy sensitivity separately in order to recommend the most appropriate treatment.

PREDICTION OF PROGNOSIS IN NODE-NEGATIVE BREAST CANCER

Prognostic models for node-negative breast cancer that rely on tumor size and histological grade are useful but imperfect. At least two distinct gene-expression profiling-based tests were recently developed which may improve prognostic prediction for these patients. One of these – Mammaprint[TM] (Agendia Inc, Amsterdam, the Netherlands) – was recently cleared by the US Food and Drug Administration (FDA) to aid prognostic prediction in node-negative breast cancer, and it may become available commercially shortly. This assay measures the expression of 70 genes and calculates a prognostic score which can be used to categorize patients into good or poor prognostic risk groups. This test was evaluated on two separate cohorts of patients that received no systemic adjuvant therapy. The first cohort included 295 patients and showed that those with the good prognosis gene signature had 95% (±2 % standard error (SE)) and 85% (±4% SE) distant metastasis-free survival at 5 and 10 years, respectively, compared to 60% (±4% SE) and 50% (±4.5% SE) in the poor prognostic group.[5] A second validation study ($n = 307$) confirmed these findings, and showed that patients with the good prognosis signature had 90% (85–96% confidence interval (CI) 95%) distant metastasis-free survival at 10 years compared to 71% (65–78%) in the poor prognosis group.[6] Importantly, the gene signature could restratify patients within clinical risk categories defined by the Adjuvant Online program. In other words, some of the clinically low-risk patients were correctly recategorized as high risk based on their gene signatures, and some clinically high-risk patients were correctly predicted to be low risk by the genomic test.

Other investigators also identified genes which were associated with relapse in node-negative breast cancer; markers were selected separately from ER-negative and ER-positive tumors, and were combined into a single 76-gene prognostic signature (VDX2, Veridex LLC, Warren, NJ, USA). This test was also evaluated on two separate cohorts of patients that received no systemic adjuvant therapy and were not included in the development of the test. The first cohort included 180 patients, and showed 5- and 10-year distant metastasis-free survival rates of 96% (89–99%) and 94% (83–98%), respectively, for the good prognosis group. The 5- and 10-year distant metastasis-free survival rates were 74% (64–81%) and 65% (53–74%) for the poor prognosis group.[7] A second independent validation of this 76-gene signature included 198 node-negative cases, and demonstrated again that the 5- and 10-year distant metastasis-free survival rates were 98% (88–100%) and 94% (83–89%), respectively, for the good prognosis group, and 76% (68–82%) and 73% (65–79%) for the poor prognosis group.[8] In this instance too, the gene signature could restratify patients within clinical risk categories defined by the Adjuvant Online program, and recurrence hazard ratios remained similar after adjusting for tumor grade, size and ER status.[8]

Both of these microarray-based assays provide prognostic prediction with moderately high precision (see CI around outcome estimates), and seem to have at least complementary value to tumor size- and grade-based predictions. However, what constitutes low enough risk to forgo systemic adjuvant chemotherapy is influenced not only by the absolute risk of relapse but also by the risk of adverse events, the probability of benefit from therapy, and also by personal preferences. Many patients seem to be willing to accept adjuvant chemotherapy for rather small gains in survival.[2] Molecular prognostic markers may provide little clinical value for these individuals because no predictive test is accurate enough to completely rule out the risk of relapse and some potential benefit from adjuvant therapy. However, many other patients are reluctant to accept the toxicities, inconvenience and costs of chemotherapy for small and uncertain benefit. For these individuals, more precise prediction of risk of recurrence and sensitivity to adjuvant therapy with genomic tests can assist in making a more informed decision.

SELECTION OF SYSTEMIC ADJUVANT THERAPY FOR ESTROGEN RECEPTOR-POSITIVE BREAST CANCER

One of the most pressing questions for patients with stage I–II ER-positive breast cancer is whether to take adjuvant endocrine therapy alone or to also receive adjuvant chemotherapy in addition to the endocrine treatment. Recently, a novel multigene diagnostic assay, Oncotype Dx (Genomic Health Inc, Redwood City, CA, USA), became commercially available to assist decision-making in this situation. This RT-PCR-based assay represents an important conceptual advance in the diagnosis of ER-positive breast cancers. Oncotype Dx measures the expression of 21 genes at the mRNA level from formalin-fixed paraffin-embedded specimens. In addition to ER mRNA, several downstream ER-regulated genes are also measured which may contain information on ER functionality. The assay also quantifies HER2 expression and several proliferation related genes, and combines these into a genomic recurrence score. A seminal study examined the correlation between the Oncotype Dx recurrence score and distant relapse in 668 ER-positive, node-negative, tamoxifen-treated patients who were enrolled in the National Surgical Adjuvant Breast and Bowel Project (NSABP) clinical trial B14.[9] The 10-year distant recurrence rates were 6.8% (4–10%), 14.3% (8–20%) and 30.5% (24–37%) for the low-, intermediate- and high-risk categories, respectively, based on the recurrence score (p <0.001). These results suggest that ER-positive patients with a high recurrence score may not be treated optimally with 5 years of tamoxifen. Similar results were observed in a community-based patient population.[10] In multivariate analysis, the genomic test predicted relapse and overall survival independently of age and tumor size, indicating an at least complementary value.

The value of the recurrence score for predicting benefit from adjuvant cyclophosphamide methotrexate, 5-fluorouracil (CMF) chemotherapy in ER-positive, node-negative breast cancers was also examined. A study that included 651 patients who were enrolled in the NSABP B20 randomized study showed that a higher recurrence score was associated with greater benefit from adjuvant CMF chemotherapy when used in combination with tamoxifen therapy.[11] The absolute improvement in 10-year distant recurrence-free survival was 28% (60% vs 88%) in patients with a recurrence score >31, while there was no benefit in patients with a recurrence score <18 (test for interaction p = 0.038). The hazard ratio for distant recurrence after CMF chemotherapy was 1.31 (0.46–3.78 CI 95%) for patients with recurrence scores <18 and it was 0.26 (0.13–0.53) for patients with scores >31. These data indicate that a high recurrence score identifies a subset of women with ER-positive and node-negative breast cancer at high risk of recurrence despite 5 years of tamoxifen therapy, and this risk can be reduced with the administration of adjuvant chemotherapy.

Oncotype Dx can be useful when the decision regarding adjuvant chemotherapy is not straightforward based on routine clinical variables. However, some important caveats must also be noted. Oncotype Dx is not appropriate to risk stratify ER-negative patients because all patients are categorized as high risk.[12]

The predictive performance of this test in patients who receive aromatase inhibitor therapy or more modern anthracycline- or taxane-containing chemotherapy regimens remains to be studied.[12] In particular, the magnitude of benefit that patients with a low or medium recurrence score experience when treated with third-generation adjuvant chemotherapy regimens is unknown.

Other gene signatures are also emerging in the literature which may in the future assist selection of endocrine therapy or chemotherapy for ER-positive breast cancers. A 200-gene endocrine sensitivity index was recently reported which could identify patients with excellent survival after 5 years of tamoxifen therapy. The same index had limited prognostic value in the absence of endocrine therapy, indicating a true predictive marker.[13] An antibody-based prognostic panel (Mammostrat™, Applied Genomics Inc, Burlingame, CA, USA) is also currently being developed using samples from the NSABP B14 and B20 studies to risk stratify ER-positive patients, somewhat similar to what can be accomplished by Oncotype Dx.[14]

EMERGING CHEMOTHERAPY RESPONSE PREDICTORS

The clinical importance of predicting who will and who will not respond to chemotherapy is intuitively obvious. If a test could predict who will respond to a given drug, the treatment could be administered only to patients who benefit, and others could avoid the unnecessary treatment and its toxicity. However, the practical development of chemotherapy response prediction tests poses several challenges. There are theoretical limits to the accuracy of any response predictor which measures the characteristics of the cancer only. Host characteristics which are not easily measured in cancer tissue, including the rate of drug metabolism, can have an important impact on response to therapy. Also, there is considerable uncertainty as to what level of predictive accuracy would be clinically useful. In fact, different levels of predictive accuracy may be required for different clinical situations.

For instance, the clinical utility of a chemotherapy response prediction test that has 60% positive predictive value (PPV; i.e. 60% chance of response if the test is positive) and 80% negative predictive value (NPV; i.e. 20% chance of response if the test is negative) will depend not only on these test characteristics but also on the availability and efficacy of alternative treatment options, as well as the frequency and severity of adverse effects, and the risks of exposure to ineffective therapy (i.e. rapid disease progression with life-threatening complications). A test with the above performance characteristics may be of limited value in the palliative setting, when alternative treatment options are limited and generally ineffective. Patients and physicians may want to try a drug even if the expected response rate is only 10% (well within the range of test negative cases), particularly if side-effects are uncommon or tolerable. On the other hand, in the setting of potentially curative therapy, when multiple treatment options are available, a test with the same performance characteristics may be helpful to select the best regimen from the several treatment options. In addition, a test developed to predict response to a given treatment in previously untreated patients may not predict response sufficiently accurately when the same drug is used as second- or third-line treatment.

Considering these complexities, not surprisingly many of the recent predictive marker studies that employed high-throughput analytical tools focused on the preoperative (neoadjuvant) treatment setting in breast cancer. Neoadjuvant chemotherapy provides a unique opportunity to identify molecular predictors of response to therapy. Pathologic complete response (pCR) to chemotherapy indicates an extremely chemotherapy-sensitive disease and represents an early surrogate of long-term benefit from therapy. Histological type, tumor size, nuclear grade and ER status all influence the probability of response to neoadjuvant chemotherapy, and these clinical variables can be combined into a multivariable model to predict probability of pCR (http://www.mdanderson.org/care_centers/breastcenter/dIndex.cfm?pn=448442B2-3EA5-4BAC983100 76A9553E63).[15] However, these clinical variables lack regimen-specific predictive value and represent features of general chemotherapy sensitivity.

Several small studies provided "proof-of-principle" that the gene expression profile of cancers which are highly sensitive to chemotherapy are different from tumors which are resistant to treatment.[16] The largest study so far included 133 patients with stage I–III breast cancer who all received preoperative weekly paclitaxel and 5-fluorouracil, doxorubicin, cyclophosphamide (T/FAC) chemotherapy.[17] The first 82 cases were used to develop a multi-gene signature predictive of pCR and the remaining 52 cases were used to test the accuracy of the predictor. The overall pCR rate was 26% in both cohorts. A 30-gene predictor correctly identified all but one of the patients who achieved pCR (12 of 13) and all but one of those who had residual cancer (27 of 28) in the validation set. It showed significantly higher sensitivity (92% vs 61%) than a clinical variable-based predictor including age, grade and ER status. The high sensitivity indicates that the predictor correctly identified almost all of the patients (92%) who actually achieved pCR. The PPV of the pharmacogenomic predictor was 52% (95% CI 30–73%); however, the lower bound of the 95% CI did not overlap with the 26% pCR rate observed with this regimen in unselected patients. This indicates that the predictor could define a patient population that is more likely to achieve pCR than unselected patients. The NPV of the test was also high, 96% (95% CI 82–100%), which indicates that <5% of test-negative patients (i.e. predicted to have residual disease) achieved pCR. These performance statistics are similar, with regard to the NPV and better with regard to PPV, than those seen with ER immunohistochemistry or HER2 gene amplification as predictive markers to endocrine or trastuzumab therapies, respectively. However, to what extent this genomic predictor of sensitivity is specific to T/FAC therapy rather than being a generic marker of chemotherapy sensitivity is yet to be determined.

WHEN IS A NEW DIAGNOSTIC TEST READY FOR ROUTINE CLINICAL USE?

One of the most commonly asked questions about novel diagnostic tests is: When is it ready for clinical use? Unlike drugs, where there are clear regulatory milestones that need to be met before a novel treatment is approved for clinical use by the US FDA, the regulations which apply to laboratory diagnostic assays is less uniform. Currently, a novel diagnostic assay may become available for clinical use through two distinct mechanisms. One is a "diagnostic kit" manufactured by a company and sold to end-users (pathology laboratories) to perform the assay. These types of diagnostic tests are regulated by the FDA and require some level of approval before marketing (www.fda.gov/cdrh). The second route to the clinic is through the CLIA (Clinical Laboratory Improvement Amendment of 1988) certification process. CLIA can classify tests based on its level of complexity. A test classified as "waived" is considered relatively simple, requiring no medical background to analyze. These tests can be administered in a doctor's office or even prescribed for home use. Other CLIA classifications require that more complex tests such as multigene assays be performed in laboratories meeting CLIA certification standards. CLIA certified laboratories (private or academic) can perform complex and new diagnostic assays using reagents which are not necessarily approved or regulated by the FDA, but this may change in the future (see www.fda.gov/OHRMS/DOCKETS/98fr/ch064 1.pdf). However, currently, when a company or an academic group becomes convinced that its favored test provides some clinical value it can start offering it for clinical use through a CLIA certified laboratory. This requires that the assay is reproducible, stable over time, and the laboratory must meet several other quality control measures, including a clear sample and data tracking process. Several of the prognostic/predictive tests discussed above are commercially available through CLIA certified laboratories.

Irrespective of the regulatory requirements that a test needs to meet before it is offered as a test in the clinic, physicians must decide what value the test provides in medical decision-making. It is important to consider that even if a test is not indicated for every patient with breast cancer, it could provide clinical value for some. Many existing and well-accepted diagnostic tests fall into this category. For example, magnetic resonance imaging (MRI) is not performed on all patients with newly diagnosed breast cancer or with a suspicious lump in the breast; however, it is a very useful test for a subset of woman with these conditions. Many of the emerging molecular prognostic and predictive tests also fall into this category. Sometimes decisions can be made about risk of recurrence relatively easily based on clinical characteristics of the disease and the currently available *moderately* accurate molecular predictors add little further value. Patient preference for aggressive therapy, even if the risk of recurrence is low and particularly if the risk of adverse events from treatment is modest (e.g. endocrine therapies), may trump the value of any prognostic marker that is currently available. However, for many patients who are undecided, molecular prognostic assays could assist in decision-making. Similarly, tests which predict the probability of response (with moderate accuracy) may be of limited value if the choice of treatments is limited, or if a patient prefers to take a particular treatment even if the probability of benefit is small. On the other hand, when alternative treatment choices are available, predicting the probability of benefit from a particular treatment, before or soon after it is started, could be helpful.

What is the minimum standard that a test needs to meet before it could be considered for clinical use? The assay needs to be technically robust and reproducible. The performance characteristics of the test, including its predictive values, for a clinically relevant outcome need to be defined with reasonably narrow confidence intervals. If these criteria are met, the test may be considered for clinical use because it is assumed to be reliable and it predicts a relevant clinical outcome with a known degree of uncertainty. Therefore, in

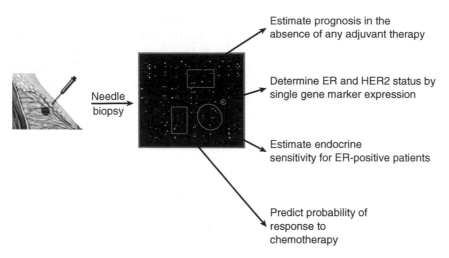

Estimate prognosis in the absence of any adjuvant therapy

Needle biopsy

Determine ER and HER2 status by single gene marker expression

Estimate endocrine sensitivity for ER-positive patients

Predict probability of response to chemotherapy

Figure 11.2 It is currently possible to determine estrogen- and HER-receptor status, make prognostic predictions and estimate chemotherapy and endocrine therapy sensitivity from a single microarray experiment.

clinical situations when the prediction result is expected to assist decision-making the assay could be helpful. However, one would also like to see proof that such "more informed" medical decision-making actually results in improved patient outcome (e.g. increased survival, better quality of life). To conduct such studies to demonstrate clinical utility is time consuming but important.

CONCLUSIONS

At least one novel genomic diagnostic test is now available in the USA to estimate the prognosis of ER-positive, lymph-node negative patients who are to receive 5 years of tamoxifen therapy. This test could help identify individuals who are at low risk (or high risk) for recurrence with endocrine therapy alone and could assist in recommending chemotherapy more appropriately for ER-positive patients. Another genomic prognostic assay was recently cleared by the FDA, and it may help in refining prognostic estimates for node-negative patients and could particularly be helpful for stage I–II ER-negative patients who are undecided about adjuvant chemotherapy. This test requires fresh-frozen tissue for analysis. The advent of multigene assays in the clinic also offers a new opportunity to package multiple prognostic and predictive tests into a single diagnostic product in the not too distant future (Figure 11.2).

It is important to realize that no prospective randomized studies have been completed to demonstrate improved patient outcome with the use of any of the new tests compared to decision-making based on clinical parameters only. Two such studies are currently under way including the MINDACT trial in Europe that tests Mammaprint™ and the TAILORX study in the USA that tests Oncotype Dx™. Survival results from these studies will not be available for several years. However, some forms of clinical benefit from novel tests may be more subtle than improvements in survival. It may be argued that additional information which helps patients (and physicians) feel more comfortable with a particular treatment recommendation is of value on its own.

REFERENCES

1. Ann G Carmichaelm, Richard M Ratzan, eds. Medicine, A Treasury of Art and Literature. New York, NY: Beaux Arts Editions, 1991: 29.
2. Ravdin PM, Siminoff IA, Harvey JA et al. Survey of breast cancer patients concerning their knowledge and expectations of adjuvant therapy. J Clin Onc 1998; 16: 515–21.
3. Olivotto IA, Bajdik CD, Ravdin PM et al. Population-based validation of the prognostic model ADJUVANT! for early breast cancer. J Clin Oncol 2005; 23: 2716–25.
4. Pusztai L. Chips to bedside: incorporation of microarray data into clinical practice. Clin Cancer Res 2006; 12(24): 7209–14.

5. Van de Vijver MJ, Yudong DH. A gene-expression signature as a predictor of survival in breast cancer. N Engl J Med 2002; 347: 1999–2009.

6. Buyse M, Loi S, van't Veer L et al. Validation and clinical utility of a 70-gene prognostic signature for women with node-negative breast cancer. J Natl Cancer Inst 2006; 98: 1183–92.

7. Foekens JA, Atkins D, Zhang Y et al. Multicenter validation of a gene expression-based prognostic signature in lymph node-negative primary breast cancer. Clin Oncol 2006; 24: 1665–71.

8. Desmedt C, Piette F, Loi S et al. Strong time dependence of the 76-gene prognostic signature for node-negative breast cancer patients in the TRANSBIG multicenter independent validation series. Clin Cancer Res 2007; 13: 3207–14.

9. Paik S, Shak S, Tang G et al. A multi gene assay to predict recurrence of tamoxifen-treated, node-negative breast cancer. N Engl J Med 2004; 351: 2817–26.

10. Habel LA, Shak S, Jacobs MK et al. A population-based study of tumor gene expression and risk of breast cancer death among lymph node-negative patients. Breast Cancer Res 2006; 8(3): R25.

11. Paik S, Tang G, Shak S et al. Gene expression and benefit of chemotherapy in women with node-negative, estrogen receptor-positive breast cancer. J Clin Oncol 2006; 24: 3726–34.

12. Goldstein LJ, Gray R, Childs B et al. Prognostic utility of the 21-gene assay in hormone receptor (HR) positive operable breast cancer and 0–3 positive axillary nodes treated with adjuvant chemo-hormonal therapy: an analysis of Intergoup trial E2197. Proc Am Soc Clin Oncol Annual Meeting 2007 [Abs 526].

13. Symmans WF, Hatzis C, Sotiriou C et al. A genomic index of estrogen receptor reporter genes predicts benefit from adjuvant endocrine therapy independent of baseline prognosis. Breast Cancer Res Treat 2006; 100(1): S47 [Abs 1027].

14. Ring BZ, Seitz RS, Beck R et al. Novel prognostic immunohistochemical biomarker panel for estrogen receptor-positive breast cancer. J Clin Oncol 2006; 24: 3039–47.

15. Rouzier R, Pusztai L, Delaloge S et al. Nomograms to predict pathologic complete response and metastasis-free survival after preoperative chemotherapy for breast cancer. J Clin Oncol 2005; 23: 8331–9.

16. Pusztai L, Gianni L. Prediction of response to preoperative chemotherapy in operable breast cancer. Nature Clin Practice Onc 2004; 1: 44–50.

17. Hess KR, Anderson K, Symmans W et al. Pharmacogenomic predictor of sensitivity to preoperative chemotherapy with paclitaxel and fluorouracil, doxorubicin, and cyclophosphamide in breast cancer. J Clin Oncol 2006; 24: 4236–44.

18. Gong Y, Yan K, Lin F et al. Determination of oestrogen-receptor status and ERBB5 status of breast carcinoma: a gene-expression profiling study. Lancet Oncol 2007; 8: 203–11.

p53 and breast cancer

12

Oliver Staples, Sonia Lain, Dorin Ziyaie and Alastair M Thompson

INTRODUCTION

p53 was first discovered in 1979 as a cellular protein of approximately 53-kDa binding to the large T antigen in cells transformed by Simian Virus 40 (SV40), at a time when oncogenic DNA viruses were a popular tool for inducing experimental malignant transformation to study neoplasia. For 10 years the p53 gene was thought to be an oncogene before the finding that it was mutated in a range of cancers, suggesting p53 had a role as a tumor suppressor. This was confirmed by evidence that wild-type, normal p53 could suppress transformation of cells caused by mutant p53 and oncogenes. In 1992, using mice with non-functional p53 which had a higher propensity to develop spontaneous tumors, p53 was firmly established as a tumor suppressor gene. It is now estimated that a wide range of cancer types and some 50% of all human tumors have specific p53 mutations (www.iarc.fr/p53).

p53, "guardian of the genome",[1] is regarded as a tumor suppressor gene with tumor development frequently attributed either to p53 deletion, p53 mutation or aberrant p53 function. p53 is involved in distinct functions at the cellular level, including regulation of normal cell growth and division, gene transcription, DNA repair, and genomic stability. Hence, p53 is regarded as a crucial regulatory protein which integrates an array of signals, in response to which it turns on a host of biochemical responses at the level of the cell and ultimately the whole organism (Figure 12.1).[2] p53 activation, resulting in cell cycle arrest or apoptosis, prevents the perpetuation of genetic defects which would otherwise go unrecognized.[1]

The p53 gene, located at 17p13.3, was long thought to produce only one protein, but it has recently been discovered that, via alternative splicing and an internal promoter, the gene can in fact make up to nine different protein isoforms.[3,4] The main protein product of the p53 gene is a phosphoprotein comprising 393 amino acid residues (Figure 12.2), with at least four recognized, highly conserved "boxes" or "domains": the N-terminal (amino-terminal) transactivation domain;[2] central DNA-binding domain; a tetramerization domain; and the C-terminal negative regulatory domain. Although each domain is involved in distinct and independent functions, overall they are interdependent in the sense that alterations within one domain can profoundly influence the functions of the other domains.[5] The biological relevance of the p53 isoforms is actively being investigated, and the expression of the different isoforms could determine cell fate in response to cellular stress[4] and may be related to prognosis in breast cancer.

Two homologues of p53 – p63 and p73 – share many structural similarities (including splice variants) and functional overlap with p53, and may cooperate with p53 in tumor suppressor effects. Indeed, p73 may replace the function of p53 in anthracyclin-treated p53-deficient cells triggering apoptosis,[6] and p63 may control a pathway for p73-dependent cisplatin sensitivity in triple-negative (estrogen receptor (ER), progesterone receptor (PR) and human epidermal growth factor receptor 2 (HER2) negative) breast cancers.[7]

The p53 protein in normal cells is in a latent form, with a low steady state due to the rapid rate of proteolytic degradation, but p53

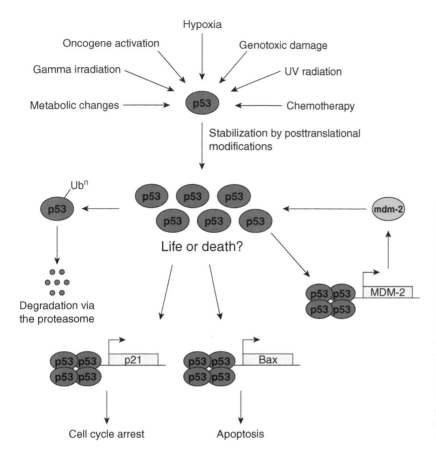

Figure 12.1 p53 integrates the cellular response to noxious stimuli including DNA damage, hypoxia, heat shock, radiation, and drugs. As part of the response, p53 tetramers activate pathways eliciting a range of responses including resulting in cell cycle arrest (involving the p21 protein) or apoptosis (involving the Bax protein). p53 also enhances Mouse Double Minute (MDM)-2 and is regulated via MDM-2, which targets p53 for destruction via polyubiquitination (Ub^n) and proteosomal degradation.

accumulates in response to multiple stimuli. This is mediated through posttranslational modification involving phosphorylation of mainly the amino-terminus by the DNA–protein kinases (PK), or the carboxy-terminus by the cyclin-dependent kinases leading to an increase in the half-life of the protein.[9] Mutations can potentially alter the conformation of p53 leading to increased stability and hence accumulation of the protein.[5,10] Since the half-life of wild-type p53 is about 20 minutes, p53 may be virtually undetectable in normal cells. Mutated p53 protein has a longer half-life and, unlike the wild-type protein, tends to accumulate in tumor cells, allowing detection by immunohistochemistry.

P53 FUNCTION

p53 has been ascribed functions as: a transcription factor; in maintaining genomic integrity; as a tumor suppressor gene mediating cell cycle arrest and/or apoptosis; and in a range of developmental and physiological roles[2,11,12] through its transcriptional and non-transcriptional functions. Indeed, p53 is central to the balance between aging and the development of cancer.[10]

p53 as a transcription factor

The cardinal feature of wild-type p53 is as a sequence-specific transcriptional activator via DNA-binding and -activation domains, which bind to specific DNA sequences of some 300 "target genes", promoting or suppressing their activities in response to DNA damage. In human cancers it is in this critical DNA-binding domain where the majority of the p53 mutations occur, termed "hot spot" mutations (www.iarc.fr/p53). A number of target-genes containing p53-binding sites, both in the

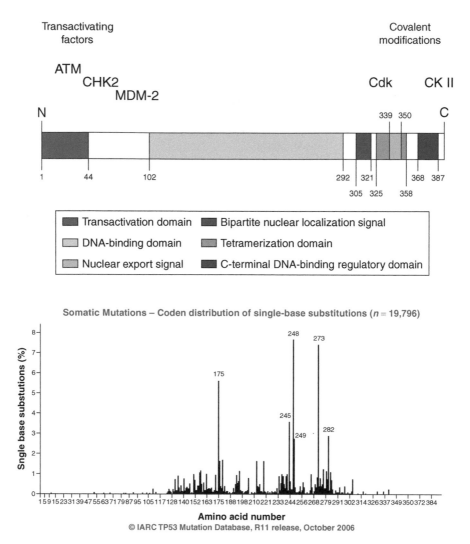

Figure 12.2 p53 comprises a 393 amino acid protein including transactivation, DNA binding, oligomerization, and negative regulatory domains. At the N-terminal end of the molecule, ATM, CHK2 and Mouse Double Minute (MDM)-2 are amongst the many proteins that interact with p53; at the C-terminus, covalent modification (phosphorylation, acetylation) and interactions with cyclin-dependent kinases (Cdk) and casein kinase II (CK II) affect the function of p53.

The mutations detected in p53 predominantly occur in the DNA-binding domain (lower panel) with specific sites being more common in human cancer (numbered amino acids, e.g. 175, versus frequency).

promoter and intron regions, have been identified, including p21^{WAF1}, MDM-2 and BAX (Figure 12.2).

p53 maintaining genomic integrity

p53 appears to have a direct effect on maintaining genomic integrity through monitoring DNA damage by activating genes which facilitate, but also regulate, DNA repair. p53 actively participates in various processes of DNA repair and DNA recombination by interaction with the repair and recombination machinery, respectively. This suggests that p53 exerts its role as the guardian of the genome at two levels. In the activated form, p53 will exert tumor-suppressor activities in response to exogenous DNA damage and cellular stress. In the noninduced form, p53 remains active through inherent exonuclease activity engaged in prevention and repair of endogenous DNA damage, thus maintaining genomic integrity.

p53 as a tumor suppressor

As a tumor suppressor, p53 plays a pivotal role as a mediator between stressful stimuli and the final cellular outcome (Figure 12.1). The two main cellular responses to DNA damage mediated through p53 are growth arrest, which prevents propagation and accumulation of cells with genetic alterations, and apoptosis (programed cell death) achieving elimination of the target cell.

Growth arrest

p53 mediates growth arrest through regulation of crucial checkpoints during both the G1 and G2 phases of cell cycle. p53-dependent G1 arrest is mediated by transactivation of the waf1 gene that codes for the small kinase inhibitor p21[waf1]. This protein in turn prevents entry to the S phase in the cell cycle by blocking the activity of the cyclin-dependent kinases (Cdk). Inhibition of this G1-phase-specific Cdk activity maintains a hypophosphorylated retinoblastoma protein (pRb), which in turn blocks the E2F-mediated transcription of genes required for entry into S phase, therefore blocking cell cycle progression and hence resulting in the accumulation of cells in the G1 phase.[13] p53-mediated G1 arrest can also be induced independent of p21.

p53-dependent G2 arrest is mediated through at least two target genes: the 14-3-3σ gene through sequestering phosphatases of the cyclinB/cdc2 complex; and, to a lesser extent, the GADD45 gene which interacts directly with cdc2 and therefore disrupts the cyclinB/cdc2 complex, which is required for the G2/M transition.

Apoptosis

While cell cycle arrest can function to inhibit growth in normal cells, cells that have undergone malignant transformation are less susceptible to growth arrest and favor apoptosis. The apoptotic pathway is characterized by the activation of caspases (cell death proteases), which are themselves activated by catalytic cleavage. This results in the disruption of the function of essential regulatory proteins and as a result cells are committed to enter the "cell death" pathway.[14] Activation of caspases is followed by characteristic structural changes within the cell, nuclear condensation and destruction, membrane blebbing, loss of cellular volume, and ultimately loss of membrane integrity. The two roles of p53 in apoptosis can be described as transcription-dependent p53-mediated apoptosis or transcription-independent mediated apoptosis.

For transcription-dependent p53-mediated apoptosis, there are two groups of regulatory genes involved in regulation, pro-apoptotic genes such as Bax, which has p53 binding sites in its promoter site and is upregulated in response to DNA damage and antiapoptotic genes such as Bcl-2 and Bcl-x.[15]

Introduction of Bax into cells results in rapid cell death which can be inhibited by coexpression of either Bax-binding proteins or death-inhibiting proteins Bcl-2 and Bcl-x. On the other hand, p53 is also known to transcriptionally repress expression of other genes such as the death-inhibiting gene Bcl-2.[15] The combination of Bcl-2 repression with induction of the death-promoting gene Bax would therefore result in cell death.[16]

Additional protein–protein interactions also play a role in directing p53 towards apoptosis with the apoptosis-stimulating protein of p53 (ASPP) family of proteins being one of the best examples. This family contains three proteins: ASPP1 and f-2, which stimulate p53-dependant apoptosis by promoting p53 binding to pro-apoptotic genes promoters; and iASPP, which inhibits p53-mediated apoptosis by antagonizing pro-apoptotic gene expression.[17]

p53 can also induce apoptosis via nontranscriptional functions, where p53 interacts with pro-apoptotic and antiapoptotic proteins belonging to the Bcl-2 family in the cytosol causing an induction of mitochondrial membrane permeabilization, cytochrome c release and subsequent caspase activation. An important aspect to this work has been the identification of differences between two polymorphic variants of p53. Within the proline-rich domain of p53, there is a polymorphism at codon 72 (pro/arg), which correlates with the apoptotic potential of the p53 proteins and their affinity for localizing to the mitochondrial outer membrane.[18] The importance of this proline-rich region in mediating apoptosis independent of p53 sequence-specific transactivation has been particularly highlighted in Li–Fraumeni[19] patients where a germ-line mutation within this region (proline-82) has been clearly identified and characterized, and in which female members have a high risk of breast cancer.

Choice between growth arrest and apoptosis

In response to DNA damage (Figure 12.1), whether the cells undergo growth arrest or apoptosis is usually dependent on the integration of signals in a cell-specific manner. The cell type and oncogenic status, the intensity and strength of the stimuli, the basal p53 levels, and the degree of p53 interaction with other cellular proteins which are directly or indirectly involved in the induction of growth arrest or apoptosis all contribute to the response.

In cancer cells, the key factors are the efficacy of the DNA repair mechanisms and the level of p53 expression in response to DNA damage. Whilst p53 at high levels promotes apoptosis, p53 expressed at low levels protects cells against apoptosis. p53 remains active as long as DNA damage persists, but if the DNA is repaired rapidly the period of p53 expression/activation is short and hence little p53 accumulates. When DNA damage is extensive the period of p53 expression is prolonged.

In addition, the balance of the regulatory mechanisms against apoptosis also play an important role: Bax (pro-apoptotic) versus Bcl-2 (antiapoptotic), the Rb–E2F pathway that mediates p53-dependent G1 cell cycle arrest, and growth/survival factor cytokines which protect cells from apoptosis in favor of growth arrest are all important factors when deciding cellular outcome in response to stress.[20]

Posttranslational modification of p53 involving phosphorylation at serine 315 by the Cdks is said to alter the specific DNA-binding affinities of p53.[21] Similar effects are seen in the interaction of p53 with other proteins such as p300, which is essential for both p21 and Mouse Double Minute (MDM)-2 induction and thyroid hormone receptor $\beta 1$, which upon binding to p53 inhibits Bax and growth arrest and DNA damage inducible gene (GADD45).

Finally, the intensity of the DNA-damaging signal, along with the time period to which cells are exposed to the stressful stimuli, has a major role in determining the cellular outcome. Thus, apoptosis is induced in response to a higher intensity and longer period of damage-inducing signals, whereas the reverse is true for induction of growth arrest.

Regulation of p53 activity

Acting as the central coordinator between the stressful stimuli and the final outcome of the cell (Figure 12.1), p53 can be subject to extensive and complex regulation. Molecular mechanisms responsible for conversion of the latent p53 in normal cells to the active form are complex but comprise a series of posttranslational modifications of p53, interaction of p53 protein with other proteins, and a series of noncovalent regulators all of which provide therapeutic opportunities.[5]

p53 regulation through the N-terminal transactivation domain

Posttranslational modifications result in conformational changes within the p53 molecule and hence activation of p53. These modifications include p53 regulation through phosphorylation sites in the N-terminal transactivation domain (residues 1–44) (Figure 12.2). While the phosphorylation sites have not yet been fully characterized, serine (Ser) 4, Ser6 and Ser9 for the casein kinase (CK) I site, and Ser15 and Ser37 for the DNA-protein kinase (PK) site appear to be important.[9]

The interaction of the N-terminal domain of p53 with other proteins within the transcriptional machinery is pivotal to its role as a transcriptional activator. p53-interacting proteins belonging to the transcription machinery include MDM-2, the DNA sequence of Ts and As where transcription factors bind (TATA) box-binding protein (TBP), TBP-associated factor (TAF), the p62 component of transcription factor IIH (TFIIH) and p300/CPB (CREB Binding Protein).[15] Amongst the key p53 N-terminal-interacting proteins, in which altered expression is demonstrated in many cancers – including breast cancer – is the MDM-2 protein.[22] MDM-2 controls the biological activity of p53 and targets p53 for destruction, acting as an E3 ligase to conjugate ubiquitin to p53, which provides a signal for p53 to be degraded by the proteasome. MDM-2 is a target gene of p53 and is therefore upregulated when p53 is activated, thus providing an inbuilt negative-feedback loop mechanism whereby p53 expression is controlled at the cellular level. The p53–MDM-2 protein interaction is of physiological relevance, as evidenced by over-expression of MDM-2 protein inactivating wild-type p53 in soft tissue sarcomas.[23] In addition, early embryonic lethal phenotype of an MDM-2 knockout mouse is rescued when crossed into a p53 null phenotype.[24]

Changes within the N-terminal domain, through interactions with other proteins, can quantitatively increase DNA binding, whereas the opposite is true for changes brought about through phosphorylation of the N-terminal sites in p53.[8] Posttranslational modification of the p53 N-terminus at Ser15 by DNA–PK has been shown to reduce the ability of p53 and MDM-2 to bind, and since MDM-2 is a strong promoter of p53 degradation this results in p53 stabilization and hence accumulation.[8] The role of MDM-2 in p53 protein stabilization is further supported by the fact that the tumor suppressor p19ARF (alternating reading frame spliced product of the murine p16INK4A locus) induces p53 stabilization through its interaction with MDM-2.

p53 regulation through the central core domain

Amongst the five conserved regions of p53, regions II–V map within the central core DNA-binding domain (residues 102–292; Figure 12.2) where the majority of mutations observed in human cancers have been identified (www.iarc.fr/p53).

Specific DNA binding of the central core domain is essential for the role of p53 as a tumor suppressor. Mutations in the cysteine residues block p53 transactivation and tumor-suppression function. Many of these residues are specifically mutated in numerous naturally occurring human cancers (www.iarc.fr/p53).

p53 regulation through the tetramerization domain

Maintaining the active p53 molecule in the form of a tetramer enhances p53's DNA sequence-specific binding properties. The altered folding and conformational structure of p53 in tumors is highlighted by using antibodies specific for denatured p53 in tumor cells. Maintaining p53 in a tetrameric structure is ensured by the p53 tetramerization domain: alterations in this domain can reduce, or indeed prevent, DNA binding of the p53 protein. As an example, in the Li–Fraumeni syndrome altered thermal stability of the tetramerization domain results in ineffective MDM-2 binding to p53.

The group of cellular proteins known as "heat shock proteins" (HSPs) also play a pivotal role in maintaining the conformational structure of p53. HSPs (mainly HSP70, HSP40, and HSP90) contribute to p53 inactivation and oppose apoptosis in some cell lines undergoing drug or radiation-induced apoptosis.[25] This effect contributes to tumor cell survival, consistent with the observed increase in the HSP–mutant p53 complex in some cancers. Conversely, HSPs are involved in protecting proteins from unfolding and aim to refold denatured proteins, in addition to targeting the irreversibly "damaged" ones for destruction.

p53 regulation through the C-terminal domain

The C-terminal regulatory domain (Figure 12.2) effects the DNA-binding ability of the central core domain either through interactions with other proteins or as the result of direct modification.[5] This domain acts both as a negative regulatory region, controlling the DNA sequence-specific binding of the central core domain, and as a separate functional domain.

Alongside regulation of the central core domain, the p53 C-terminus can also be regarded as a damage-recognition region. The p53 C-terminus is able to bind DNA ends and strands, DNA mismatches, Holliday junctions, and irradiated DNA. In addition, a number of proteins involved in the DNA repair mechanisms can also interact with and regulate p53, presumably through the C-terminus.

The significance of these interactions and their probable effect on the p53 sequence binding transactivation function have yet to be fully explored. However, it is clear that the relationship between p53 and the DNA-repair processes is not only through stimulation and signaling after DNA damage but also through its multiple direct interactions with the proteins involved in the DNA-repair mechanisms.

Posttranslational modification of p53 involving phosphorylation

Posttranslational modifications involving phosphorylation affect p53 turnover and accumulation,[8] particularly within the N- and C-terminal domains of the protein.

p53 protein can be phosphorylated by PKs at various sites along the length of the molecule. These include kinases such as CK I (at the transactivation domain), DNA–PK, c-Jun N-terminal kinase (JNK), mitogen-activated protein (MAP) kinase, and CK II.[9] Radiation can alter phosphorylation status of at least two key regulatory sites in the p53 molecule, which in turn alters its activity as a transcription factor, and phosphorylation of the carboxyl terminal can alter the sequence-specific DNA binding.[26] Thus, p53 modification by phosphorylation may alter the functional balance of this key cellular regulation pathway and the relative efficacy of activation of different p53 target genes.[9]

p53 can also undergo posttranslational modification via acetylation, sumolyation, neddylation, and methylation. Such modifications mediate the transactivation potential of p53 either by enhancing or repressing direct DNA binding by p53, or influencing the affinity of p53 for regulatory partners. More recently the in vivo importance of acetylation, sumolyation and neddylation has been called into question via the use of mice models, and thus further investigation will be required to determine how important modifications other than phosphorylation are in vivo.[27]

P53 INDUCING OR SUPPRESSING THE FUNCTION OF OTHER GENES

Amongst some of the key p53 transactivated target genes containing p53-binding sites, in which altered expression is demonstrated in many cancers, are MDM-2[22] and p21.[28]

The MDM-2 gene encodes the mdm-2 protein that controls the biological activity of p53 and targets p53 for destruction,[22] and therefore provides an inbuilt mechanism whereby p53 expression is controlled at the cellular level. p21 mediates the tumor-suppressing effects of p53 by inhibiting Cdk complex activity, therefore blocking the transition from G1 to S phase in cell cycle progression, mediating p53-dependent growth arrest.[29]

Mouse Double Minute-2

There are at least seven different transcripts of the human MDM-2 gene, coding for the MDM-2 protein. The largest human MDM-2 protein consists of 491 amino acids and has several conserved features. These include the amino-terminus domain which interacts with p53, inhibiting transcriptional activity, the nuclear localization sequence (NLS) and the nuclear export signal (NES) sequence which mediate MDM-2 shuttling between the nucleus and the cytoplasm, the highly acidic domain which constitutes a second p53 interaction site, the zinc-finger domain and a further two zinc fingers in a ring conformation (RING-finger domain) which mediate sequence-specific RNA binding and is also involved auto-ubiquitination and ubiquitination of p53, necessary for degradation by the proteasome.

A single nucleotide polymorphism (SNP) of MDM-2 at position 309 has been suggested as a predisposing factor in breast cancer,[30] but a large meta-analysis of the 5000 cases examined in the literature has failed to confirm any linkage to early onset of breast cancer.[31]

MDM-2–p53 interaction

p53 and MDM-2 form an autoregulatory feedback loop in that p53 upregulates MDM-2 levels whilst MDM-2 negatively regulates p53 levels and hence p53 activity. In response to DNA damage, there is a fall in both the MDM-2 mRNA and protein levels, with a subsequent rise in p53 levels. This is followed by an increase in the transcriptional activity of p53 and initiation of the relevant cellular response to DNA damage. The high levels of transcriptionally active p53 increase MDM-2 gene transcription which results in inhibition of p53's transcriptional activity and promotion of p53 degradation.[32]

MDM-2 as an oncogene

MDM-2 was first regarded as an oncogene when it was realized that cell lines overexpressing MDM-2 show tumorigenic properties in nude mice. In addition, targeted MDM-2 overexpression in the mammary tissue of mice during lactation has been shown to not only induce cellular changes similar to the phenotypes with inactive or defective p53 but also to progress to the development of mammary gland tumors by the time the mice reach 18 months of age.[33]

The oncogenic properties of MDM-2 were further suggested in a range of tumor types including breast cancers,[22] where overexpression of MDM-2 was found either through gene amplification, increased transcription, or increased translation. In some individuals with Li–Fraumeni syndrome, who have two alleles of p53 without the capacity to express p21, show overexpression of MDM-2 in their normal tissues. Overexpression of MDM-2 in the absence of p21 expression (which is transcriptionally induced by p53) suggests that MDM-2 overexpression is p53 independent and may be a direct cause of the high tumor incidence (including breast cancer) in these families.[34]

Mouse Double Minute-4

MDM-4 (MDMX) was identified as a binding partner of p53 and shows structural homology to MDM-2, and is thus a potentially important regulator of p53. When bound to p53 it inhibits p53 transactivation, but does not appear to target p53 for degradation as it lacks the E3 ubiquitin ligase function of MDM-2. MDMX overexpression can protect p53 from MDM-2-mediated degradation while still maintaining suppression of p53 transactivation.[35] The gene for MDMX is overexpressed or amplified in 10–20% of diverse tumor types including breast cancer.[27] Like MDM-2, MDMX knockout mice are embryonic lethal, although this can be rescued by being in a p53-deficient background. It has been suggested that to fully activate p53 both MDM-2 and MDMX need to be inactivated, which adds another level of complexity when trying to discover ways of exploiting p53 for therapeutic gain.

p21

In mammalian cells, the cell cycle is positively regulated by a series of stable and unstable proteins termed Cdks and cyclins, respectively. This regulation is mediated through the phosphorylation of specific substrates which are inhibited by the so-called cyclin kinase inhibitors (CKIs), which therefore negatively regulate cell cycle progression.[36] p21[CIP1/WAF1] was the first CKI identified in mammalian cells.

To ensure genomic integrity and prevent the propagation of damaged DNA onto future generations of cells, eukaryotic cells have developed a series of "checkpoint-response pathways". These are controlled through the damage-suppressor genes, either acting directly or indirectly, mediating specific target genes. p21 is regarded as one of the major target genes in p53-mediated cell cycle growth arrest in both normal and the tumor cells.

Inhibition of cell cycle progression, mediated through p21 activity, occurs at two main regulatory checkpoint-response pathways: G1 arrest and G2 arrest.

p53-dependent G1 arrest

In response to DNA damage, p53-induced G1 arrest is mediated through transactivation of the WAF1 gene that codes for the small kinase inhibitor p21^{WAF1}. By blocking the activity of the Cdks (namely, Cdk2, Cdk4, and cdc2 cyclin complexes), p21 blocks the entry into the S phase at G1.[13] Arrest of the cell cycle at G1 through inhibition of the G1-specific kinases results in the maintenance of the hypophosphorylated form of the protein product of the retinoblastoma susceptibility gene pRb. The hypophosphorylated pRb blocks the E2F-mediated transactivation of the genes which is required for the entry into S phase, which results in the accumulation of the cells at G1.

Accumulation of the cells in S phase is also mediated through proliferating-cell nuclear antigen (PCNA). In the process of DNA replication, PCNA forms a complex with replication factor C (RF-C), which together promote recognition of a primer-template junction which facilitates the uptake of DNA polymerase δ. The "trimeric" protein complex PCNA–RF-C–polymerase δ induces DNA replication. Direct binding of p21 to PCNA dissociates the PCNA–RF-C–polymerase δ complex, which arrests the replicating DNA.[37]

p53-independent G2 arrest

Cell cycle arrest mediated by p21 can also occur at the later stages of the cell cycle, namely the G2 phase. p21^{WAF1} mRNA upregulation as well as peaking in G1 is also seen to be transiently elevated at the G2/M phase. This is said to be through p21 association with cyclin A and B complexes.[38] In late G2, nearly half of the Cdk2/cyclin A is in a complex with p21. The inhibition of Cdk2/cyclin A can either be as the result of the direct inhibition of the activated kinase by p21, indirectly through inactivation of the Cdk-activating kinase (CAK) by p21 or, indeed, through blocking the interaction of other cyclin substrates with the Cdk2/cyclin A complex.

LESSONS FROM IN VIVO STUDIES OF P53

As a step towards understanding the role of p53 in breast cancer, the development of mouse models has been crucial in defining the function of p53 as a tumor-suppressor gene and in examining the effect on downstream genes.

Through gene targeting technology, p53 has been inactivated in mouse models by disrupting the DNA-binding domain[39] or through inducing point mutations at regions mainly involving the crucial coding sequences in the p53 gene.[40] When these mice were bred to homozygosity, a high proportion showed a tendency towards rapid development of tumors by 6 months and almost all died or developed tumors by 10 months. Heterozygous mice (p53+/−), which model the genetics of the Li–Fraumeni syndrome, also show similar tendencies but with a slightly longer latency time to tumor development.[39] The concept of tumor development by loss of one normal allele, loss of heterozygosity (LOH), followed by mutation of the second allele highlights the importance of normal p53 function in protection against carcinogenesis.

The role of p21 as one of the major components in p53-mediated cell cycle arrest came to light when mice with homozygous deletion for p21^{WAF1} were shown to be able to go through normal development but failed to demonstrate cell cycle arrest at the G1 checkpoint.[41] Similarly, the function of MDM-2 as both a p53 transcriptionally activated gene and p53 degradation regulator gene came to light and was confirmed through studies on the mouse models. This was demonstrated through an example of "phenotype rescue" when MDM-2-deficient mice were crossed to p53-deficient mice. It was observed that though MDM-2 null mice resulted in early embryonic lethality, when MDM-2 heterozygous mice were crossed with p53-deficient mice the double null p53 and

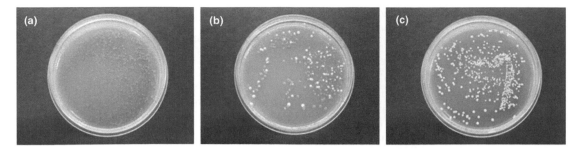

Figure 12.3 Methods used to detect p53 aberrations include: (a) the yeast functional assay where mutation in p53 appears as red colonies on the agar plate, (b)yeast colonies with wild-type p53 as white colonies and a tumor sample demonstrates a mix of red colonies from cancer cells with mutant p53 and (c)white colonies from the normal tissue in the biopsy specimen (after Duddy et al 2000).

MDM-2 mice were completely viable with no developmental abnormalities. The so-called "rescue of the embryonic lethality" highlighted the primary function of MDM-2 in development is to inactivate the p53 activity that coincides with a high level of cell cycle progression activity. This therefore suggests that the lethality of the MDM-2 null mice was due to unregulated activity of p53 which would otherwise have been controlled by MDM-2.[24]

More recently, mouse models of tumor formation have become more advanced and have been used to test whether reactivation of p53 in developed tumors can lead to tumor suppression. In elegant experiments it was shown that if p53 could be reintroduced into established tumors then the tumors were subject to massive apoptosis of cell growth arrest, depending on tumor type.[42,43] This has lead to the increased enthusiasm for the development of novel p53-activating drugs for cancer therapy.

METHODS TO DETECT P53

The detection of p53 in breast cancer can be at the genomic level (DNA), as transcribed messenger RNA, or as the p53 protein (Figure 12.3). Studies of p53 DNA can be classed as looking for mutations or polymorphisms by DNA sequencing, yeast functional assay or Chip-based technology; allele loss (LOH)/allelic imbalance, resulting in wild-type p53 gene haplo-insufficiency, which can be sufficient to predispose to malignancy. The yeast functional assay uses a reporter system in S cerevisiae and can detect <10% of breast cancer cells bearing mutant p53 in a tissue sample, supplemented by direct sequencing to locate the precise mutation.[44] This combination can point to the functional significance of individual gene mutations but avoids the problem of directly sequencing breast cancer tissue DNA and hence missing mutations where the cancer tissue is outnumbered by normal cells. The clinical utility of the yeast functional assay in predicting response to taxane- or anthracyclin-based therapy is currently under study in a randomized trial of neoadjuvant chemotherapy (EORTC trial 10094). Direct DNA sequencing, supplemented by laser-capture microscopy to isolate the relevant tumor tissue, is a useful research tool, but both techniques may be supplanted by the Affymetrix platform-based p53 mutation Chip (Roche Diagnostics, Pleasanton, CA, USA), which can detect mutations and polymorphisms across the p53 gene from a single DNA sample.

While detection of p53 mRNA by Northern blotting, polymerase chain reaction (PCR) techniques or in situ techniques can indicate levels of p53 expression in breast tissue, there appears to be little correlation between mRNA expression and p53 protein activity in breast cancer.[45] This may be further compounded by differential expression of p53 isoforms at the mRNA and protein level.[3]

The majority of studies of p53 in breast cancer have been based on antibodies to various domains or individual amino acid residues in p53, both in Western blots and by immuno-histochemistry utilizing either paraffin-fixed tissue or frozen samples depending on the antibody in question. Incorrect assumptions that simple detection of p53 in tumor tissues reflects the presence of mutant p53, disregarding tissue processing and the effect that has on p53 protein, p53 localization within the tissues or the specificity of the antibody has led to a confused picture as to the value of p53 protein studies in response to therapy or as a prognostic marker.

P53 AND BREAST CANCER

p53 mutation is uncommon in breast cancer families accounting for approximately only 1% of breast cancer predisposition.[46] p53 protein overexpression or mutation is rare in normal breast or in benign breast conditions, although p53 protein accumulation has been linked to an increased risk of breast cancer in women with benign breast disease.[47] Abnormalities in p53 function appear to be more common than specific p53 gene mutations in breast cancer, unlike many other cancer types. Loss of p53 normal function as the result of LOH (loss of one allele) is more common than the homozygous deletion (loss of both alleles), and is seen in up to 61% of the primary breast cancers[45] and may precede the invasive phenotype (particularly in high-grade or comedo-type ductal carcinoma in situ (DCIS).[48] The observation of p53 mutation or overexpression of p53 protein in up to 52% of primary breast cancer specimens, along with increasing knowledge of the characteristics of p53, has focused the attention in recent years into two areas:

- using p53 as a potential marker for studying the relationship between mutant p53 expression and tumor development, progression, response to treatment, and disease outcome;
- designing alternative treatment strategies specifically aiming at restoring p53 function to normal.

p53 as a diagnostic marker

Specific p53 mutations are only observed in 15–35% of breast cancers. Mutant p53 as a diagnostic marker for familial breast cancers has been most promising in the Li–Fraumeni syndrome,[19] an autosomal dominant familial disorder characterized by the development of bone/soft tissue sarcomas, leukemia, adrenocortical, brain and breast cancers. The expected disease penetrance is 50% by the age of 30 and 90% by the age of 60. Typically, p53 mutation in one allele is accompanied by loss of the other allele (LOH) in the tumors arising in family members. Thus, somatic cells lack normal p53 function, in the Li–Fraumeni patients who have inherited one defective copy of p53.[49]

p53 germ-line mutations have been observed in a large proportion of these families, with some reports finding them in up to 70%.[50] While Li–Fraumeni families are uncommon, the detection of p53 mutation represents a clinically useful diagnostic tool since p53 mutations matching the "codons" or the "hot spots" which are seen in these tumors can be sought by examining the DNA obtained from a peripheral blood sample in family members.

For sporadic breast cancer, there is conflicting data on the clinical relevance of polymorphisms in codon 72 of p53.[30] For example, an increased risk of developing breast cancer; in particular, the arg/arg phenotype[51] contrasts with an association between the pro/pro phenotype with poorer disease-free survival in patients who went on to receive adjuvant chemotherapy;[52] the value of the codon 72 p53 polymorphism has, at present, uncertain clinical utility.

p53 as a predictor for treatment strategy or disease response

Endocrine therapy, systemic chemotherapy and breast radiotherapy have been shown to significantly reduce disease relapse and prolong survival in patients with breast cancer. However, it has not been possible to confidently identify the patients in whom treatment is of benefit or those for whom such treatments ought to be avoided.

The function of a number of anticancer agents is directed towards inducing cell death or apoptosis. Loss of normal p53 function can potentially result in relative resistance of breast cancers to chemotherapeutic agents, due to loss of the apoptotic properties of p53. This has been of particular significance in the use of preoperative, neoadjuvant chemotherapy whereby poorer outcome has been observed in those tumors with higher p53 accumulation rates, as demonstrated by immunohistochemistry,[53] while patients with tumors containing wild-type p53 show a more dramatic positive response rate to the preoperative chemotherapy.[54] The importance of p53 in response to chemotherapy may depend both on the chemotherapy agent(s) themselves and on the tumor subtype, since mutant p53 containing inflammatory breast cancer[55] or the basal histological subtype[56] may be more responsive to chemotherapy.

Several studies have suggested that p53 status is an important determinant of tumor responsiveness to antineoplastic agents in breast cancer, including Cyclophosphamide, Methotrexate and 5-fluorouracil (CMF) chemotherapy[57] and anthracycline-based chemotherapy where specific mutations in p53 have been associated with poor response to primary systemic therapy,[58,59] response to neoadjuvant therapy,[60] and overall survival.[61] However, a differential effect of anthracyclines and taxanes on breast cancers based on the p53 status of the tumor underpins the EORTC 10094 trial testing the hypothesis that taxanes may have a greater efficacy against p53 mutant breast cancer than anthracyclines.[59,62]

Although there have been suggestions that p53 immunohistochemistry may be a poor prognostic factor for some forms of chemotherapy but of less apparent value for others, in general, most studies suggest p53 immunohistochemistry does not predict drug sensitivity in breast cancer.

For systemic endocrine therapy, the pro72 polymorphism appears to be associated with improved disease-free survival in patients with an ER-positive cancer given adjuvant tamoxifen.[63] Node-positive patients with primary breast cancer positive for p53 mutation have a poorer response rate to adjuvant tamoxifen treatment,[64] further supported by the reduced response to tamoxifen associated with p53 protein accumulation in cytosolic extracts.[65] p53 protein accumulation in breast cancer is also associated with time to endocrine failure,[66] poor response to endocrine therapy in the metastatic setting,[67] and reduced postrelapse survival.[67]

The relationship between radiotherapy and p53 in breast cancer also appears to be complex. There are series which have shown that tumors with wild-type p53 have a better response to radiotherapy, than for chemotherapy,[54] but others suggest that tumors harboring p53 mutations should be more susceptible to postoperative radiotherapy than those with normal p53.[68] One explanation of this could be that having been exposed to radiation damage, cells with mutant p53 cannot activate p53-dependent repair mechanisms.[69] However, more recent microarray expression studies suggest that p53 mutation does influence gene expression patterns following radiotherapy.[70]

The value of p53 as an independent marker for treatment response and prognosis has also been related to the clinical stage at the time of presentation. p53 nuclear accumulation in early breast cancer (stage I), may be of significant prognostic value,[71,72] whereas in locally advanced breast cancer (stage IIIA/IIIB), p53 may not have the same independent prognostic significance.[73]

p53 mutation alone may not be sufficient to predict response to systemic therapy in clinical settings, since both in vitro and in vivo studies[74] have suggested that p53 function may be dissociated from drug resistance and other cellular factors are likely to play an important role. Whether p53 is a significant independent predictor for response to treatment remains unclear and is the subject of clinical trials; currently, there are insufficient data to support the routine assessment of p53 status as a marker of response to treatment in breast cancer. p53 has been shown to affect apoptosis by regulating the expression of Bcl-2 and Bax, which inhibit and promote apoptosis, respectively.[16,75] The reduced Bcl-2 and increased Bax expression, and hence increased cell death observed in a p53-dependent manner following treatment with systemic chemotherapy, suggest that analysis of the Bcl-2:Bax ratio as well as p53 status offers more practical information on tumor response following systemic chemotherapy.

p53 as a prognostic factor

Alteration of the p53 gene in breast cancer is associated with an unfavorable prognosis.[76–79] Accumulation of nuclear p53, or expression of mutant p53, is associated with a number of histological, biological and clinical adverse prognostic factors including developing metastasis and reduced disease-free survival.[80] Microarray approaches have identified a 32-gene expression signature which distinguishes mutant from wild-type p53 and outperforms sequence-based assessment of p53 in predicting prognosis,[62] underlining that not all mutations are equal.[81] p53 network changes may occur without mutation and the role of p53 in different therapeutic settings may vary. However, p53 overexpression may be a predictor of local recurrence in operable breast cancer.[82]

p53 aberrations vary between different histological types of breast cancers. They are more common in the invasive ductal carcinomas as opposed to lobular carcinomas, and less common in the well-differentiated types with more favorable prognosis.[77] Recent microarray techniques have identified the basal phenotype of breast cancer where p53 mutation features.[80] There are exceptions: poorly differentiated medullary carcinomas displaying p53 gene mutations ironically have a more favorable prognosis.[77] However, p53 abnormalities are generally associated with the higher grade cancers, aneuploid tumors and those with a high S-phase fraction (mitotic rate).[72] Therefore, the histology of a specific breast tumor should be considered as an adjunct to p53 status when using p53 as a prognostic marker.

p53 expression is considered to be a marker of more aggressive cancer[76,77] both for locally advanced and inflammatory cancers. There are reports of a higher tumor proliferation rate, early disease recurrence and early death in node-negative breast cancers,[72] and correlation with tumor size, axillary nodal involvement and low hormone-receptor content for patients with breast cancer containing p53 mutation.[77] p53 aberrations are associated with low levels of ER and PR, which are known to be markers of less aggressive tumors with better response rate to systemic hormonal therapies.[45,72,77]

The prognostic power of p53 may be best combined with other cellular and biological parameters. These include a p53-positive Bcl-2-negative phenotype independently associated with poor prognosis,[83] c-erb-2 (HER2/neu), Ki67 antigen, and tumor cell characteristics such as microvessel density and tumor cell proliferation rate.[71] Concurrent p53 and c-erb-2 protein overexpression are associated with poor overall survival and metastasis-free interval[74] in node-negative tumors, particularly those with missense mutations.[84,85]

With the appreciation of p53 as an independent biological marker for response to treatment and disease outcome, at least when p53 mutations have been detected,[77] detecting p53 antibodies or p53 mutations in patient serum has been proposed as a diagnostic tool since such techniques may identify breast cancer patients.[86]

STRATEGIES FOR MANIPULATION OF THE P53 PATHWAY IN THE TREATMENT OF BREAST CANCER

The insights provided by p53 laboratory research over three decades are now moving to clinical applications for enhanced diagnostic, prognostic, and therapeutic intervention. The detailed strategies for engaging and manipulating the p53 pathway have been comprehensively reviewed in the literature for a wide range of human cancers.[5,10,86] For breast cancer, where not only p53 mutation but also aberrations of the p53 pathway occur commonly, many of these strategies hold promise.

Strategies which target tumors with mutant p53

Gene therapy

The addition of the wild-type p53 gene back into tumors which have mutated p53 or which are null for p53 is possible by the use of gene therapy. Using virus-based vectors which are replication defective it has been possible to demonstrate a significant clinical effect of stabilizing tumor growth or causing tumor regression in a fraction of patients with no significant toxicity.[87] This form of gene therapy has been tested in clinical trials in a range of cancers based on the concept that the combined use of these vectors with chemotherapy or radiotherapy may have an enhanced clinical effect.[86] One recent phase II trial of intratumoral adenoviral vector containing wild-type p53 (AdCMV-p53) combined with chemotherapy[88] has shown enhanced p53 activity, local immunomodulatory effects and objective clinical response in locally advanced breast cancer.

Selective replication of oncolytic virus

A different approach uses a defective adenovirus, Onyx-O15, which can selectively divide in p53-null cells.[89] Onyx-O15 harbors a deletion in its E1B gene, the protein product of which binds to p53 and selectively replicates in and subsequently lyses cells that are p53 null, whilst leaving normal cells with wild-type p53 unaffected. This virus has been shown to work in vivo via xenograft models but the mechanism of action in relation to p53 has remained controversial. Though the potential of this selective replication and destruction approach is promising, the ability of the virus to reach metastatic sites remains problematic since the replicating virus may evoke an immune response and be destroyed by the immune system. This, combined with the variability in clinical trial data, means that much work remains to be done to elucidate the precise mechanism of action in different tissue contexts.[86]

Small molecule reactivators of mutant p53

One of the most attractive opportunities for exploiting p53 for therapeutic gain comes from the observation that tumor cells containing mutant p53 have a large amount of inactive p53 contained within them, which constitutes a "loaded gun" of tumor-suppressor function.[90] Coupled to the fact that only tumor cells have mutant p53, drugs which could reactivate mutant p53, should kill or arrest the growth of tumor cells but not affect normal cells. This has been demonstrated using monoclonal antibodies which specifically recognize a C-terminus epitope of p53 or short peptides derived from the C-terminus of p53. Following this rationale, screens have been carried out to identify small drug-like molecules which can reactivate mutant p53 causing it to function as wild-type p53 or to preferentially kill mutant p53 cell lines over wild-type p53 cell lines.[90]

Several structurally unrelated compounds have been discovered including ellipticine, CP-31398, WR1065, PRIMA-1 (and PRIMA-1MET), and MIRA.[87,90] Perhaps the most developed of these molecules is the PRIMA-1MET (for *p53 reactivation and induction of massive apoptosis, methylated analogue*), although the direct mechanism of action of this compound has not been elucidated. It is possible that PRIMA-1MET induces the expression of chaperone protein such as the HSPs, which could then bind to p53 and facilitate correct folding of p53. In fact, PRIMA-1 has been shown to induce the expression of HSP90 and enhance its binding to p53 supporting this mechanism. However, elucidating the mechanism of action of molecules which may help in the refolding of proteins is possibly more challenging than discovering the target, for example, of a kinase-domain inhibitor.[86]

Rescue of p53 function

In vivo studies have shown that posttranslational modification of the p53 C-terminus can act as a rate-limiting step for p53 activation, and thus interfere with the specific DNA-binding activity and hence the tumor-suppressor properties.[91] Ablation of the negative regulatory domain at the p53 C-terminus has been achieved by using synthetic short peptides derived from the p53 C-terminus, or antibodies

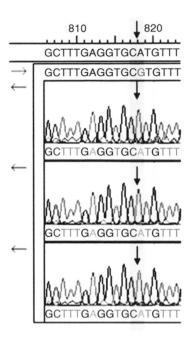

Figure 12.4 Sequencing the p53 gene DNA: in this instance there is mutation of guanosine to adenine at base 818 in the p53 gene (amino acid 273, a common mutation).

to the C-terminus which induce a p53-dependent response in some cell lines with mutant p53.[92] Alternatively, compounds which maintain and stabilize the DNA-binding domain in the active conformation have been shown to not only promote the stability of the wild-type p53 but also to allow the mutant p53 to retain an active conformation.[93]

Reactivation of wild-type p53

In the majority of breast cancers where the p53 gene is not mutated, the p53 protein is often kept at very low levels by excessive negative regulation, even under cellular stress. Since MDM-2 binds to and inhibits p53 directly, it has been possible to screen for small molecules which disrupt this binding, leading to reactivated p53. Molecules capable of doing just this have been identified and include the Nutlins,[94] potent p53-reactivating molecules, which have been shown to work in vivo by reducing tumor growth in mice xenograft

models, but confirmatory clinical data is awaited. Other molecules which reactivate wild-type p53 include RITA, shown to work in vivo via xenograft mice models, which may bind to the N-terminus of p53 causing a conformational change in the protein and preventing MDM-2 binding.[95] Screening chemical libraries for p53-reactivating compounds has identified other compounds, such as Sangivamycin, but their mechanism of action in relation to p53 reactivation has not been elucidated and their in vivo activity remains to be determined.[96]

p53 can also be reactivated by preventing the E3 ubiquitin ligase function of MDM-2, thus preventing p53 targeting for degradation. This strategy has identified a family of compounds called HLI98. The effect of these compounds on p53 transcriptional activity is weak, as they also lead to the stabilization of MDM-2.[97]

Other aspects of p53 regulation can also be targeted for therapeutic gain, such as preventing the nuclear–cytoplasmic shuttling of p53 by MDM-2 leading to an increase in active p53 in the nucleus. This has been shown by the use of the CRM-1 nuclear exportin inhibitor Leptomycin B, with potent in vivo antitumor activity and in early phase trials for the treatment of malignancies where local administration is possible.[10]

Although the theory of reactivating p53, mutant or wild type, for cancer treatment holds great promise there is a noticeable lack of clinical data, even in breast cancer, to support this as a viable therapeutic avenue at present. A further approach is to explore the differential responses of normal and tumor tissues. Conventional chemotherapy and radiotherapy may be limited by p53-dependent toxicity in normal tissues. Using a small molecule (pifithrin-α), which allows normal cell growth but inhibits p53-induced transcription following activation by doxorubicin, may protect against the side-effects of current therapies by acting as a p53 regulator.[98] The use of a drug such as this would require close scrutiny as it could also enhance side-effects of the chemotherapeutic agent.

Activation of p53 by Nutlins may also have a protective effect on cells with wild-type p53 when treated with mitotic-inhibiting

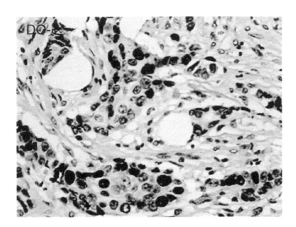 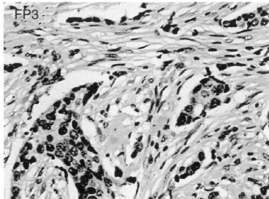

Figure 12.5 Immunohistochemical staining of a cancer for p53 using the antibodies DO-1 (binds to the N-terminal end of p53) and FP3 (binds to the phosphorylated serine 392 residue at the C-terminus). Nuclear p53 staining of most cells for p53 (DO-1) and many cells for activated, phosphorylated p53 (FP3) is demonstrated.

chemotherapeutics but does not protect cells with mutant p53. This has lead to speculation that pretreatment with p53 activators could protect normal cells from mitotic inhibitors leaving mutant p53 tumors increasingly susceptible to the chemotherapeutic agent, but conversely could protect wild-type p53 tumors from the therapy.[99] Thus, if used clinically, the p53 mutational status of the tumor would require confirmation prior to treatment.

Upstream targets

Since mutation in upstream signaling kinases have been seen to ablate the p53 response, the role of ATM and CHK2 kinases in signaling DNA damage to p53 also presents an attractive target. Activation of these kinases blocks p53 degradation by phosphorylating both p53 and MDM-2.

Simulating lost function of the p53-dependent target genes

p53 conveys its activity as a tumor-suppressor gene via downstream target genes, activities of which are lost if p53 is inactive or mutant. Replacing or simulating the function of these genes, for example p21, which mediates p53-dependent growth arrest, would provide the potential of restoring lost functions. Finding

molecules which can replace or mimic p21 function could potentially provide the basis for the design of novel anticancer drugs.[100] Altering the balance between Bax/Bcl-2, or selective and specific toxicity against cells which over express Bcl-2, is another therapeutic option and drugs such as antimycin A are being actively pursued to this end.[101]

Immunotherapy

The altered proteins coded by mutant p53 can potentially be used as targets for the immune system, which if recognized accurately could provide a nontoxic tumor specific treatment. Most of the in vivo work in this area has been carried out on mice and the potential of using this treatment in human cancers, in a way analogous to growth factor receptor therapies such as Lapatanib and Herceptin, has yet to be explored.[102] One promising phase II trial of vaccination with p53 peptide pulsed dendritic cells did result in associated with disease stabilization in 40% of patients with p53 expression in advanced breast cancer.[103]

CONCLUSIONS

The p53 gene is a complex protein at the center of a network of cellular pathways with multiple interactions involved in the response to cell-damaging agents including radiotherapy and chemotherapy. Through pleiotropic actions – including regulation of cell growth and division, gene transcription, DNA repair, and genomic stability – p53 behaves as a guardian of the genome. Aberrations of p53, including alterations in the upstream and downstream pathways (e.g. MDM-2, p21, and Bax), mutation, and modifications of protein expression and activation make p53 a key target for anticancer therapy. The precise clinical importance of p53 in human breast cancer as a diagnostic marker, predictor of disease response or poor prognostic factor remains controversial. However, therapeutic strategies to bolster the function of normal p53 or substitute for its function where p53 is mutant, are yielding in vitro and in vivo clinical advances. While much remains to be understood and developed into clinically useful strategies in the field of p53 in breast cancer, substantial progress in our understanding has been achieved and therapeutic benefits are awaited.

REFERENCES

1. Lane DP. Cancer. p53, guardian of the genome. Nature 1992; 358: 15–16.
2. Vousden KH, Lane DP. p53 in health and disease. Nat Rev Mol Cell Biol 2007; 8: 75–83.
3. Bourdon JC, Fernandes K, Murray-Zmijewski F et al. p53 isoforms can regulate p53 transcriptional activity. Genes Dev 2005; 19: 2122–37.
4. Bourdon JC. p53 and its isoforms in cancer. Br J Cancer 2007; 97: 277–82.
5. Hupp TR, Lane DP, Ball KL. Strategies for manipulating the p53 pathway in the treatment of human cancer. Biochem J 2000; 352: 1–17.
6. Vayssade M, Haddada H, Faridoni-Laurens L et al. P73 functionally replaces p53 in adriamycin-treated, p53 deficient breast cancer cells. Int J Cancer 2005; 116: 860–9.
7. Leong CO, Vidnovic N, DeYoung MP et al. The p64/p73 network mediates chemosensitivity to cisplatin in a biologically defined subset of primary breast cancers. J Clin Invest 2007; 117: 1370–80.
8. Shieh SY, Ikeda M, Taya Y et al. DNA damage-induced phosphorylation of p53 alleviates inhibition by mdm2. Cell 1997; 91: 325–34.
9. Meek DW. Post-translational modification of p53. Sem Cancer Biol 1994; 5: 203–10.
10. Lane DP, Lain S. Therapeutic exploitation of the p53 pathway. Trends in Molecular Medicine 2002; 8: No 4 (Suppl).
11. Vogelstein B, Lane D, Levine AJ. Surfing the p53 network. Nature 2000; 408: 307–10.
12. Balint E, Vousden KH. Activation and activities of the p53 tumour suppressor protein. Br J Cancer 2001; 85: 1813–23.
13. EL-Deiry WS, Tokino T, Velculescu VE et al. WAF1, a potential mediator of p53 tumour suppression. Cell 1993; 75: 817–25.
14. Martin S, Green D. Protease activation during apoptosis: death by a thousand cuts? Cell 1995; 82: 349–52.
15. Ko LJ, Prives C. p53: puzzle and paradigm. Genes Dev 1996; 10: 1054–72.
16. Miyashita T, Harigai M, Hanaka M et al. Identification of a p53-dependent negative response element in the bcl-2 gene. Cancer Res 1994; 54: 3131–5.
17. Bergamaschi D, Samuels Y, O'Neil NJ et al. IASPP oncoprotein is a key inhibitor of p53 conserved from worm to human. Nat Genet 2003; 33: 162–7.
18. Moll UM, Wolff S, Speidel D, Deppert W. Transcription-independent pro-apoptotic functions of p53. Curr Opin Cell Biol 2005; 17: 631–6.
19. Li FP, Fraumeni Jr JF. Soft-tissue sarcomas, breast cancer and other neoplasms. A familial syndrome? Ann Intern Med 1969; 71: 747–52.
20. Vousden KH, Lu X. Live or let die: the cell's response to p53. Nat Rev Cancer 2002; 2: 594–604.
21. Wang Y, Prives C. Increased and altered DNA binding of human p53 by S and G2/M but not G1 cyclin-dependent kinases. Nature 1995; 376: 88–91.
22. O'Neill M, Campbell SJ, Save V et al. An immuno-chemical analysis of mdm-2 expression in human breast cancer and the identification of a growth-regulated cross-reacting species p170. J Pathol 1998; 186: 254–61.
23. Lane DP, Hall PA. MDM2-arbiter of p53's destruction. Trends Biochem Sci 1997; 22: 372–4.
24. Jones SN, Roe AE, Donehower LA et al. Rescue of embryonic lethality in Mdm2-deficient mice by absence of p53. Nature 1995; 378: 206–8.
25. Gordon SA, Hoffman RA, Simmons RL et al. Induction of heat shock protein 70 protects thymocytes against radiation-induced apoptosis. Arch Surg 1997; 132: 1277–82.
26. Hupp TR, Sparks A, Lane DP. Small peptides activate the latent sequence specific DNA binding function of p53. Cell 1995; 83: 237–45.
27. Toledo F, Wahl GM. Regulating the p53 pathway: in vitro hypotheses in vivo veritas. Nat Rev Cancer 2006; 6: 909–23.
28. Jiang M, Shao ZM, Wu J et al. p21/waf1/cip1 and mdm-2 expression in breast carcinoma patients as related to prognosis. Int J Cancer 1997; 74: 529–34.
29. Harper JW, Adami GR, Wei N et al. The p21 Cdk-interacting protein Cip1 is a potent inhibitor of G1 cyclin-dependent kinases. Cell 1993; 75: 805–16.
30. Pietsch EC, Humbey O, Murphy ME. Polymorphisms in the p53 pathway. Oncogene 2006; 25: 1602–11.
31. Wilkening S, Bermejo JL, Hemminki K. MDM2 SNP309 and cancer risk: A combined analysis. Carcinogenesis 2007 Sep 7 (e-pub ahead of print; www.iarc.fr/p53).

32. Chen J, Lin J, Levine AJ. Regulation of transcription functions of the p53 tumour suppressor by the mdm-2 oncogene. Mol Med 1995; 1: 142–52.

33. Lundgren K, Montes de Oca Luna R, Mcneill YB et al. Targeted expression of MDM2 uncouples S phase from mitosis and inhibits mammary gland development independent of p53. Genes Dev 1997; 11: 714–25.

34. Picksley SM, Spicer JF, Barnes DM et al. The p53-MDM2 interaction in a cancer-prone family, and the identification of a novel therapeutic target. Acta Onc 1996; 35: 429–34.

35. Jackson MW, Berberich SJ. MdmX protects p53 from Mdm2-mediated degradation. Mol Cell Biol 2000; 20: 1001–7.

36. Harper JW. Cyclin dependent kinase inhibitors. Cancer Surv 1997; 29: 91–108.

37. Waga S, Hannon GJ, Beach D et al. The p21 inhibitor of cyclin-dependent kinases controls DNA replication by interaction with PCNA. Nature 1994; 369: 574–8.

38. Li R, Waga S, Hannon GJ et al. Differential effects by the p21 CDK inhibitor on PCNA-dependent DNA replication and repair. Nature 1994; 371: 534–7.

39. Donehower LA, Harvey M, Slagle BL et al. Mice deficient for p53 are developmentally normal but susceptible to spontaneous tumors. Nature 1992; 356: 215–21.

40. Jacks T, Remington L, Williams BO et al. Tumor spectrum analysis in p53-mutant mice. Curr Biol 1994; 4: 1–7.

41. Deng C, Zhang P, Harper JW et al. Mice lacking p21$^{CIP1/WAF1}$ undergo normal development, but are defective in G1 checkpoint control. Cell 1995; 82: 675–84.

42. Martins CP, Brown-Swigart L, Evan GI. Modeling the therapeutic efficacy of p53 restoration in tumors. Cell 2006 Dec 29; 127(7): 1323–34.

43. Ventura A, Kirsch DG, McLaughlin ME et al. Restoration of p53 function leads to tumour regression in vivo. Nature 2007; 445(7128): 661–5.

44. Duddy PM, Hanby AM, Barnes DM et al. Improving the detection of p53 mutations in breast cancer by use of the FASAY, a functional assay. J Mol Diagn 2000; 2: 139–44.

45. Thompson AM, Anderson TJ, Condie A et al. P53 allele losses, mutations and expression in breast cancer and their relationship to clinico-pathological parameters. Int J Cancer 1992; 50: 528–32.

46. Ansari B, Thompson AM. Genetic risk factors in breast cancer. Adv Breast Cancer 2006; June: 27–32.

47. Rohan TE, Li SQ, Hartwick R, Kandel RA. p53 alterations and protein accumulation in benign breast tissue and breast cancer risk: a cohort study. Cancer Epidemiol Biomarkers Prev 2006 Jul; 15(7): 1316–23.

48. O'Malley FP, Vnencak-Jones CL, Dunpont WD et al. p53 mutations are confined to the comedo type ductal carcinoma in situ of the breast: Immunohistochemical and sequencing data. Lab Invest 1994; 71: 67–72.

49. Malkin D. p53 and the Li-Fraumeni syndrome. Cancer Genet Cytogenet 1993; 66: 83–92.

50. Varley JM, McGown G, Thorncroft M et al. Germline mutations of TP53 Li-Fraumeni families: an extended study of 39 families. Cancer Res 1997; 57: 3245–52.

51. Damin AP, Frazzon AP, Damin DC et al. Evidence for an association of TP53 codon 72 polymorphism with breast cancer risk. Cancer Detect Prev 2006; 30: 523–9.

52. Toyama T, Zhang Z, Nishio M et al. Association of TP53 codon 72 polymorphism and the outcome of adjuvant therapy in breast cancer patients. Breast Cancer Res 2007; 9(3): R34.

53. Clahsen PC, van de Velde CJ, Duval C et al. p53 protein accumulation and response to adjuvant chemotherapy in pre-menopausal women with node-negative early breast cancer. J Clin Oncol 1998; 16: 470–9.

54. Fromenti SC, Dunnington G, Uzieli B et al. Original p53 status predicts for pathological response in locally advanced breast cancer patients treated preoperatively with continuous infusion 5-fluorouracil and radiation therapy. Int J Radiat Oncol Biol Phys 1997; 39: 1059–68.

55. Bertheau P, Plassa F, Espié M et al. de Thé effect of mutated TP53 on response of advanced breast cancers to high-dose chemotherapy. Lancet 2002; 360: 852–4.

56. Bertheau P, Turpin E, Rickman DS et al. de Thé HExquisite sensitivity of TP53 mutant and basal breast cancers to a dose-dense epirubicin-cyclophosphamide regimen. PLoS Med 2007 Mar; 4(3): e90.

57. Andersson J, Larsson L, Klaar S et al. Worse survival for TP53 (p53)-mutated breast cancer patients receiving adjuvant CMF. Ann Oncol 2005; 16: 743–8.

58. Aas T, Borresen AL, Geisler S et al. Specific p53 gene mutations are associated with de novo resistance to doxorubicin in breast cancer patients. Nat Med 1996; 2: 811–14.

59. Kandioler-Eckersberger D, Ludwig C, Rudas M et al. TP53 mutation and p53 overexpression for prediction of response to neoadjuvant treatment in breast cancer patients. Clin Cancer Res 2000; 6: 50–6.

60. Geisler S, Børresen-Dale AL, Johnsen H et al. TP53 gene mutations predict the response to neoadjuvant treatment with 5-fluorouracil and mitomycin in locally advanced breast cancer. Clin Cancer Res 2003; 9: 5582–8.

61. Borresen AL, Andersen TI et al. TP53 mutations and breast cancer prognosis: particularly poor survival rates for cases with mutations in the zinc-binding domains. Genes Chromosome Cancer 1995; 14: 71–5.

62. Miller LD, Smeds J, George J et al. An expression signature for p53 status in human breast cancer predicts mutation status, transcriptional effects, and patient survival. Proc Natl Acad Sci USA 2005; 102: 13,550–5.

63. Wegman P, Stal O, Askmalm MS et al. p53 polymorphic variants at codon 72 and the outcome of therapy in randomized breast cancer patients. Pharmacogenet Genomics 2006; 16: 347–51.

64. Bergh J, Norberg T, Sjogren S et al. Complete sequencing of the p53 gene provides prognostic

information in breast cancer patients, particularly in relation in adjuvant systemic therapy and radiotherapy. Nat Med 1995; 1: 1029–34.

65. Berns EM, Klijn JG, van Putten WL et al. p53 protein accumulation predicts poor response to tamoxifen therapy of patients with recurrent breast cancer. J Clin Oncol 1998; 16: 121–7.

66. Kai K, Nishimura R, Arima N et al. p53 expression status is a significant molecular marker in predicting the time to endocrine therapy failure in recurrent breast cancer: a cohort study. Int J Clin Oncol 2006; 11: 426–33.

67. Yamashita H, Toyama T, Nishio M et al. p53 protein accumulation predicts resistance to endocrine therapy and decreased post-relapse survival in metastatic breast cancer. Breast Cancer Res 2006; 8(4): R48.

68. Jansson T, Inganas M, Sjogren S et al. p53 status predicts survival in breast cancer patients treated with or without postoperative radiotherapy: a novel hypothesis based on clinical findings. J Clin Oncol 1995; 13: 2745–51.

69. Silvestrini R, Veneroni S, Benini E et al. Expression of p53, glutathione S-transferase-π, and bcl-2 proteins and benefit from adjuvant radiotherapy in breast cancer. J Natl Cancer Inst 1997; 89: 639–45.

70. Helland S, Johnsen H, Frøyland C et al. Radiation-induced effects on gene expression: an in vivo study on breast cancer. Radiother Oncol 2006; 80: 230–5.

71. Isola J, Visakorpi T, Holli K et al. Association of overexpression of tumour suppressor protein p53 with rapid cell proliferation and poor prognosis in node-negative breast cancer patients. J Natl Cancer Inst 1992; 84: 1109–14.

72. Allred DC, Clark GM, Elledge R et al. Association of p53 protein expression with tumour cell proliferation rate and clinical outcome in node-negative breast cancer. J Natl Cancer Inst 1993; 85: 200–6.

73. Honkoop AH, van Diest PJ, de Jong JS et al. Prognostic role of clinical, pathological and biological characteristics in patients with locally advanced breast cancer. Br J Cancer 1998; 77: 621–6.

74. MacGrogan G, Mauriac L, Durand M et al. Primary chemotherapy in breast invasive carcinoma: predictive value of the immunohistochemical detection of hormonal receptors, p53, c-erB-2, MiB1, pS2 and GST pi. Br J Cancer 1996; 74: 1458–65.

75. Miyashita T and Reed JC. Tumor suppressor p53 is a direct transcriptional activator of the human bax gene. Cell 1995; 80: 293–9.

76. Elledge RM, Fuqua SA, Clark GM et al. The role and prognostic significance of p53 gene alterations in breast cancer. Breast Cancer Res Treat 1993; 27: 95–102.

77. Olivier M, Langerød A, Carrieri P et al. The clinical value of somatic TP53 gene mutations in 1794 patients with breast cancer. Clin Cancer Res 2006; 12: 1157–67.

78. Kyndi M, Alsner J, Hansen LL et al. LOH rather than genotypes of TP53 codon 72 is associated with disease-free survival in primary breast cancer. Acta Oncol 2006; 45: 602–9.

79. Langerød A, Zhao H, Borgan Ø et al. TP53 mutation status and gene expression profiles are powerful prognostic markers of breast cancer. Breast Cancer Res 2007; 9(3): R30.

80. Overgaard J, Yilmaz M, Guldberg P et al. TP53 mutation is an independent prognostic marker for poor outcome in both node-negative and node-positive breast cancer. Acta Oncol 2000; 39: 327–33.

81. Kato S, Han SY, Liu W et al. Understanding the function-structure and function-mutation relationships of p53 tumor suppressor protein by high-resolution missense mutation analysis. Proc Natl Acad Sci USA 2003; 100: 8424–9.

82. de Roos MA, de Bock GH, de Vries J et al. p53 overexpression is a predictor of local recurrence after treatment for both in situ and invasive ductal carcinoma of the breast. J Surg Res 2007; 140: 109–14.

83. Rolland P, Spendlove I, Madjd Z et al. The p53 positive Bcl-2 negative phenotype is an independent marker of prognosis in breast cancer. Int J Cancer 2007; 120: 1311–17.

84. Ozcelik H, Pinnaduwage D, Bull SB et al. Type of TP53 mutation and ERBB2 amplification affects survival in node-negative breast cancer. Breast Cancer Res Treat 2007, 2006 Jul; 15(7): 1316–23.

85. Balogh GA, Mailo DA, Corte MM et al. Mutant p53 protein in serum could be used as a molecular marker in human breast cancer. Int J Oncol 2006; 28: 995–1002.

86. Wiman KG. Strategies for therapeutic targeting of the p53 pathway in cancer. Cell Death Differ 2006; 13: 921–6.

87. Bykov VJ, Wiman KG. Novel cancer therapy by reactivation of the p53 apoptosis pathway. Ann Med 2003; 35: 458–65.

88. Cristofanilli M, Krishnamurthy S, Guerra L et al. A nonreplicating adenoviral vector that contains the wild-type p53 transgene combined with chemotherapy for primary breast cancer: safety, efficacy, and biologic activity of a novel gene-therapy approach. Cancer 2006; 107: 935–44.

89. Heise C, Sampson-Johannes A, Williams A et al. ONYX-015, an E1B gene-attenuated adenovirus, causes tumor-specific cytolysis and antitumoral efficacy that can be augmented by standard chemotherapeutic agents. Nat Med 1997; 3: 639–45.

90. Selivanova G, Wiman KG. Reactivation of mutant p53: molecular mechanisms and therapeutic potential. Oncogene 2007; 26: 2243–54.

91. Hupp TR. Regulation of p53 protein function through alterations in protein-folding pathways. Cell Mol Life Sci 1999; 55: 88–95.

92. Selivanova G, Kawasaki T, Ryabchenko L et al. Reactivation of mutant p53: a new strategy for cancer therapy. Seminar Cancer Biol 1998; 8: 369–78.

93. Foster BA, Coffey HA, Morin MJ et al. Pharmacological rescue of mutant p53 conformation and function. Science 1999; 286: 2507–10.

94. Vassilev LT, Vu BT, Graves B et al. In vivo activation of the p53 pathway by small-molecule antagonists of MDM2. Science 2004; 303: 844–8.

95. Issaeva N, Bozko P, Enge M et al. Small molecule RITA binds to p53, blocks p53-HDM-2 interaction and activates p53 function in tumors. Nat Med 2004; 10: 1321–8.

96. Berkson RG, Hollick JJ, Westwood NJ et al. Pilot screening programme for small molecule activators of p53. Int J Cancer 2005; 115: 701–10.

97. Yang Y, Ludwig RL, Jensen JP et al. Small molecule inhibitors of HDM2 ubiquitin ligase activity stabilize and activate p53 in cells. Cancer Cell 2005; 7: 547–59.

98. Komarov PG, Komarova EA, Kondratov RV et al. A chemical inhibitor of p53 that protects mice from the side effects of cancer therapy. Science 1999; 285: 1733–7.

99. Carvajal D, Tovar C, Yang H et al. Activation of p53 by MDM2 antagonists can protect proliferating cells from mitotic inhibitors. Cancer Res 2005; 65: 1918–24.

100. Ball KL, Lain S, Fahraeus R et al. Cell-cycle arrest and inhibition of Cdk4 activity by small peptides based on the carboxy-terminal domain of p21WAF1. Curr Biol 1997; 7: 71–80.

101. Tzung SP, Kim KM, Basanez G et al. Antimycin A mimics a cell-death-inducing Bcl-2 homology domain 3. Nat Cell Biol 2001; 3: 183–91.

102. Gabrilovich DI, Cunningham HT, Carbone DP. IL-12 and mutant P53 peptide-pulsed dendritic cells for the specific immunotherapy of cancer. J Immunother Emphasis Tumor Immunol 1996; 19: 414–8.

103. Svane IM, Pedersen AE, Johansen JS et al. Vaccination with p53 peptide-pulsed dendritic cells is associated with disease stabilization in patients with p53 expressing advanced breast cancer; monitoring of serum YKL-40 and IL-6 as response biomarkers. Cancer Immunol Immunother 2007; 56: 1585–99.

Assessment of human epidermal growth factor receptor 2 in breast cancer

13

EA Rakha, RS Rampaul, JMS Bartlett and IO Ellis

INTRODUCTION

The human epidermal growth factor receptor 2 (HER2) gene, localized to chromosome 17q21, encodes a 185 kDa transmembrane tyrosine kinase receptor and is overexpressed in about 20–25% of invasive carcinomas of the breast[1–3] as a result of gene amplification.[4] HER2 is important for cell differentiation and adhesion, induces cell division and stimulates factors facilitating cell motility and tumor metastasis.[5] The clinical consequences of HER2 overexpression or gene amplification, henceforth referred to as "HER2 positivity", are widely documented.[6–9] HER2 positivity is associated with worse prognosis (higher rate of recurrence and mortality) in patients with newly diagnosed breast cancer who do not receive any adjuvant systemic therapy. Therefore, some countries incorporate HER2 status into clinical decision-making along with other prognostic factors when considering whether to give adjuvant systemic therapy. There is also preliminary evidence of the predictive value of HER2 status in relation to systemic chemotherapies.[6,9,10] Most critically, several studies have now shown that agents which target HER2, especially Herceptin and Lapatinib, are remarkably effective in the metastatic and adjuvant settings.[11–14]

HER2 remains an important target in the development of a variety of new cancer therapies, which include monoclonal antibody (mAb)-based therapy, small-molecule drugs directed at the internal tyrosine kinase portion of the HER2 oncoprotein, and vaccines. The most widely known HER2-directed therapy is trastuzumab (Herceptin; Genentech, South San Francisco, CA, USA). Trastuzumab is a humanized recombinant mAb that specifically targets the HER2 extracellular domain. Recently, the US Food and Drug Administration (FDA) also approved Lapatinib (Tykerb; GSK, Philadelphia, PA, USA) for clinical use.[15]

There are a variety of techniques available to determine HER2 status in breast cancer, some of which are employed for research purposes only.[9,10,16] In diagnostic pathology laboratories, HER2 status is routinely assessed either by immunohistochemistry (IHC), which assesses expression of the HER2 oncoprotein, and in situ hybridization (FISH), which measures the number of HER2 gene copies or gene amplification.[17,18] Modifications of ISH using colorimetric detection are increasingly being developed including chromogenic in situ hybridization (CISH) or silver enhanced in situ hybridization (SISH).[19–24]

This chapter reviews the various methods used to detect HER2 expression as well as HER2 gene status as a prognostic and predictive factor, paying particular attention to criteria for robust and accurate HER2 diagnostics. Future prospects for novel HER2 biodirected therapies are also briefly considered.

METHODS FOR HER2 TESTING

Diagnostic tests must be robust, reproducible, accurate and reliable, as well as being applicable to routinely fixed tissue samples. For this reason, many techniques which are either not applicable to fixed tissues (e.g. Southern, Northern and Western blotting[3,17,25–28]) or which disrupt tissue architecture (e.g. polymerase chain reaction (PCR) based methods[29]) are not at present regarded as appropriate for clinical diagnosis of HER2 status.[9]

Current guidelines for HER2 testing[1,30] specify the use of in situ methods of detecting either the HER2 protein (by IHC) or gene amplification (using FISH or other in situ methods). Guidelines stress the need for stringent, reproducible and consistent criteria for testing [reviewed in refs.[1,9,30] However, Wolff et al[1] also recommend that attention is given to accuracy: "A precise definition of accuracy is how close the measured values are to a supposed true value." We have therefore reviewed data on test accuracy below and included this in the discussion of the relative merits of current diagnostic methods.

Immunohistochemistry for HER2 testing

Among the methods in use for determining HER2 status, IHC has become predominant. However, several factors can adversely affect IHC process, especially when performed on formalin-fixed paraffin-embedded tissues. Previous studies have demonstrated a significant loss of tumor marker-immunostaining intensity on stored paraffin slides of breast cancer[31] and that different fixatives impact on HER2 immunostaining.[32] In studies employing various commercially available antibodies, a wide variety of sensitivity and specificity in fixed paraffin-embedded tissues is seen.[33,34] Antigen retrieval techniques are also nonstandardized and so introduce the potential for false-positive staining. Nonetheless, IHC does possess many advantages to support widespread adoption: (1) it allows for the preservation of tissue architecture and so can be used to identify local areas of overexpression within a heterogeneous sample, and can distinguish between in situ and invasive cancer; and (2) it is applicable to routine patient samples facilitating use as a diagnostic test, and in performing prospective and retrospective research studies

of HER2 status including the high-throughput tissue microarray (TMA) technology.

However, many studies have highlighted the potential for error and inconsistency in HER2 IHC when nonstandardized methods and multiple antibodies are used. Following the introduction of trastuzumab, the Task Force for Basic Research of the EORTC–GCGC[35] began the drive towards a consensus on immunohistochemical staining interpretation. Two FDA-approved IHC tests for determining HER2 status are available: HercepTest (DAKO, Carpeteria, CA, USA), based upon a polyclonal antibody; and CB11 (Pathway, Ventana Medical Systems, Tucson, AZ, USA), based upon a monoclonal antibody. The National Comprehensive Cancer Network guidelines[18] classified an IHC score of 0 or 1+ as representing HER2-negative status, 3+ as positive, while 2+ is equivocal. Positive staining was defined as strong, continuous membranous expression of HER2 in at least 10% of tumor cells. However, a joint report from the American Society of Clinical Oncology (ASCO) and the College of American Pathologists (CAP),[1] specified a threshold of >30% strong circumferential membrane staining for a positive result. If both uniformity and a homogeneous, dark circumferential pattern are seen (Figure 13.1), the resultant cases are likely to be amplified by FISH as well as positive for HER2 protein expression. The equivocal range for IHC (score 2+), which may include up to 15% of samples,[36] is defined as complete membrane staining that is either nonuniform or weak in intensity, but with obvious circumferential distribution in at least 10% of cells. Equivocal or inconclusive results should be tested by FISH. Consistent with previous guidelines, a negative HER2 test is defined as either an IHC result of 0 or 1+ for cellular membrane protein expression (no staining or weak, incomplete membrane staining in any proportion of tumor cells).

In situ hybridization for HER2 testing

FISH and CISH directly measure the number of HER2 genes, and when there is a chromosome

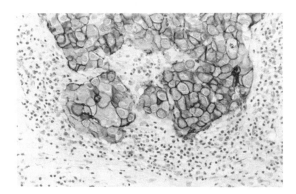

Figure 13.1 Overexpression of the HER2 protein by immunohistochemistry.

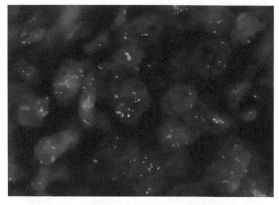

Figure 13.2 Amplification of the HER2 gene detected by fluorescence in situ hybridization (FISH) using a Vysis Kit with an inbuilt control (chromosome 17 probe).

centromeric enumeration probe (CEP) included also the copy number of chromosome 17.[17,33,37] Gene amplification is defined as an increase in HER2:CEP17 ratio >2.0. Some laboratories have used copy number cut-offs as a surrogate for amplification but this may lead to diagnostic inaccuracy. ISH results are semiquantitative, counting the number of signals in nonoverlapping interphase nuclei of the lesion using either single-colour (HER2 probe only, e.g. Ventana Inform) or dual-colour hybridization (using HER2 and chromosome 17 centromere probes simultaneously (e.g. Abbott, Chicago, USA, DAKO, Copenhagen, Denmark etc), the latter making it easier to distinguish true HER2 amplification from chromosomal aneuploidy. ISH allows simultaneous morphologic assessment, where evaluation of gene amplification can be restricted to invasive carcinoma cells. Many studies have compared FISH and IHC in the evaluation of HER2[36,38–40] demonstrating variable concordance between the two techniques of up to 91%. Two studies have shown that FISH more accurately predicts HER2 positivity[41,42] than IHC when applied to molecularly characterized breast cancers. Further studies suggest that FISH results in fewer equivocal results[42] and is markedly more reproducible than IHC.[41,43,44] These results suggest that FISH may be a more appropriate first-line test than IHC in line with standards defined by the ASCO/CAP guidelines.[1]

Three FISH tests are FDA-approved for selecting patients for treatment with trastuzumab. The Path Vysion (Vysis Inc, Downers Grove, IL, USA) and PharmDx (Dako) tests require a ratio of HER2:CEP17 ≥2.0 for the sample to be considered amplified, and both include an HER2 gene probe and a chromosome 17 probe (Figure 13.2). The INFORM test (Ventana Medical Systems) requires that at least 5.0 gene copies of HER2 be present if a sample is to be considered amplified as this kit uses a single HER2 gene probe without a chromosome 17 probe.

A small number of cases are diagnosed with an average HER2 gene: CEP17 ratio of between 1.8 and 2.2[45] due to the variation in scores between observers;[9] some recommendations have suggested these cases be regarded as "borderline". However, for the vast majority of these cases scoring additional cells will result in a clear diagnosis.

Accuracy and reproducibility of diagnostic assays

Despite considerable efforts devoted to standardizing methods to determine HER2 status by IHC or FISH, there are still several conditions which can result in false-positive or false-negative results for these techniques: antigen loss may occur in up to 20% of HER2-positive samples.

Several other conditions can contribute to false-positive or false-negative IHC results, including tissue processing, reagent variability, antigen retrieval methods, scoring interpretation, tumor heterogeneity, and the semiquantitative nature of the test.[18,21,44,46]

In addition, discrepancies in HER2 status can be laboratory dependent. For example, Perez et al[44] reported that when HER2 status determined by IHC and FISH were compared between local pathology laboratories and central laboratories, a high degree of discordance was found to exist in HER2 between them. They also confirmed that FISH results were significantly more consistent between local and central laboratories (see ref[70]). Also, in cases of discordance between local and central laboratories, there was a high degree of agreement between the central laboratory and reference laboratories. Reddy et al[46] concluded that use of high-volume HER2 testing reference laboratories will improve the process of selecting patients who are likely to benefit from trastuzumab by accurate determination of HER2 status.

RECOMMENDED GUIDELINES FOR HER2 ASSESSMENT

Recently, guidelines for HER2 assessment have been published,[1,18,30] which recommended the following.

1. There should be standardized fixation: Breast specimens, after appropriate gross inspection and designation of margins, should be promptly sliced at 5–10 mm intervals and fixed in 10% neutral buffered formalin. Fixation should be for at least 6 hours (needle core biopsies) to no more than 48 hours. Fixation masks protein antigen expression and changes the requirements for enzymatic digestion. Prolonged fixation may result in false-negative IHC results.
2. Prolonged storage of glass slides with cut sections of tissue should be avoided.
3. For both IHC- and FISH-based HER2 testing, comprehensive standardization of

methodology and the inclusion of validated controls are mandatory.
4. Excessive antigen retrieval can be monitored by an evaluation of normal breast epithelial cells as an internal control. The inclusion of a recommended positive control, or controls, producing results close to important decision-making points and a negative control are recommended.

A two-phase testing algorithm based on IHC assay as the primary screen with reflex to FISH reserved for equivocal cases is currently recommended. This is based on evidence showing very good concordance between IHC and FISH results on breast carcinomas from 37 laboratories when tested in experienced reference centers.[40]

For the assessment of both IHC and FISH preparations, training and experience in the interpretation of histological characteristics of breast tissue are essential. The recognition of different histological tumor types is required. HER2 status should be determined only on the invasive portion of the tumor.

Participation in external quality assessment schemes are essential, as there is evidence to show increased reproducibility of results by laboratories over time when participating in external quality assessment for HER2. The United Kingdom National External Quality Assessment Scheme (UK-NEQAS) schemes are open to laboratories across Europe.

Guidelines for HER2 testing

Although published data support the use of FISH for the selection of patients most likely to respond to trastuzumab,[20,45,47] the current UK licence for this agent allows the treatment of patients with tumors strongly staining by IHC. Worldwide, there remains an ongoing debate as to whether laboratories should switch to the use of FISH for all specimens, removing the need for a second tier of testing to identify HER2-positive cases, or adopt the two-tier testing strategy currently in use in the UK. Increasingly, FISH testing is seen as the optimal method for determining HER2 status in breast cancer.

IHC recommendations

1. Antigen retrieval must be standardized and follow strict protocols. The antibody used and its titre should be predefined. Standardization can be assisted using commercial assays. For inhouse assays no single antibody has consistently been shown to offer superior specificity and sensitivity. However, choice of antibody can affect decision-making. Fornier et al[48] reported that 95% of patients evaluated using mAb CB11 were found to be 2+/3+, but only 84% of patients evaluated using the polyclonal Herceptest antibody were 2+/3+. Such variation in results has important implications for patients. Test conditions (temperature, exposure time, etc.) should be standardized.

2. It is recommended that the sensitivity of the IHC method should be set below that which detects normal amounts of HER2 protein in benign or normal breast epithelial cells. Observers should be aware of the range of common artefacts, including edge artefacts, which can be problematic in small biopsy samples, and the effects of variation in method sensitivity, such as excessive antigen retrieval, leading to background staining and normal cell membrane reactivity.

3. Membrane staining must only be scored positive if circumferential regardless of the percentage of positive cells.

4. Only invasive tumor should be considered when scoring HER2 tests.

5. The scoring method recommended is a semiquantitative system based on the intensity of the reaction product and the percentage of membrane-positive cells, giving a score range of 0–3+.

FISH recommendations

1. To appropriately diagnose HER2 gene amplification inclusion of a chromosome 17 control probe is essential, either in a single assay or in a two-step progress. Over 50% of breast cancers have chromosome 17 aneusomy and this can markedly affect the HER2 result.[49]

2. Adequate quality assurance, both internal and external, by participation in national external quality assurance schemes; this is regarded as mandatory by both local UK and international guidelines.

3. For FISH, there is no evidence that prolonged storage of blocks leads to deterioration of signal; however, cut sections should be processed within 12 months. Methods should be standardized to maintain nuclear morphology and should follow strict protocols. Areas of invasive tumor should be located for scoring as ductal carcinoma in situ (DCIS) will often be amplified even when adjacent invasive tumor cells are negative.

4. Scoring by FISH should including analysis of 20–60 cells from at least three invasive tumor areas; areas of in situ carcinoma should not be counted. HER2 FISH results are conventionally expressed as the ratio of HER2 signal to chromosome 17 signal or the HER2 gene copy number. In most cases, where either clear amplification is observed or the ratio is <1.5, scoring of 20 cells is sufficient. In cases where either tumor heterogeneity is seen (1–2% of cases) or the ratio is close to 2.0 more cells should be scored (up to 60). If genomic heterogeneity of HER2 gene amplification is found, it must be specifically reported;[50] however, no current consensus recommendations exist for handling of genomic heterogeneity.

QUALITY ASSURANCE

All clinical laboratories using assays for HER2 as predictive or prognostic tests must participate in an appropriate external quality assurance (EQA) program, such as that run by the UK NEQAS for IHC (UK NEQAS-ICC). In the USA, the CAP Laboratory Accreditation Program now requires that every CAP-accredited laboratory performing HER2 testing participates in a guideline-concordant proficiency testing program for that testing. In the future, it is expected that all accrediting agencies will require guideline-concordant proficiency testing and laboratory accreditation requirements for HER2 testing.

OTHER APPROACHES IN HER2 TESTING

Tissue microarray technology enables a large number of cancers to be analyzed under identical conditions in a highly economical and efficient manner. Using this technology in assessing HER2 status in primary breast cancers[51,52] there was a highly significant correlation of HER2 scores between whole sections and corresponding tissue microarrays (94% ($p < 0.0001$)).[51,53]

The use of automated image analysis systems, which removes bias in colour grading, has been suggested as a means to improve the reporting of IHC-stained HER2[54–56] and FISH tests.[57,58] Other studies have applied high-throughput semiautomated assessment of HER2 status by assessing the feasibility of profiling HER2 by combining tissue microarray technology and the image analysis.[39]

Chromogenic in situ hybridization

CISH and SISH are colorimetric methods to detect gene amplification which can be viewed using a standard light microscope. Most studies report concordance between FISH and CISH of 83–100%.[21,22] In a recent study of comparison between FISH and SISH for the validation of HER2 gene status,[23] the overall concordance between the two techniques was 96.0% (kappa=0.754, 95% confidence interval (CI). Most of the discrepancies were seen in tumors with intratumoral heterogeneity of HER2 amplification. There was a low interobserver variability in the interpretation of SISH, suggesting that SISH is equally reliable in determining HER2 amplification as FISH. Our results were also consistent with the only previous study that compared the two techniques,[24] and showed a high rate of concordance between SISH and FISH. Therefore, we can conclude that HER2 gene copy status can be reliably determined by SISH. Although SISH combines bright-field microscopy with molecular analysis and full automation, has

showed a high rate of concordance with FISH, and appears to be particularly suited for routine application in surgical pathology, it is still of research interest and has yet to be approved for diagnostic use.

PRIMARY AND METASTATIC BREAST CANCER

Currently, treatment of metastatic breast cancer patients with HER2-positive tumors is based on HER2 status derived from the primary tumor, which was generally removed many years previously and stored as paraffin-embedded blocks. In a report by Zidan et al,[59] it was pointed out that HER2 status of the primary tumor may not accurately reflect the HER2 status of the metastatic tumour, and that this should be taken into account when making treatment decisions. Those investigators demonstrated 14% discordance between primary and metastatic tumors by IHC. Edgerton et al,[60] employing IHC and FISH, reported 20% discordance between the primary and metastatic tumor, which was due to normal HER2 expression in the primary tumor and HER2 overexpression in the metastatic tumor. Gancberg et al[61] compared HER2 status of the primary breast tumor with that of at least one distant metastatic tumor in 107 patients using both IHC and FISH. There was a 6% (6/100) rate of discordance with IHC between the primary and metastatic tumor. In the six cases of discordance, there was greater HER2 staining in the metastatic tumor tissue than in the primary tumor tissue. By FISH analysis, 7% (5/68) of the cases were discordant. Although evidence is limited at present, and more research is needed, we have suggested that, where available, metastatic deposits of breast cancer should be tested for HER2 status in addition to the primary site.

ASSESSMENT OF HER2 IN BREAST CORE NEEDLE BIOPSIES

Several reports have shown that the assessment of HER2 status on needle core biopsies (NCBs) in breast cancer is accurate and reliable.[62-65] A study of 325 primary breast cancer patients investigated the accuracy of HER2 status using IHC and FISH on NCBs, and compared the result with surgical specimens.[66] They found that the accuracy of IHC assessment of HER2 in NCBs was 92% and increased to 96% with additional FISH analysis, which was applied to all strongly positive cases. Therefore, they recommended performing FISH analysis for cases with strong IHC positivity on NCBs in order to minimize the number of false-positive results. Although NCBs have the advantage of good fixation, there can be crushing that makes it difficult to interpret the pattern of staining, and there may be staining at the edge of the cores (edge artefact). In addition, more care should be taken to differentiate between DCIS staining and invasive tumor staining for HER2 in NCBs, and a comparison with hemotoxylin and eosin (H&E) may be helpful in this regard. There is no data available to indicate whether repeating staining on resected specimens in cases where HER2 is 1+ or 2+ on NCBs is of value, but this may be appropriate until evidence-based data are available.

CLINICAL VALUE OF HER2 TESTING

Prognostic significance and association with other prognostic factors

The seminal work by Slamon et al[3] in 1987 showed that HER2 gene amplification independently predicted overall survival (OS) and disease-free survival (DFS) in a multivariate analysis in node-positive patients.[3] Since then most large studies have confirmed this relationship in multivariate analysis.[7,52] Thus, it is now well established that there is a significant correlation between HER2 overexpression/amplification and poor prognosis for patients with nodal metastasis. There is, at present, no consensus on the prognostic value of HER2 in node-negative breast cancer patients; a group most often diagnosed through screening programs and representing a subgroup which could potentially benefit highly from appropriate adjuvant therapy. Rilke et al[67] reported on the prognostic significance of HER2

expression and its relationship with other prognostic factors. Using specimens from 1210 consecutive patients treated between 1968 and 1971 at a single institution (National Cancer Institute of Milan), with no systemic adjuvant therapy and 20-year follow-up, they found overexpression of HER2 in 23% of cases and showed a negative impact on survival of node-positive but not node-negative patients. Some studies have also reported lack of prognostic significance in node-negative group;[68-70] however, others have found a prognostic value for HER2 in node-negative patients in selected subgroups.[71-73] This plethora of conflicting results may be explained by low numbers of patients evaluated in some studies and the diversity of methods used.

There is, at present, no agreement on the association between HER2 and other prognostic factors. Several studies suggest a lack of association between HER2 status and increasing tumor size,[3,74] yet some do find a correlation.[70,75] Most studies have failed to find an association between patient age at diagnosis and HER2 status.[3,70,76] Similar inconsistencies have been reported for aneuploidy, grade, and proliferation index.[67,76,77]

Prediction of response to therapy

Selection of adjuvant treatment for patients with breast cancer based on HER2 status was initially addressed by Clark et al.[78] Since then there have been numerous studies but results have not been consistent, and interpretation of these data is complicated and open to discussion.[79]

Endocrine therapy

Transfection of normal breast cancer cells with the HER2 gene has been shown to result in acquisition of estrogen-independent growth which is insensitive to tamoxifen.[80,81] A number of clinical studies, using various endpoints, have reported an association between HER2 positivity and resistance to endocrine therapy.[82-84] Some reports have described specific resistance to tamoxifen in HER2-overexpressing tumors.[82,84] The recently reported 20-year update of the Naples GUN Trial[82] found that HER2 overexpression not only predicted resistance to tamoxifen, but that HER2-positive patients had a worse outcome on tamoxifen therapy compared to those who were untreated.

Several studies have also shown a reduction in response rates to endocrine therapy. Metastatic breast cancer which overexpressed HER2, measured by high plasma levels of the extracellular domain, demonstrated a substantial reduction in response rate to endocrine therapy.[85] Cheung et al[86] have examined marker levels [CA 15.3, CEA, ESR and serum HER2] in 15 patients receiving docetaxel-based regimes from two multicenter trials. Measurement of serum HER2 showed a correlation with tissue HER2 (Herceptest) in the primary tumor ($p < 0.003$); and, more importantly, among those patients with positive tissue staining, sequential changes in serum HER2 paralleled initial response.

Other studies have failed to find an association or even a trend between HER2 status and response to endocrine therapy.[87–89] Elledge et al[89] examined the response to tamoxifen in 205 tumors with estrogen receptor (ER)-positive disease. In HER2-positive compared to HER2-negative patients, they found no significant evidence for a poorer response, time to treatment failure, or survival. In another study, the relationship between HER2 overexpression and response to tamoxifen was examined in the adjuvant setting in 741 (650 ER-positive, 91 ER-negative/progesterone receptor (PR) positive) of the total 1572 patients in the CALGB 8541 Trial who had HER2 measured.[87] Tamoxifen significantly improved response, DFS and OS irrespective of HER2 status. However, it is important to appreciate that tamoxifen was not randomized within this trial and that all patients had received one of three regimens of doxorubicin, and response to this was related to HER2 status. Thus, this data on tamoxifen resistance has some limitations in interpretation.

Chemotherapy

Initial studies examining the role of HER2 in predicting response to chemotherapy looked at regimens containing cyclophosphamide, methotrexate and 5-fluorouracil (5-FU) (CMF). Results from these analyses demonstrated a reduced benefit from CMF therapy in HER2-positive as against HER2-negative patients;[83,90,91] however, other authors do not support this.[92] Thus, whilst HER2 status may be predictive of response to CMF therapy, it must again be remembered most of these studies were based on use of archival material obtained for retrospective analysis using multiple techniques and scoring methods.

A potential relationship between HER2 status and response to anthracycline-based chemotherapy, usually doxorubicin combined with cyclophosphamide and 5-FU (CAF), has been addressed in several studies.[93] In the first described analysis of an interaction between expression of HER2 and adjuvant therapy with doxorubicin-containing regimens using results from the Cancer and Leukaemia Group B (CALGB) study, Muss et al[87] found that tumors which overexpressed HER2 responded well to dose-intensive CAF. Additional studies have confirmed these results.[94,95] The NSABP study B-11 was originally designed to compare regimens of L-phenylalanine mustard plus 5-FU with or without doxorubicin.[94] In this trial the addition of doxorubicin improved outcomes in HER2-positive patients to the extent that they were equivalent to those with HER2-negative tumors. These data suggest a significant interaction between HER2 overexpression and chemosensitivity to anthracyclines. There are, however, several studies which have demonstrated no predictive value in response to anthracycline-based therapy.[96,97] However, it is important to note that most of these studies had fewer patients than those showing a positive predictive value. Also, in the study by Clahsen et al,[96] the patients received only one cycle of perioperative chemotherapy rather than the standard four or more cycles. Thus, HER2 overexpression may indicate a relative sensitivity to optimal versus suboptimal anthracycline dosage. The predictive potential between HER2 overexpression and response to other forms of treatment has been investigated in several studies, but the results are not definitive and further studies are required before conclusions can be drawn.

Anticancer approaches using monoclonal antibodies

The HER2 receptor has an extracellular part and binds to a putative growth factor for activation, which suggests that one or both may be possible therapeutic targets. Research studies have demonstrated that the extracellular domain of the HER2 receptor tyrosine kinase is readily accessible to systemically administered antibody-based therapeutics, including growth-inhibiting monoclonals such as rhuMAbHER2 (trastuzmab/Herceptin®) as well as anti-HER2 immunotoxins, antibody-dependent enzyme prodrug therapy (ADEPT), and immune cell recruiting bispecific antibodies.

Several studies have described the development of murine monoclonal antibodies directed against various epitopes of the extracellular domain of HER2. These antibodies were found to inhibit the proliferation of tumors and transformed cells which overexpressed HER2.[98-100] A murine anti-HER2 antibody (4D5) has been investigated and found to inhibit the growth of human breast cancer cell lines both in vitro and in xenograft models which overexpress the HER2 extracellular domain.[101,102] Additionally, the antibody was shown to enhance the antitumor effect of paclitaxel and doxorubicin against HER2-positive human breast cancer xenografts,[103] and the effects of cisplatin against breast and ovarian cancer cell lines.[104] The ability of anti-HER2 antibodies to interfere with repair of cisplatin-induced DNA damage has been postulated as a possible mechanism.[105]

A major limiting factor with the use of murine monoclonal antibodies in humans is the development of neutralizing human anti-mouse antibodies (HAMA), which is why most have remained in experimental use. However, this recurring problem can be circumvented by humanizing chimeric antibodies. The humanization of the murine 4D5 monoclonal antibody has lead to developing the resulting recombinant human anti-HER2 monoclonal antibody (trastuzumab). Trastuzumab was the first of the monoclonal antibodies to be used in the treatment of those patients who have HER2-positive metastatic breast cancer. It is most effective when combined with cytotoxics, such as the taxanes and vinorelbine.[106-108] It is well tolerated but associated cardiotoxicity makes use with anthracyclines, and in patients with cardiac dysfunction, problematic. A further adverse observation is that the rate of development of cerebral metastases is more than double in patients who have received trastuzumab as part of the treatment regimens.[109,110] Trastuzumab has been combined with cytotoxics, hormones, other monoclonal antibodies (such a pertuzumab and bevacizumab), and targeted small molecules such as lapatinib, and it can be conjugated with cytotoxics to deliver them to cancer cells.[111-113] The dosage, duration of therapy and optimal combinations in advanced and early stage breast cancer, and use after relapse, are still being defined. Although no overall survival advantage has been reported in these trials, nonetheless, adjuvant trastuzumab has demonstrated a benefit in prolonged DFS and reduction of risk of recurrence by up to 50% in early stage breast cancer.

Other HER2-directed therapy

Immunotherapy and immunization

Vaccine strategies are being investigated as another method of targeting HER2 overexpressing cancer cells. Patients with HER2-positive tumors have been shown to develop an immune response against the protein,[114-116] which suggests that antireceptor vaccines may be successful in mounting an anticancer response. With a large difference in levels of expression between HER2-positive tumors and normal tissues, there exists a potential therapeutic window for such cancers with no residual autoimmune toxicity. Some of the first described investigations of targeting and treating by immunization were murine tumors overexpressing the rat oncogenic neu. These cancers were immunized with a vaccinia virus recombinant of the protein's extracellular domain.[117] Both intracellular and extracellular portions of the HER2 receptor have been shown to elicit specific responses from cytotoxic T-lymphocytes (CTL). Immunizing rats with peptides derived from the self-rat Neu, but not with the whole protein, is known to promote antibody and T-cell responses against the native protein.[118] Nagata et al[119] have subsequently shown that similar peptides, derived from the murine ErbB-2 receptor, can induce CTL activity, which results in the suppression of growth of HER2 overexpressed cells in syngeneic hosts.

Gene therapy

HER2 overexpression is significantly influenced by transcriptional upregulation in human cancers.[120] This suggests that manipulation of the promoter activity could be used as a therapeutic approach. Selective expression of suicide genes driven by regulatory regions of the HER2 promoter renders cells sensitive to gancyclovir.[121] Adenovirus type 5 early region 1A gene product (E1A) has been used to repress HER2 expression, thereby suppressing the tumorigenic potential of overexpressed cells.[122] More importantly, the growth of human breast cancer cells in nude mice is efficiently inhibited by the viral product using vector or liposomal delivery.[123] Anti-HER2 targeted hammerhead ribosomes, under control of a tetracycline-regulated promoter, have been shown to abrogate expression of the HER2 protein, resulting in inhibition of tumor growth in nude mice and tumor regression upon tetracycline withdrawal.[124] Adenoviral vectors have been used for the introduction of an anti-HER2 single-chain antibody (via DNA delivery) which retains the protein within the cell. When the vector was injected intraperitonially, it resulted in reduction of tumor burden in severe combined immunodeficiency mice.[125]

Immunotoxins

Advances in recombinant antibody technology have made it possible to circumvent problems inherent in chemical coupling of antibodies and toxins, and have allowed construction via gene fusion of recombinant molecules which combine antibody-mediated recognition of tumor cells with specific delivery of potent protein toxins of bacterial or plant origin. Therefore, antibodies to HER2 may also be able to play a role as vehicles for the targeting of therapeutic agents to cancers. Immunotoxins have been constructed with various anti-HER2 antibodies which have been coupled to Lys-PE40, a recombinant form of Pseudomonas exotoxin.[126] The ligands in the erbB family have also been studied as potential carriers, utilizing their binding affinity to respective receptors. Complete regression of human breast cancer xenografts in nude mice was seen when a fusion toxin of NRG 1 was administered.[127] A bispecific toxin of an anti-HER2 antibody and transforming growth factor-α also inhibited the growth of breast cancer cells in vivo.[128] Antibody targeting of drug-loaded liposomes has also been investigated as a vehicle for drug delivery. Park et al[129] showed that immunoliposomes can efficiently bind to cancer cells, and deliver cytotoxic doses of doxorubicin in a targeted manner. The development of a new class of tumor-specific killer lymphocytes which supplies a HER2-specific toxin has been described. These cells produce and secrete an antibody-targeted toxin in the region of the tumor which results in high cytotoxicity towards tumors in an athymic murine model,[130] but human trials are required to assess the clinical significance of such type of therapy.

CONCLUSION

HER2 is an oncoprotein which is overexpressed in about 20% of breast cancers, almost universally as a consequence of gene amplification. HER2 can be used as a prognostic factor, may be predictive of response to systemic chemotherapy, but is clearly predictive for response to Herceptin. It is therefore imperative that reliable and simple assays are implemented into routine practice in most hospital settings. Standardization of such assays, as well as uniform scoring systems, must be adhered to for accurate diagnosis of

HER2 status. All invasive breast carcinoma cases should be tested for HER2. A two-phase testing algorithm based on IHC assay as the primary screen, with reference to FISH reserved for equivocal cases, is currently recommended. Positive IHC HER2 staining is defined as uniform intense membrane staining of >30% of invasive tumor cells, while an equivocal result (2+) is complete membrane staining which is either nonuniform or weak in intensity but with obvious circumferential distribution in at least 10% of cells. In any equivocal cases, FISH test should be performed. Positive FISH result of amplified HER2 gene copy number is defined as average of >6 gene copies/nucleus for test systems without internal control probe or HER2:CEP17 ratio of >2.0, where CEP17 is a centromeric probe for chromosome 17 on which the HER2 gene resides. IHC and FISH are the method of choice for HER2 testing while, at present, other methods should be used for research only. Stringent quality assurance procedures should be taken to ensure a valid test is performed in clinical settings.

REFERENCES

1. Wolff AC, Hammond ME, Schwartz JN et al. American Society of Clinical Oncology/College of American Pathologists guideline recommendations for human epidermal growth factor receptor 2 testing in breast cancer. J Clin Oncol 2007; 25: 118–45.
2. Lipponen HJ, Aaltomaa S, Syrjanen S et al. c-erbB-2 oncogene related to p53 expression, cell proliferation and prognosis in breast cancer. Anticancer Res 1993; 13: 1147–52.
3. Slamon DJ, Clark GM, Wong SG et al. Human breast cancer: correlation of relapse and survival with amplification of the HER-2/neu oncogene. Science 1987; 235: 177–82.
4. Varshney D, Zhou YY, Geller SA et al. Determination of HER-2 status and chromosome 17 polysomy in breast carcinomas comparing HercepTest and PathVysion FISH assay. Am J Clin Pathol 2004; 121: 70–7.
5. Sauer T, Wiedswang G, Boudjema G et al. Assessment of HER-2/neu overexpression and/or gene amplification in breast carcinomas: should in situ hybridization be the method of choice? Apmis 2003; 111: 444–50.
6. Yamauchi H, Stearns V, Hayes DF. When is a tumor marker ready for prime time? A case study of c-erbB-2 as a predictive factor in breast cancer. J Clin Oncol 2001; 19: 2334–56.
7. Ross JS, Fletcher JA. The HER-2/neu oncogene in breast cancer: Prognostic factor, predictive factor, and target for therapy. Oncologist 1998; 3: 237–52.
8. Revillion F, Bonneterre J, Peyrat JP. ERBB2 oncogene in human breast cancer and its clinical significance. Eur J Cancer 1998; 34: 791–808.
9. Bartlett JM. Pharmacodiagnostic testing in breast cancer: focus on HER2 and trastuzumab therapy. Am J Pharmacogenomics 2005; 5: 303–15.
10. Bartlett J, Mallon E, Cooke T. The clinical evaluation of HER-2 status: which test to use? J Pathol 2003; 199: 411–17.
11. Cobleigh MA, Vogel CL, Tripathy D et al. Multinational study of the efficacy and safety of humanized anti-HER2 monoclonal antibody in women who have HER2-overexpressing metastatic breast cancer that has progressed after chemotherapy for metastatic disease. J Clin Oncol 1999; 17: 2639–48.
12. Piccart-Gebhart MJ, Procter M, Leyland-Jones B et al. Trastuzumab after adjuvant chemotherapy in HER2-positive breast cancer. N Engl J Med 2005; 353: 1659–72.
13. Smith I, Procter M, Gelber RD et al. 2-year follow-up of trastuzumab after adjuvant chemotherapy in HER2-positive breast cancer: a randomised controlled trial. Lancet 2007; 369: 29–36.
14. Romond EH, Perez EA, Bryant J et al. Trastuzumab plus adjuvant chemotherapy for operable HER2-positive breast cancer. N Engl J Med 2005; 353: 1673–84.
15. Johnston SR, Leary A. Lapatinib: a novel EGFR/HER2 tyrosine kinase inhibitor for cancer. Drugs Today (Barc) 2006; 42: 441–53.
16. Bartlett JMS, Mallon EA, Cooke TG. Molecular diagnostics for determination of HER2 status in breast cancer. Curr Diagnos Pathol 2003; 9: 48–55.
17. Kallioniemi OP, Kallioniemi A, Kurisu W et al. ERBB2 amplification in breast cancer analyzed by fluorescence in situ hybridization. Proc Natl Acad Sci USA 1992; 89: 5321–5.
18. Carlson RW, Moench SJ, Hammond ME et al. HER2 testing in breast cancer: NCCN Task Force report and recommendations. J Natl Compr Canc Netw 2006; 4 (Suppl 3): S1–S22; quiz S23–S24.
19. Isola J, Tanner M, Forsyth A et al. Interlaboratory comparison of HER-2 oncogene amplification as detected by chromogenic and fluorescence in situ hybridization. Clin Cancer Res 2004; 10: 4793–8.
20. Tanner M, Gancberg D, Di Leo A et al. Chromogenic in situ hybridization: a practical alternative for fluorescence in situ hybridization to detect HER-2/neu oncogene amplification in archival breast cancer samples. Am J Pathol 2000; 157: 1467–72.
21. Hanna WM, Kwok K. Chromogenic in-situ hybridization: a viable alternative to fluorescence in-situ hybridization in the HER2 testing algorithm. Mod Pathol 2006; 19: 481–7.

22. Dandachi N, Dietze O, Hauser-Kronberger C. Chromogenic in situ hybridization: a novel approach to a practical and sensitive method for the detection of HER2 oncogene in archival human breast carcinoma. Lab Invest 2002; 82: 1007–14.

23. Dietel M, Ellis IO, Hofler H et al. Comparison of automated silver enhanced in situ hybridisation (SISH) and fluorescence ISH (FISH) for the validation of HER2 gene status in breast carcinoma according to the guidelines of the American Society of Clinical Oncology and the College of American Pathologists. Virchows Arch 2007 (in press).

24. Tubbs RR, Pettay JD, Swain E et al. Automation of manual components and image quantification of direct dual label fluorescence in situ hybridization (FISH) for HER2 gene amplification: A feasibility study. Appl Immunohistochem Mol Morphol 2006; 14: 436–40.

25. Heintz NH, Leslie KO, Rogers LA et al. Amplification of the c-erb B-2 oncogene and prognosis of breast adenocarcinoma. Arch Pathol Lab Med 1990; 114: 160–3.

26. Slamon DJ, Godolphin W, Jones LA et al. Studies of the HER-2/neu proto-oncogene in human breast and ovarian cancer. Science 1989; 244: 707–12.

27. Naber SP, Tsutsumi Y, Yin S et al. Strategies for the analysis of oncogene overexpression. Studies of the neu oncogene in breast carcinoma. Am J Clin Pathol 1990; 94: 125–36.

28. Seshadri R, Firgaira FA, Horsfall DJ et al. Clinical significance of HER-2/neu oncogene amplification in primary breast cancer. The South Australian Breast Cancer Study Group. J Clin Oncol 1993; 11: 1936–42.

29. Deng G, Kim YS. Quantitation of erbB-2 gene copy number in breast cancer by an improved polymerase chain reaction (PCR) technique, competitively differential PCR. Breast Cancer Res Treat 1999; 58: 213–17.

30. Ellis IO, Bartlett J, Dowsett M et al. Best Practice No 176: Updated recommendations for HER2 testing in the UK. J Clin Pathol 2004; 57: 233–7.

31. Jacobs TW, Prioleau JE, Stillman IE et al. Loss of tumor marker-immunostaining intensity on stored paraffin slides of breast cancer. J Natl Cancer Inst 1996; 88: 1054–9.

32. Penault-Llorca F, Adelaide J, Houvenaeghel G et al. Optimization of immunohistochemical detection of ERBB2 in human breast cancer: impact of fixation. J Pathol 1994; 173: 65–75.

33. Ratcliffe N, Wells W, Wheeler K et al. The combination of in situ hybridization and immunohistochemical analysis: an evaluation of Her2/neu expression in paraffin-embedded breast carcinomas and adjacent normal-appearing breast epithelium. Mod Pathol 1997; 10: 1247–52.

34. Busmanis I, Feleppa F, Jones A et al. Analysis of cerbB2 expression using a panel of 6 commercially available antibodies. Pathology 1994; 26: 261–7.

35. van Diest PJ, van Dam P, Henzen-Logmans SC et al. A scoring system for immunohistochemical staining: consensus report of the task force for basic research of the EORTC–GCCG. European Organization for Research and Treatment of Cancer–Gynaecological Cancer Cooperative Group. J Clin Pathol 1997; 50: 801–4.

36. Owens MA, Horten BC, Da Silva MM. HER2 amplification ratios by fluorescence in situ hybridization and correlation with immunohistochemistry in a cohort of 6556 breast cancer tissues. Clin Breast Cancer 2004; 5: 63–9.

37. Press MF, Bernstein L, Thomas PA et al. HER-2/neu gene amplification characterized by fluorescence in situ hybridization: poor prognosis in node-negative breast carcinomas. J Clin Oncol 1997; 15: 2894–904.

38. Jacobs TW, Gown AM, Yaziji H et al. Comparison of fluorescence in situ hybridization and immunohistochemistry for the evaluation of HER-2/neu in breast cancer. J Clin Oncol 1999; 17: 1974–82.

39. Zhang D, Salto-Tellez M, Do E et al. Evaluation of HER-2/neu oncogene status in breast tumors on tissue microarrays. Hum Pathol 2003; 34: 362–8.

40. Dowsett M, Bartlett J, Ellis IO et al. Correlation between immunohistochemistry (HercepTest) and fluorescence in situ hybridization (FISH) for HER-2 in 426 breast carcinomas from 37 centres. J Pathol 2003; 199: 418–23.

41. Bartlett JM, Going JJ, Mallon EA et al. Evaluating HER2 amplification and overexpression in breast cancer. J Pathol 2001; 195: 422–8.

42. Press MF, Slamon DJ, Flom KJ et al. Evaluation of HER-2/neu gene amplification and overexpression: comparison of frequently used assay methods in a molecularly characterized cohort of breast cancer specimens. J Clin Oncol 2002; 20: 3095–105.

43. Bartlett JM, Ibrahim M, Jasani B et al. External quality assurance of HER2 fluorescence in situ hybridisation testing: results of a UK NEQAS pilot scheme. J Clin Pathol 2007; 60: 816–19.

44. Perez EA, Suman VJ, Davidson NE et al. HER2 testing by local, central, and reference laboratories in specimens from the North Central Cancer Treatment Group N9831 intergroup adjuvant trial. J Clin Oncol 2006; 24: 3032–8.

45. Press MF, Sauter G, Bernstein L et al. Diagnostic evaluation of HER-2 as a molecular target: an assessment of accuracy and reproducibility of laboratory testing in large, prospective, randomized clinical trials. Clin Cancer Res 2005; 11: 6598–607.

46. Reddy JC, Reimann JD, Anderson SM et al. Concordance between central and local laboratory HER2 testing from a community-based clinical study. Clin Breast Cancer 2006; 7: 153–7.

47. Ellis IO, Dowsett M, Bartlett J et al. Recommendations for HER2 testing in the UK. J Clin Pathol 2000; 53: 890–2.

48. Fornier MN, Seidman AD, Schwartz MK et al. Serum HER2 extracellular domain in metastatic breast

cancer patients treated with weekly trastuzumab and paclitaxel: association with HER2 status by immunohistochemistry and fluorescence in situ hybridization and with response rate. Ann Oncol 2005; 16: 234–9.

49. Watters AD, Going JJ, Cooke TG et al. Chromosome 17 aneusomy is associated with poor prognostic factors in invasive breast carcinoma. Breast Cancer Res Treat 2003; 77: 109–14.

50. Hicks DG, Tubbs RR. Assessment of the HER2 status in breast cancer by fluorescence in situ hybridization: a technical review with interpretive guidelines. Hum Pathol 2005; 36: 250–61.

51. Rampaul RS, Pinder SE, Gullick WJ et al. HER-2 in breast cancer – methods of detection, clinical significance and future prospects for treatment. Crit Rev Oncol Hematol 2002; 43: 231–44.

52. Abd El-Rehim DM, Pinder SE, Paish CE et al. Expression and co-expression of the members of the epidermal growth factor receptor (EGFR) family in invasive breast carcinoma. Br J Cancer 2004; 91: 1532–42.

53. Fitzgibbons PL, Murphy DA, Dorfman DM et al. Interlaboratory comparison of immunohistochemical testing for HER2: results of the 2004 and 2005 College of American Pathologists HER2 Immunohistochemistry Tissue Microarray Survey. Arch Pathol Lab Med 2006; 130: 1440–5.

54. Wang S, Saboorian MH, Frenkel EP et al. Assessment of HER-2/neu status in breast cancer. Automated Cellular Imaging System (ACIS)-assisted quantitation of immunohistochemical assay achieves high accuracy in comparison with fluorescence in situ hybridization assay as the standard. Am J Clin Pathol 2001; 116: 495–503.

55. Jasani B, Miller K. Cell line standards to reduce HER-2/neu assay variation and the potential of automated image analysis to provide more accurate cut points for predicting clinical response to trastuzumab. Am J Clin Pathol 2005; 123: 314; author reply 314–15.

56. Rhodes A, Borthwick D, Sykes R et al. The use of cell line standards to reduce HER-2/neu assay variation in multiple European cancer centers and the potential of automated image analysis to provide for more accurate cut points for predicting clinical response to trastuzumab. Am J Clin Pathol 2004; 122: 51–60.

57. Ciampa A, Xu B, Ayata G et al. HER-2 status in breast cancer: correlation of gene amplification by FISH with immunohistochemistry expression using advanced cellular imaging system. Appl Immunohistochem Mol Morphol 2006; 14: 132–7.

58. Ellis CM, Dyson MJ, Stephenson TJ et al. HER2 amplification status in breast cancer: a comparison between immunohistochemical staining and fluorescence in situ hybridisation using manual and automated quantitative image analysis scoring techniques. J Clin Pathol 2005; 58: 710–14.

59. Zidan J, Dashkovsky I, Stayerman C et al. Comparison of HER-2 overexpression in primary breast cancer and metastatic sites and its effect on biological targeting therapy of metastatic disease. Br J Cancer 2005; 93: 552–6.

60. Edgerton SM, Moore D 2nd, Merkel D et al. erbB-2 (HER-2) and breast cancer progression. Appl Immunohistochem Mol Morphol 2003; 11: 214–21.

61. Gancberg D, Di Leo A, Cardoso F et al. Comparison of HER-2 status between primary breast cancer and corresponding distant metastatic sites. Ann Oncol 2002; 13: 1036–43.

62. Cavaliere A, Sidoni A, Scheibel M et al. Biopathologic profile of breast cancer core biopsy: is it always a valid method? Cancer Lett 2005; 218: 117–21.

63. Burge CN, Chang HR, Apple SK. Do the histologic features and results of breast cancer biomarker studies differ between core biopsy and surgical excision specimens? Breast 2006; 15: 167–72.

64. Smyczek-Gargya B, Krainick U, Muller-Schimpfle M et al. Large-core needle biopsy for diagnosis and treatment of breast lesions. Arch Gynecol Obstet 2002; 266: 198–200.

65. Jacobs TW, Siziopikou KP, Prioleau JE et al. Do prognostic marker studies on core needle biopsy specimens of breast carcinoma accurately reflect the marker status of the tumor? Mod Pathol 1998; 11: 259–64.

66. Taucher S, Rudas M, Mader RM et al. Prognostic markers in breast cancer: the reliability of HER2/neu status in core needle biopsy of 325 patients with primary breast cancer. Wien Klin Wochenschr 2004; 116: 26–31.

67. Rilke F, Colnaghi MI, Cascinelli N et al. Prognostic significance of HER-2/neu expression in breast cancer and its relationship to other prognostic factors. Int J Cancer 1991; 49: 44–9.

68. Schlotter CM, Vogt U, Bosse U et al. C-myc, not HER-2/neu, can predict recurrence and mortality of patients with node-negative breast cancer. Breast Cancer Res 2003; 5: R30–R36.

69. Bianchi S, Paglierani M, Zampi G et al. Prognostic significance of c-erbB-2 expression in node negative breast cancer. Br J Cancer 1993; 67: 625–9.

70. Clark GM, McGuire WL. Follow-up study of HER-2/neu amplification in primary breast cancer. Cancer Res 1991; 51: 944–8.

71. Wright C, Angus B, Nicholson S et al. Expression of c-erbB-2 oncoprotein: a prognostic indicator in human breast cancer. Cancer Res 1989; 49: 2087–90.

72. Borg A, Baldetorp B, Ferno M et al. ERBB2 amplification is associated with tamoxifen resistance in steroid-receptor positive breast cancer. Cancer Lett 1994; 81: 137–44.

73. Paik S, Hazan R, Fisher ER et al. Pathologic findings from the National Surgical Adjuvant Breast and Bowel Project: prognostic significance of erbB-2 protein overexpression in primary breast cancer. J Clin Oncol 1990; 8: 103–12.

74. Yamashita J, Ogawa M, Sakai K. Prognostic significance of three novel biologic factors in a clinical trial of adjuvant therapy for node-negative breast cancer. Surgery 1995; 117: 601–8.

75. Schonborn I, Zschiesche W, Spitzer E et al. C-erbB-2 overexpression in primary breast cancer: independent prognostic factor in patients at high risk. Breast Cancer Res Treat 1994; 29: 287–95.

76. Tetu B, Brisson J. Prognostic significance of HER-2/neu oncoprotein expression in node-positive breast cancer. The influence of the pattern of immunostaining and adjuvant therapy. Cancer 1994; 73: 2359–65.

77. Gullick WJ, Love SB, Wright C et al. c-erbB-2 protein overexpression in breast cancer is a risk factor in patients with involved and uninvolved lymph nodes. Br J Cancer 1991; 63: 434–8.

78. Clark GM. Should selection of adjuvant chemotherapy for patients with breast cancer be based on erbB-2 status? J Natl Cancer Inst 1998; 90: 1320–1.

79. Piccart M, Awada A, Hamilton A. Integration of new therapies into management of metastatic breast cancer: a focus on chemotherapy, treatment selection through use of molecular markers, and newly developed biologic therapies in late clinical development. In: Perry MC, ed. Americal Society of Clinical Oncology educational book. Alexandria, VA: American Society of Clinical Oncology, 1999; 536–9.

80. Benz CC, Scott GK, Sarup JC et al. Estrogen-dependent, tamoxifen-resistant tumorigenic growth of MCF-7 cells transfected with HER2/neu. Breast Cancer Res Treat 1992; 24: 85–95.

81. Pietras RJ, Arboleda J, Reese DM et al. HER-2 tyrosine kinase pathway targets estrogen receptor and promotes hormone-independent growth in human breast cancer cells. Oncogene 1995; 10: 2435–46.

82. Blanco AR, Laurentils MD, Carlomagno C et al. 20-year update of the naples gun trial of adjuvant breast cancer therapy: evidence of interaction between c-erb-b2 expression and tamoxifen efficacy. Proc Am Soc Clin Oncol 1998; 17: 97A.

83. Berns EM, Foekens JA, van Staveren IL et al. Oncogene amplification and prognosis in breast cancer: relationship with systemic treatment. Gene 1995; 159: 11–18.

84. Newby JC, Johnston SR, Smith IE et al. Expression of epidermal growth factor receptor and c-erbB2 during the development of tamoxifen resistance in human breast cancer. Clin Cancer Res 1997; 3: 1643–51.

85. Yamauchi H, O'Neill A, Gelman R et al. Prediction of response to antiestrogen therapy in advanced breast cancer patients by pretreatment circulating levels of extracellular domain of the HER-2/c-neu protein. J Clin Oncol 1997; 15: 2518–25.

86. Cheung TH, Wong YF, Chung TK et al. Clinical use of serum c-erbB-2 in patients with ovarian masses. Gynecol Obstet Invest 1999; 48: 133–7.

87. Muss H, Berry D, Thor A et al. Lack of interaction of tamoxifen (T) use and ErbB-2/ HER-2/neu (H) expression in CALGB 8541: a randomized adjuvant trial of three different doses of cyclophosphamide, doxorubicin and fluorouracil (CAF) in node-positive primary breast cancer (BC). Proc Am Soc Clin Oncol 1999; 18: 68A.

88. Archer SG, Eliopoulos A, Spandidos D et al. Expression of ras p21, p53 and c-erbB-2 in advanced breast cancer and response to first line hormonal therapy. Br J Cancer 1995; 72: 1259–66.

89. Elledge RM, Green S, Ciocca D et al. HER-2 expression and response to tamoxifen in estrogen receptor-positive breast cancer: a Southwest Oncology Group Study. Clin Cancer Res 1998; 4: 7–12.

90. Pritchard KI, Shepherd LE, O'Malley FP et al. HER2 and responsiveness of breast cancer to adjuvant chemotherapy. N Engl J Med 2006; 354: 2103–11.

91. Stal O, Sullivan S, Wingren S et al. c-erbB-2 expression and benefit from adjuvant chemotherapy and radiotherapy of breast cancer. Eur J Cancer 1995; 31A: 2185–90.

92. Miles DW, Harris WH, Gillett CE et al. Effect of c-erbB(2) and estrogen receptor status on survival of women with primary breast cancer treated with adjuvant cyclophosphamide/methotrexate/fluorouracil. Int J Cancer 1999; 84: 354–9.

93. Tagliabue E, Menard S, Robertson JF et al. c-erbB-2 expression in primary breast cancer. Int J Biol Markers 1999; 14: 16–26.

94. Paik S, Bryant J, Park C et al. erbB-2 and response to doxorubicin in patients with axillary lymph node-positive, hormone receptor-negative breast cancer. J Natl Cancer Inst 1998; 90: 1361–70.

95. Ravin PM, Green S, Albain KS et al. Initial report of the SWOG biological correlative study of c-erbB-2 expression as a predictor of outcome in a trial comparing adjuvant CAF T with tamoxifen (T) alone. Proc Am Soc Clin Oncol 1998; 17: 97A.

96. Clahsen PC, van de Velde CJ, Duval C et al. p53 protein accumulation and response to adjuvant chemotherapy in premenopausal women with node-negative early breast cancer. J Clin Oncol 1998; 16: 470–9.

97. Rozan S, Vincent-Salomon A, Zafrani B et al. No significant predictive value of c-erbB-2 or p53 expression regarding sensitivity to primary chemotherapy or radiotherapy in breast cancer. Int J Cancer 1998; 79: 27–33.

98. Fendly BM, Winget M, Hudziak RM et al. Characterization of murine monoclonal antibodies reactive to either the human epidermal growth factor receptor or HER2/neu gene product. Cancer Res 1990; 50: 1550–8.

99. Harwerth IM, Wels W, Schlegel J et al. Monoclonal antibodies directed to the erbB-2 receptor inhibit in vivo tumour cell growth. Br J Cancer 1993; 68: 1140–5.

100. McKenzie SJ, Marks PJ, Lam T et al. Generation and characterization of monoclonal antibodies specific for the human neu oncogene product, p185. Oncogene 1989; 4: 543–8.

101. Lewis GD, Figari I, Fendly B et al. Differential responses of human tumor cell lines to anti-p185HER2 monoclonal antibodies. Cancer Immunol Immunother 1993; 37: 255–63.

102. Shepard HM, Lewis GD, Sarup JC et al. Monoclonal antibody therapy of human cancer: taking the HER2 protooncogene to the clinic. J Clin Immunol 1991; 11: 117–27.

103. Baselga J, Norton L, Albanell J et al. Recombinant humanized anti-HER2 antibody (Herceptin) enhances the antitumor activity of paclitaxel and doxorubicin against HER2/neu overexpressing human breast cancer xenografts. Cancer Res 1998; 58: 2825–31.

104. Hancock MC, Langton BC, Chan T et al. A monoclonal antibody against the c-erbB-2 protein enhances the cytotoxicity of cis-diamminedichloroplatinum against human breast and ovarian tumor cell lines. Cancer Res 1991; 51: 4575–80.

105. Pietras RJ, Pegram MD, Finn RS et al. Remission of human breast cancer xenografts on therapy with humanized monoclonal antibody to HER-2 receptor and DNA-reactive drugs. Oncogene 1998; 17: 2235–49.

106. Limentani SA, Brufsky AM, Erban JK et al. Phase II study of neoadjuvant docetaxel, vinorelbine, and trastuzumab followed by surgery and adjuvant doxorubicin plus cyclophosphamide in women with human epidermal growth factor receptor 2-overexpressing locally advanced breast cancer. J Clin Oncol 2007; 25: 1232–8.

107. Ferretti G, Papaldo P, Fabi A et al. Adjuvant trastuzumab with docetaxel or vinorelbine for HER-2-positive breast cancer. Oncologist 2006; 11: 853–4.

108. Garcia-Saenz JA, Martin M, Puente J et al. Trastuzumab associated with successive cytotoxic therapies beyond disease progression in metastatic breast cancer. Clin Breast Cancer 2005; 6: 325–9.

109. Bulut N, Harputluoglu H, Dizdar O et al. Role of trastuzumab in patients with brain metastases from Her2 positive breast cancer. J Neurooncol 2008; 86: 241.

110. Bria E, Cuppone F, Fornier M et al. Cardiotoxicity and incidence of brain metastases after adjuvant trastuzumab for early breast cancer: the dark side of the moon? A meta-analysis of the randomized trials. Breast Cancer Res Treat 2007 (in press).

111. Nishimura R, Okumura Y, Arima N. Trastuzumab monotherapy versus combination therapy for treating recurrent breast cancer: time to progression and survival. Breast Cancer 2008; 15: 57–64.

112. Viani GA, Afonso SL, Stefano EJ et al. Adjuvant trastuzumab in the treatment of her-2-positive early breast cancer: a meta-analysis of published randomized trials. BMC Cancer 2007; 7: 153.

113. Carter P, Presta L, Gorman CM et al. Humanization of an anti-p185HER2 antibody for human cancer therapy. Proc Natl Acad Sci USA 1992; 89: 4285–9.

114. Disis ML, Knutson KL, Schiffman K et al. Pre-existent immunity to the HER-2/neu oncogenic protein in patients with HER-2/neu overexpressing breast and ovarian cancer. Breast Cancer Res Treat 2000; 62: 245–52.

115. Ward RL, Hawkins NJ, Coomber D et al. Antibody immunity to the HER-2/neu oncogenic protein in patients with colorectal cancer. Hum Immunol 1999; 60: 510–15.

116. Disis ML, Bernhard H, Gralow JR et al. Immunity to the HER-2/neu oncogenic protein. Ciba Found Symp 1994; 187: 198–207; discussion 207–11.

117. Bernards R, Destree A, McKenzie S et al. Effective tumor immunotherapy directed against an oncogene-encoded product using a vaccinia virus vector. Proc Natl Acad Sci USA 1987; 84: 6854–8.

118. Disis ML, Gralow JR, Bernhard H et al. Peptide-based, but not whole protein, vaccines elicit immunity to HER-2/neu, oncogenic self-protein. J Immunol 1996; 156: 3151–8.

119. Nagata Y, Furugen R, Hiasa A et al. Peptides derived from a wild-type murine proto-oncogene c-erbB-2/HER2/neu can induce CTL and tumor suppression in syngeneic hosts. J Immunol 1997; 159: 1336–43.

120. Kraus MH, Popescu NC, Amsbaugh SC et al. Overexpression of the EGF receptor-related proto-oncogene erbB-2 in human mammary tumor cell lines by different molecular mechanisms. Embo J 1987; 6: 605–10.

121. Ring CJ, Blouin P, Martin LA et al. Use of transcriptional regulatory elements of the MUC1 and ERBB2 genes to drive tumour-selective expression of a prodrug activating enzyme. Gene Ther 1997; 4: 1045–52.

122. Yu DH, Hung MC. Expression of activated rat neu oncogene is sufficient to induce experimental metastasis in 3T3 cells. Oncogene 1991; 6: 1991–6.

123. Chang H, Riese DJ 2nd, Gilbert W et al. Ligands for ErbB-family receptors encoded by a neuregulin-like gene. Nature 1997; 387: 509–12.

124. Juhl H, Downing SG, Wellstein A et al. HER-2/neu is rate-limiting for ovarian cancer growth. Conditional depletion of HER-2/neu by ribozyme targeting. J Biol Chem 1997; 272: 29,482–6.

125. Deshane J, Siegal GP, Wang M et al. Transductional efficacy and safety of an intraperitoneally delivered adenovirus encoding an anti-erbB-2 intracellular single-chain antibody for ovarian cancer gene therapy. Gynecol Oncol 1997; 64: 378–85.

126. Batra JK, Kasprzyk PG, Bird RE et al. Recombinant anti-erbB2 immunotoxins containing Pseudomonas exotoxin. Proc Natl Acad Sci USA 1992; 89: 5867–71.

127. Groner B, Wick B, Jeschke M et al. Intra-tumoral application of a heregulin-exotoxin-a fusion protein causes rapid tumor regression without adverse systemic or local effects. Int J Cancer 1997; 70: 682–7.

128. Schmidt M, Hynes NE, Groner B et al. A bivalent single-chain antibody-toxin specific for ErbB-2 and the EGF receptor. Int J Cancer 1996; 65: 538–46.

129. Park JW, Hong K, Carter P et al. Development of anti-p185HER2 immunoliposomes for cancer therapy. Proc Natl Acad Sci USA 1995; 92: 1327–31.

130. Chen SY, Yang AG, Chen JD et al. Potent antitumour activity of a new class of tumour-specific killer cells. Nature 1997; 385: 78–80.

Index

T - #0523 - 071024 - C5 - 254/190/10 - PB - 9780367386931 - Gloss Lamination